DEVELOPMENTS IN
PSYCHOPHARMACOLOGY

DEVELOPMENTS IN
PSYCHOPHARMACOLOGY

SATISH SERIAL PUBLISHING HOUSE
403, Express Tower, Commercial Complex, Azadpur, Delhi - 110033 (INDIA)
Phone : 011-27672852 Fax : 91-11-27672046
E-mail : info@satishserial.com, hkjain1975@yahoo.com
Website : www.satishserial.com

Published by :

SATISH SERIAL PUBLISHING HOUSE
403, Express Tower, Commercial Complex, Azadpur, Delhi - 110033 (INDIA)
Phone : 011-27672852 Fax : 91-11-27672046
E-mail : info@satishserial.com, hkjain1975@yahoo.com

ISBN 81-89304-31-3

Printed at
SALASAR IMAGING SYSTEMS, DELHI-35

Dedicated
to
My Family

Foreword

It was almost four decades back that I had first seen Shrinivas Kulkarni in Bangalore and brought him with me to work in my laboratory at Jaipur in pursuit of advanced degrees in Pharmacology of the Faculty of Medical Sciences. In the six years that he spent in my laboratory, he was able to publish more than fifteen research papers mostly in reputed International Journals. One of these "**Effect of reserpine, chlorpromazine and meprobamate on stress...**" was published in *Indian Journal of Experimental Biology (IJEB)* in 1973. Little did I know then that this handsome, bright, young man will one day become a distinguished Professor of Pharmacology, a prolific writer in Medical Science literature and an invited speaker in demand both in India and at other international centres of learning. I was not surprised that as many as 50 research papers by him and his colleagues have appeared in *IJEB* in the discipline of psycho-neuro-pharmacology. These research papers include his pioneering work on GABA receptors and behavioral pharmacology carried out at a time when the whole concept of GABAergic mechanism was still evolving. His efforts in compiling these in the form of a book is highly commendable and the publishers are to be congratulated for taking up this "Science job" that may not be financially remunerative.

Not many can do such advanced science, publish it and then compile such a treatise that carries in one volume, a four decades of dedicated scientific work by more than a dozen workers. My observations of Shrinivas some 40 years ago have come true that he would be a distinguished scientist and a dedicated teacher in times to come. He has established a world class school of psychopharmacology research and trained a large number of students over the years. The work compiled in this volume is a testimony to his contributions to pharmacological sciences. While writing this foreword, I take the opportunity to congratulate him for his efforts and feel good that he thought of me to write on this unique endeavour of his. I am proud of him and of my long association with him. He has been able to produce a book of the kind I never did. He excels and makes me joyous.

P.C. DANDIYA Ph.D. (Toronto), FAMS
Emeritus Professor
Sawai Mansingh Medical College, Jaipur

Preface

In the beginning of 2006 we published our 50th research paper in the *Indian Journal of Experimental Biology* (IJEB), a NISCAIR, CSIR publications. Looking back, I realized that my firstresearch paper in IJEB had appeared in 1973, some 33 years ago. It is rather unusual for any scientist to continue to contribute to one research journal (IJEB) for such a long time. The reason was simply because IJEB was one of the few journals published from India listed in the *Current Contents* of Eugene Garfield, the scientific communication revolutionary. Therefore, initially there was an excitement of receiving reprint requests from all over the globe for our articles in IJEB.

Inspite of the revolutionary developments in scientific communication and retrieval of information, particularly online research journals and publications, we still continue to receive the reprint requests. I realized that many of the peripheral institutions in India still do not have access to internet facilities. Our research publications in IJEB are broadly related to two areas of Psychoneuropharmacology namely, *Central nervous system actions of drugs* and *Pain and inflammation.* These articles describe novel and simple techniques and pharmacological concepts which are of great utility to postgraduate and research scholars in pharmacology. With this background I thought of compiling all the 50 publications in the form of a book and approached the editors of IJEB (Mr. Rajiv Mathur) for bringing out a special compilation edition of our publications. While the idea was appreciated but for reasons best known to IJEB editorial management they allowed me to do the compilation work on my own. The first three chapters of this volume give an overview on the status GABA receptor pharmacology and its role in various behavioral paradigms, and the chapter 21 describes the basic concepts of pain and inflammation. These concepts are supported by our selected publications in IJEB.

We appreciate the permission of IJEB, NISCAIR, CSIR, New Delhi for allowing to reproduce the research papers in this volume and their continued support in our research endeavors. The selected research papers have been converted into book format without altering their contents. I appreciate the efforts of Dad's Sons Graphics, Chandigarh for their meticulous work and Mr. H. K. Jain Publications, New Delhi for bringing out the elegant book. The dedicated efforts of Mr. Ashish Dhir, Research Fellow in Pharmacology to complete the work in time is highly appreciated.

It is indeed a great sense of gratification for me as Professor P.C. Dandiya, my revered teacher with whom I published the first paper in IJEB has kindly written the foreword.

Chandigarh
August 14, 2006

S.K. KULKARNI

Contents

1

γ - Amino butyric acid receptor pharmacology: From concepts to application

S. K. KULKARNI
Pharmacology Division, University Institute of Pharmaceutical Sciences,
Panjab University, Chandigarh 160 014, India

Introduction

γ-Amino butyric acid (GABA) is quantitatively the major inhibitory neurotransmitter of the mammalian central nervous system[1]. Almost 60-75 % of the neurons in the central nervous system are GABAergic in nature and they are virtually absent outside the brain and the spinal cord. The early ionotophoretic studies with GABA indicated that it generally produced inhibitory hyperpolarizing response on neurons, which was competitively blocked by the alkaloid bicuculline. The hyperpolarizing response is due to an increase in the chloride conductance of the neuronal membrane allowing chloride ions to flow down their electrochemical gradient into the cell. GABA controlled the state of excitability of the brain areas and the ongoing level of neuronal activity is regulated by the balance between excitatory inputs (mostly glutamatergic) and inhibitory GABAergic activity. Increased levels of GABAergic activity produce CNS depression, sedation, amnesia and ataxia. Any attenuation of the GABAergic system, on the other hand results in arousal response, anxiety, restlessness, insomnia and excitation[1]. A typical GABAergic synapse is shown in Fig.1

GABA receptors

GABA is known to act on three distinct receptors i.e. $GABA_A$, $GABA_B$ and $GABA_C$ respectively.

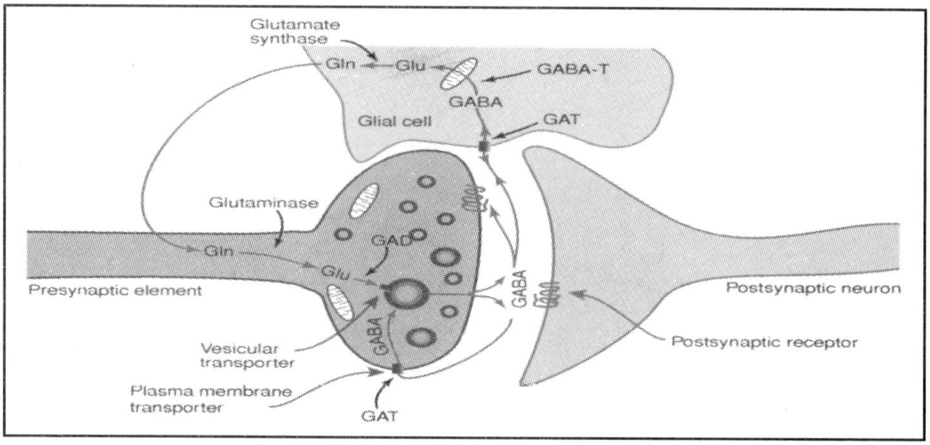

Fig. 1. GABA ergic synapse

The $GABA_A$ receptor is a member of a superfamily of ligand-gated ion channels of the type of nicotinic acetylcholine, glycine, and 5-HT_3 receptors. $GABA_A$ receptor is a hetero-oligomeric (pentameric protein) complex in its native state, composed of subunits with molecular weight of ~ 40-60 kDa[2]. At least 18 different receptor subunit genes have been separated into the sequence homology subfamilies alpha (α_1- α_6), beta (β_1 to β_3), gamma (γ_1- γ_3), delta, pi, epsilon, and theta, building a ligand gated chloride channel[3]. Furthermore, two additional subunits (β_4, γ_4) of GABA receptors in chick brain and five isoforms of the rho-subunits in the retina of the white perch have been identified. Most functional subtypes of $GABA_A$ receptor contain alpha, beta and gamma subunits. The preferred pentameric combination is either of two alpha, one beta and two gamma-subunits ($\alpha_2\beta\gamma_2$) or two alpha, two beta and one gamma ($\alpha_2\beta_2\gamma$) subunit. But one can expect a large number of combinatorial possibilities of $GABA_A$ receptors (Fig.2).

In the 1980's Bowery and his colleagues[4], observed that application of GABA reduced the evoked release of noradrenaline in the rat heart and this effect was not blocked by bicuculline. This action of GABA was mimicked by baclofen, 4-amino-3- (4-chlorophenyl) butanoic acid, a compound that had no effect on chloride conductance in central nervous system. This receptor was subsequently named as $GABA_B$ to differentiate it from its more familiar cousin, $GABA_A$ receptor $GABA_B$ receptor is a metabotropic receptor, which are widely distributed within the central nervous system and also in peripheral autonomic terminals. The activation of $GABA_B$ receptors causes an inhibition of both basal and forskolin stimulated adenyl cyclase activity together with a

α1	β1	γ1	δ	ε
α2	β2	γ2		
α3	β3	γ3		
α4	β4			
α5				
α6				

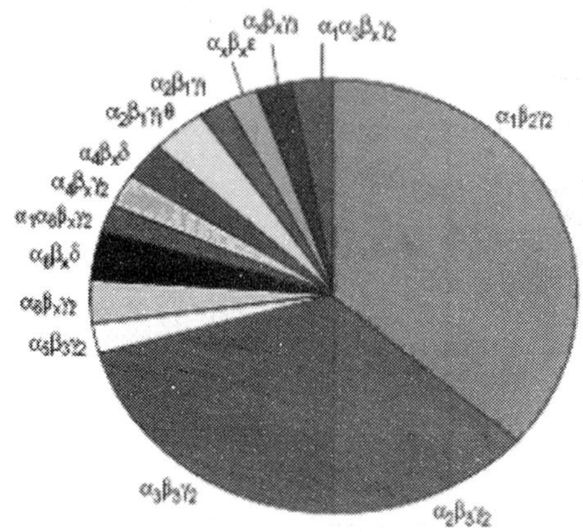

Fig. 2. Different protein subunits of $GABA_A$ receptor and various possible pentameric combinations of α, β and γ subunits of the receptor

decrease in Ca^{2+} and an increase in K^+ conductance in neuronal membranes. These receptors are activated by baclofen, and inhibited by phaclofen and saclofen. The $GABA_B$ receptor agonists are useful in the treatment of spasticity, pain and to reduce the craving for drugs of addiction. There is limited information on the therapeutic potential of $GABA_B$ receptor antagonists. The $GABA_B$ receptors are also functionally classified after the heterodimerization of $GABA_{(B1)}$ and $GABA_{(B2)}$ (previously known as GBR1 and GBR2). Both subunits are G-protein coupled receptors, a family of 7-transmebrane receptor family that shows a 30 % sequence homology to the metabotropic glutamate receptors[5, 6].

The third type of receptors namely $GABA_C$ are a distinct class of ligand gated ion channels that are activated by GABA. $GABA_C$ receptors are not blocked by bicuculline and do not recognize the benzodiazepines, barbiturates or the neuroactive steroids but, like $GABA_A$ receptors they are blocked by picrotoxin. The Table-1 summarizes the characteristics of different GABA receptor agonists and antagonists.

Functional consequences of $GABA_A$ receptors

The $GABA_A$ receptor complex is one of the most versatile drug-responsive mechanisms in the body. Each subunit possesses a large extracellular N-terminus with a cysteine bridge (beta-loop transmembrane domains) (M1-M4), a large variable intracellular loop

Table 1. Classification of GABA receptors: Molecular mechanism, Agonists and antagonists

	$GABA_A$	$GABA_B$	$GABA_C$
Effector Pathway	Ionotropic (ion channel) Cl^- ionophore	G- protein coupled (metabotropic). ↓ in Ca^{2+} and ↑ in K^+ conductance	Ion-channel receptor
Agonist	GABA, muscimol, many allosteric +ve modulators like benzodiazepines, barbiturates, neurosteroids, alcohol, general anesthetics, hypnotics, zolpidem	(-) Baclofen	Cis-4-aminocrotonic acid
Antagonists	Bicuculline, picrotoxin, pentylenetetrazol	Saclofen, phaclofen, CGP-35348, CGP55845A, CGP 54626	1,2,5,6-tetra hydropyridine-4-yl phosphinic acid (TPMPA)

between M3 and M4 and a short extracellular C-terminus. The extracellular N-terminus region contains three sites for N-linked glycosylation and the two-cysteine residues, which form the beta loop and may function in binding GABA and other ligands. The ends of the membranes spanning domains (M1-M4) are characterized by an abundant occurrence of positive charged amino acids, which are possibly involved in the regulation of chloride channels. The M2 domain, which is composed of several hydrophilic residues, is thought to line the channel pore. The extremely variable (length and composition) intracellular loop between M3 and M4 of some subunits contains consensus sequences for phosphorylation by protein kinase A and the tyrosine protein kinase (Fig. 3)

Activation of $GABA_A$ receptor by GABA leads to increased influx of chloride ions, resulting in membrane hyperpolarisation and neuronal inhibition.

A great number of distinct drug binding sites of the chloride channel have been characterized, each with its own set of agonists and antagonists (Fig. 4). The common pharmacological properties of three important $GABA_A$ receptor modulators are tabulated below (Table 2).

Benzodiazepine receptors coupled to $GABA_A$ receptor

The benzodiazepine receptors coupled to $GABA_A$ receptor domain are the site for at least three different types of ligand i.e. (1) diazepam-

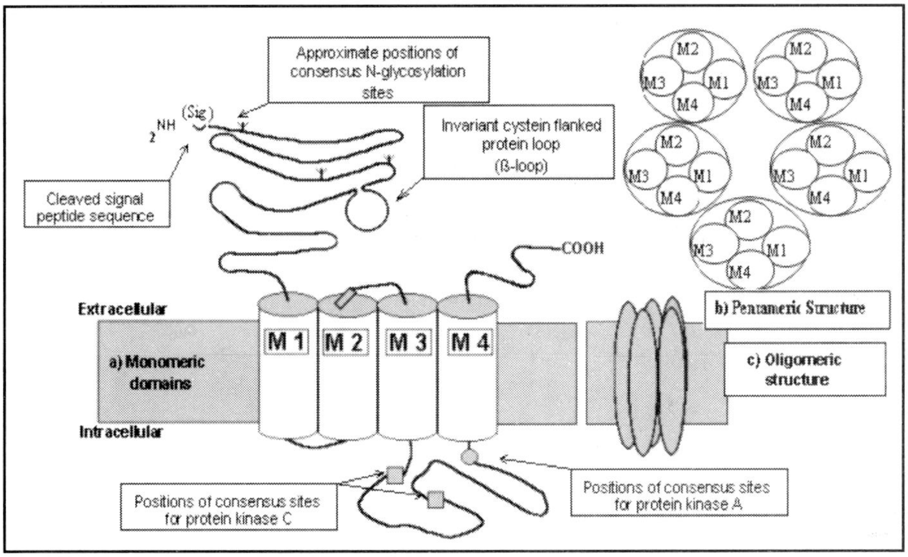

Fig. 3. Model of $GABA_A$ receptor (for details see text)

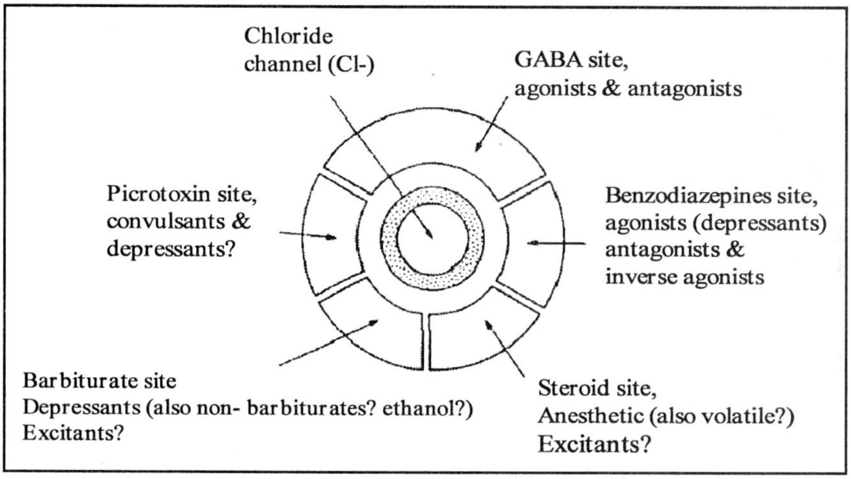

Fig. 4. Various binding sites on the $GABA_A$ receptor Cl^- ionophore complex

Table 2- Common Pharmacological Properties of three modulators of $GABA_A$ receptors

Drugs	Anti-convulsant	Hypno-sedative	Muscle relaxant	Withdrawal reaction
Benzodiazepines	++	+++	+++	++
Barbiturates	+++	+++	±	++
Alcohol	+	++	+	+++

like (agonists) (2), opposite to diazepam (inverse agonists), and (3) neutral, having no direct effect, but antagonize diazepam effects (antagonists). The bidirectionality (agonists and inverse agonists) at the benzodiazepine receptor concept has been widely accepted and attempts have been made to explore the biological and clinical significance of endogenous ligands as well as drugs that modulated these two receptors state of benzodiazepines (Fig. 5a and Fig. 5b)[7,8].

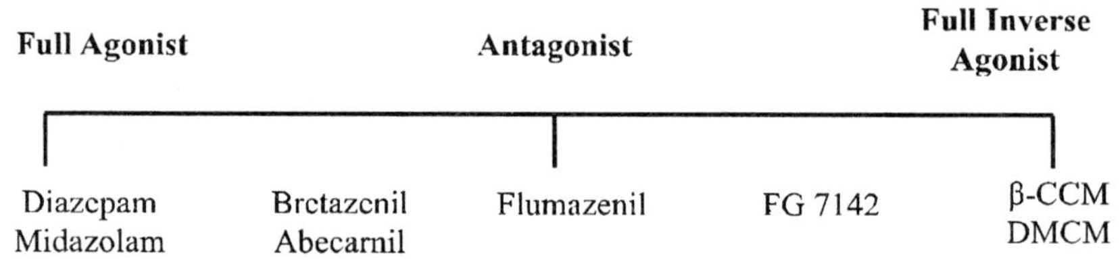

Fig. 5a. Spectrum of activity of compounds acting at the benzodiazepine receptor

Inverse agonist concept

The beta-carbolines, methyl-β-carboline-3-carboxylate (β-CCM), 6, 7-dimethoxy-4-ethyl-beta-carboline-3-carboxylic acid methyl ester (DMCM), and N-methyl-beta-carboline-3-carboxamide (FG-7142) act as inverse agonists or partial inverse agonists. These inverse agonists have the pharmacological effects that are opposite to full agonist namely diazepam, i.e. inverse agonists are anxiogenic, pro-conflict and pro-convulsants[9].

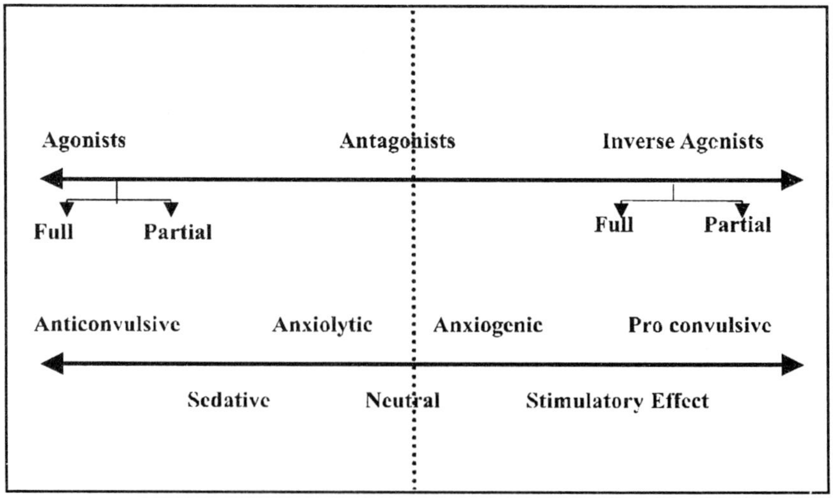

Fig. 5b. Benzodiazepine receptor ligands and their functional consequences

Benzodiazepines and beta carboline (inverse agonist) recognition sites are located in the alpha subunits of the $GABA_A$ receptor and are organized into an allosteric modulatory centre[10,11]. This centre appears to exist in two interconvertible transitional states. One prefers anxiogenic beta carbolines & other prefers anxiolytic benzodiazepines. Injection of beta carbolines in humans causes a panic-anxiety disorder. GABA downregulates the binding of beta carbolines. When the centre is occupied by beta carbolines, the probability of action of GABA at $GABA_A$ receptor is reduced. Flumazenil, an imidazobenzodiazepine, a benzodiazepine antagonist, antagonizes the action of beta carbolines as well as benzodiazepines. Fig. 6 illustrates the modulation of benzodiazepine receptor by agonists, inverse agonists and antagonist.

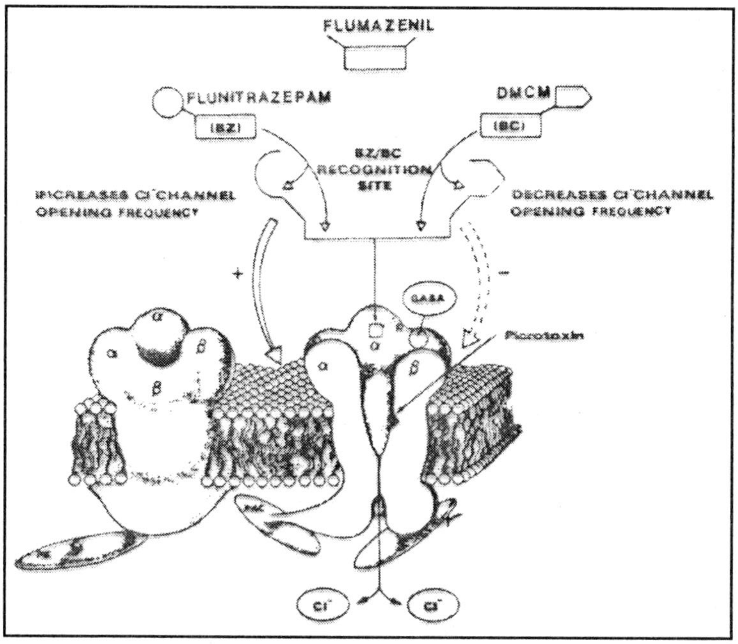

Fig. 6. Modulation of benzodiazepine receptor by different ligand molecules

Partial allosteric modulators

Imidazenil and bretazenil are new class of partial allosteric modulators (PAM) of $GABA_A$ receptors with high potency but low efficacy. Unlike alprazolam which is a full allosteric modulator (FAM) of $GABA_A$ receptors, these drugs i.e. imidazenil or bretazenil do not produce ataxia and sedation in rats and also do not potentiate the effects of ethanol or thiopental (Fig. 7). Further, when given along with diazepam imidazenil antagonizes the side effects of diazepam.

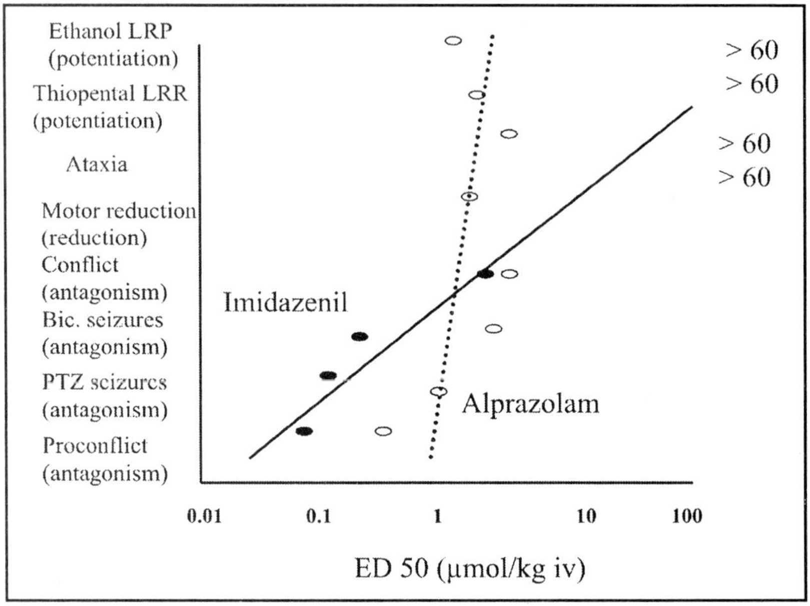

Fig. 7. Pharmacological profiles of PAM imidazenil (PAM) and alprazolam (FAM) in different behavioral tests in rats. Closed circles refer to the experiments with imidazenil and open circles refer to the experiments with alprazolam. Note that imidazenil fails to potentiate the effects of ethanol. LRR-Loss of Righting Reflex.

Ethanol and $GABA_A$ receptors

Ethanol has been reported to potentiate certain behavioral effects of GABA. Ethanol is also known to exert a number of behavioral effects such as sedation, ataxia, antianxiety, amnesia, muscle relaxation and anticonvulsant properties (Table 3) similar to diazepam. It has been speculated that the GABA-benzodiazepine receptor-coupled Cl^- channel could be the site of action of ethanol in the brain[7].

Ethanol is reported to potentiate GABA mediated Cl^- conductance. The formation of beta-carbolines is increased following ethanol and the urinary excretory pattern of these substances is correlated well with ethanol withdrawal syndrome, particularly anxiety and withdrawal convulsions. The inverse agonists favor the reversal of acute central nervous system depressant effect of ethanol and other depressants.

With this background, several inverse agonists, both beta-carbolines and other benzodiazepines have been extensively investigated for their useful effect in reversing the acute intoxicating

Table 3. Anticonvulsant effect of ethanol when studied against different chemoconvulsants in mice

Treatment (mg/kg, i.p.)	Onset (min ± SD)	Total seizure duration (min ± SD)	Mortality (%)
Bicuculline (4)	1.8 ± 0.8	6.4 ± 1.4	100
Picrotoxin (10)	5.0 ± 1.8	15.8 ± 3	100
Strychnine (4)	2.5 ± 0.5	5.2 ± 0.8	100
Ethanol (2 g/kg) + Bicuculline	2.3 ± 0.6	-	0
Ethanol (2 g/kg) + Picrotoxin	16 ± 1.0**	17.0 ± 3	70
Ethanol (2 g/kg) + Strychnine	2.3 ± 0.5	48 ± 27.0*	75

**P<0.01 and **P<0.001 as compared to corresponding per se effect of convulsant respectively*

effects of alcohol. These compounds were thought to produce sobering effect in individuals intoxicated with ethanol[8].

Of particular interest is the imidazobenzodiazepine, R015-4513, a structural analogue of benzodiazepine receptor antagonist, flumazenil (R015-1788) which has been extensively investigated for anti-alcohol effects.

Reversal of ethanol effect by R015-4513, an inverse agonist

R015-4513 is the azido analogue of the classic benzodiazepine receptor antagonist R015-1788 with ability to bind to benzodiazepine receptors. R015-4513 antagonized both *in vitro* ability of ethanol to stimulate $^{36}Cl^-$ uptake in rat brain synaptoneurosomes and *in vivo*, the anticonflict activity of low dose of ethanol as well as sedative effect of higher dose of ethanol in rats and mice. However, when administered alone, R015-4513 lowered seizure threshold to bicuculline, pentylenetetrazol, and R0 5-3663 and reduced explorative behavior in a hole-board apparatus.

Anti-alcohol pill: A myth or reality

Drugs possessing alcohol antagonistic properties have far reaching clinical application in the management of acute alcohol effect in man. The recent research findings with R015-4513 have raised wide speculations regarding the possible clinical use of this as well as other related drugs for sobering effects in alcohol intoxication. Rats passed out from alcohol intoxication acted sober within two minutes of R015-

4513 administration. However, the possible clinical use of R015-4513 is limited due to its proconvulsant property (Table 4)[7], since it may precipitate withdrawal symptoms in alcoholics and also it has short duration of action.

Table 4. Proconvulsant effects of R015-4513 as studied against bicuculline

Treatment (mg/kg, i.p.)	Onset (sec ± SEM)	Mortality time (min ± SEM)	Mortality (/n)	Severity of convulsions
Bicuculline (1)	-	-	-	No convulsions
Bicuculline (4)	59 ± 5.77	14 ± 1.62	4/7	++
Bicuculline (8)	36 ± 2.32	8 ± 0.63	10/10	+++
R015-4513 (1) + Bicuculline (4)	28 ± 2.25	15 ± 1.75	4/4	++
R015-4513 (1) + Bicuculline (8)	13 ± 3.0**	6 ± 0.84	6/6	+++
R015-4513 (4) + Bicuculline (8)	16 ± 1.35	2.8 ± 0.20*	5/5	+++

GABA$_A$ receptors and neurosteroids

Neurosteroids are the steroids that are synthesized within the brain either from cholesterol or from peripheral steroid hormones[12]. Steroid hormones have long been recognized as possessing sedative and anaesthetic properties in animals and humans[13]. Deoxycorticosterone, the first adrenal steroid isolated by Von Steiger in 1937[14], has profound effect on CNS excitability besides having weak mineralocorticoid action. This neurosteroid can act as an endogenous anticonvulsant substance. Stress-induced hypothalamic corticotropin releasing hormone (CRH) stimulates adrenocorticotrophic hormone (ACTH), which in turn stimulates synthesis and release of cortisol and deoxycorticosterone from the adrenal cortex. During the course of stress response, the increased levels of tetrahydrodeoxycorticosterone (THDOC) synthesized in liver and brain from circulating deoxycorticosterone, activates GABAergic inhibitory transmission in neuronal networks in hippocampus, amygdala, and cerebral cortex and controls seizure susceptibility (Fig. 8).

Studies indicate that antiseizure activity of deoxycorticosterone is due to its conversion to allotetrahydrodeoxycorticosterone (THDOC), a neurosteroid (Fig 8). Allopregnanolone and THDOC are generally viewed to share common physiological and pharmacological effects (anxiolytic, antiseizure, antistress, antidepressant, amnesic, and neuroprotection). Several studies have shown that neurosteroids are

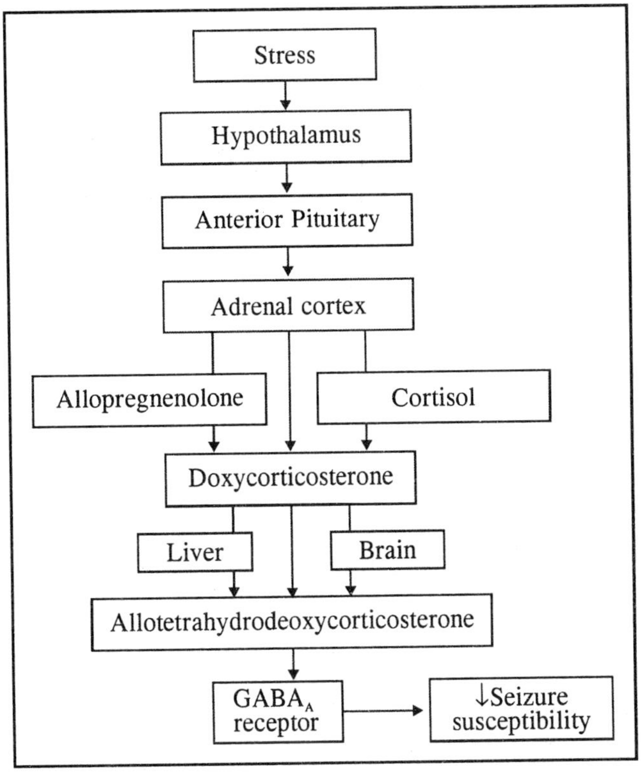

Fig. 8. Stress and activation of neurosteroids

shown to produce pharmacological action by acting on GABA$_A$ receptors[15]. The proposed molecular site for neurosteroid on GABA$_A$ receptor is shown in Fig. 9.

THDOC binds to GABA$_A$ receptor at site different from GABA, benzodiazepine or barbiturate. Several studies indicate that THDOC acts as positive allosteric modulator of GABA$_A$ receptor function and increases the inhibitory post-synaptic potential. THDOC potentiated the $^{36}Cl^-$ flux stimulated by GABA$_A$ receptor agonists. Neurosteroids enhancement of submaximal GABA$_A$ receptor function occurs through increase in both channel open frequency and open duration[16,17].

Ganaxolone (3α-hydroxy-3β-methyl-5α-pregnane- 20-one), the synthetic 3β-methyl analog of the natural neurosteroid allopregnanolone, is a potent positive allosteric modulator of GABA$_A$ receptors and is an effective anticonvulsant in the pentylenetetrazol (PTZ) seizure test as well as in other animal models used in the evaluation of antiepileptic drugs. Unlike allopregnanolone, which has

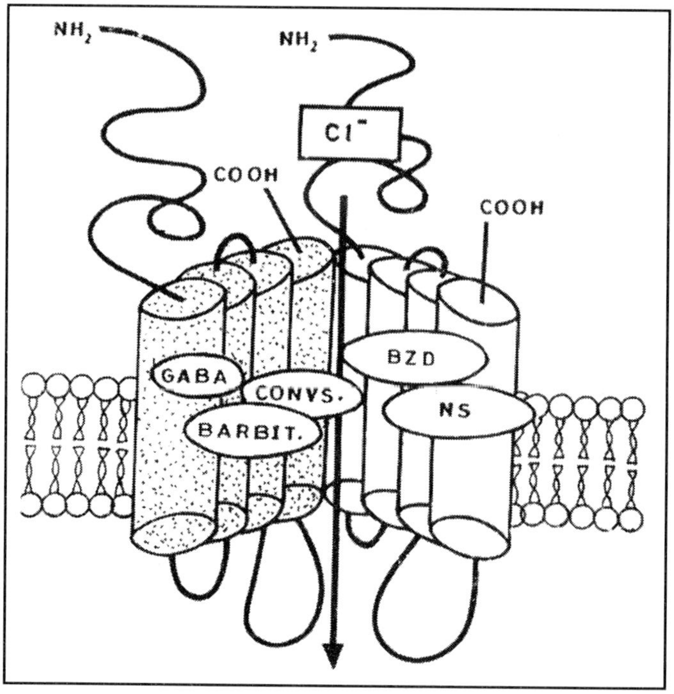

Fig . 9. The possible binding site of neurosteroids (NS) on $GABA_A$ receptor

a short duration of action, ganaxolone is orally active and adequate blood levels can be maintained in human subjects with two or three times daily dosing.

Summary

γ-Amino butyric acid (GABA) is the major inhibitory neurotransmitter in the mammalian central nervous system. Almost 60-75 % of the neurons in the central nervous system are GABAergic in nature and they are virtually absent outside the brain and the spinal cord. GABA produces inhibitory hyperpolarizing response by increasing the chloride (Cl^-) conductance of the neuronal membrane. Increased GABAergic activity produces CNS depression, sedation, ataxia and amnesia. Any loss in GABAergic tone would lead to arousal response, insomnia and excitation. GABA is known to act on three distinct receptor subtypes, of which $GABA_A$ receptors are widely studied. The $GABA_A$ receptor is a ligand gated ion channel receptor and is influenced by diverse chemical ligands. Many drugs including benzodiazepines, alcohol, neurosteroids and inverse agonists modulated $GABA_A$ receptor mediated physiological functions. Such diversity provides many avenues for the design and development of new chemical entities acting on $GABA_A$ receptors.

REFERENCES

1. Kulkarni SK & Sharma A, GABA-B receptors and nociception, *Drugs of Today* 30 (1994) 459.
2. Schofield PR, Darlison MG, Fujita N, Burt DR, Stephenson FA, Rodriguez H, Rhee LM, Ramachandran J, Reale V, & Glencorse TA, Sequence and functional expression of the GABA A receptor shows a ligand-gated receptor super-family. *Nature,* 328 (1987) 221.
3. Bormann J, The 'ABC' of GABA receptors. *Trends Pharmacol Sci,* 21(2000) 9
4. Bowery NG, Doble A, Hill DR, Hudson AL, Shaw JS, Turnbull MJ & Warrington R, Bicuculline-insensitive GABA receptors on peripheral autonomic nerve terminals. *Eur J Pharmacol,* 71(1981)53.
5. Kulkarni SK, GABAB receptors and Phaclofen. *Meth Find Exp Clin Pharmacol,* 11(1989) 129.
6. Billinton A, Ige AO, Bolam JP, White JH, Marshall FH & Emson PC, Advances in the molecular understanding of GABA (B) receptors. *Trends Neurosci,* 24 (2001)277.
7. Ticku MK & Kulkarni SK, Molecular interactions of ethanol with GABAergic system and potential of Ro 15-4513 as an ethanol antagonist. *Pharmacol Biochem Behav,* 30(1988)501.
8. Kulkarni SK, Development of an anti-alcohol pill: a myth or reality. *The Eastern Pharmacist,* 1988(1988) 51.
9. Kulkarni SK & Mehta AK, Benzodiazepine receptor antagonists and inverse agonists. *Drugs of Today* 21(1985) 145.
10. Costa E & Guidotti A, Molecular mechanisms in the receptor action of benzodiazepines. *Annu Rev Pharmacol Toxicol,* 19(1979)531.
11. Costa E, Polytypic signaling at GABAergic synapses. *Life Sci* 42(1988)1407.
12. Baulieu EE, Neurosteroids: A novel function of the brain. *Psychoneuroendocrinology,* 23(1998)963.
13. Selye H, Correlations between the chemical structure and the pharmacological actions of the steroids. *Endocrinology,* 3(1942)437
14. Von Steiger M & Reichstein T. Dexoxycorticosterone (21-oxyprogesterone) aus DELTA5- 3- oxy-atio-cholensaure. *Helv Chim Acta,* 20 (1937) 1164.
15. Kulkarni SK & Reddy DS, Neurosteroids: A new class of neuromodulators. *Drugs of Today,* 6 (1995) 433-435.
16. Reddy DS & Kulkarni SK, Development of neurosteroid-based novel psychotropic drugs. *Prog Med Chem,* 37(2000) 135.
17. Reddy DS, The clinical potentials of endogenous neurosteroids. *Drugs of Today,* 38 (2002) 465.

2

γ- Amino butyric acid (GABA) mediated behavioral studies

S.K. KULKARNI AND ASHISH DHIR
Pharmacology Division, University Institute of Pharmaceutical Sciences,
Panjab University, Chandigarh 160 014, India

Introduction

γ- Amino butyric Acid (GABA) is a non-essential amino acid found ubiquitously in the mammalian brain. It is an inhibitory neurotransmitter. Its inhibitory action results from a hyperpolarization of the synaptic transmembrane potential of the neuron. GABA is referred to as the "brain's natural calming agent". At least three receptors have been characterized on which GABA acts to bring about the physiological response. These include $GABA_A$ (ionotropic receptors), $GABA_B$ (metabotropic receptors) and $GABA_C$ (ionotropic receptors), respectively *(for details see earlier section)*. As discussed in the previous chapter GABA agonists or modulators have profound clinical applications in a variety of CNS disorders namely anxiety, stress, sleep, memory, epilepsy, depression, and drug addiction. In this chapter the role of GABA modulators in various neurological disorders has been discussed. Attempt has also been made to correlate CNS effects of herbals with GABAergic modulation. The last part of the chapter briefly discusses about the stress and the neuroendocrine system of the body.

Epilepsy

The word "Epilepsy" is derived from a Greek word ***epilamvanein*** meaning "a condition of being overcome, seized, or attacked." It is an age old disease, considered as a curse and described as a "disease of lightning-struck down by a bolt from the sky". Many famous historical figures such as Alexander the Great, Julius Caesar, Napoleon Bonaparte, Charles Dickens, and Vincent Van Gogh were affected by epilepsy[1]. Epilepsy is a nonhomogenous group of neurological disorder, including primary generalized (tonic clonic or absence) epilepsy and myoclonic seizure disorders. John H. Jackson, considered as father of modern concepts of epilepsy (in the late 1880s) described epilepsy as "occasional, sudden, excessive, rapid and local discharges of the gray matter". The epidemiological studies indicate that one in 200 in the general population suffered from epilepsy. The etiology of epilepsy is multifactorial, and the exact cause is often unknown. Head trauma, stroke, birth injury, brain tumors or infections are some of the causes of epilepsy (Fig 1)[2]. Abnormal and massive electric discharges in the brain are now considered as the basis for differential diagnosis of the disease. The incidence of epilepsy varies considerably with age; the greatest being in early childhood, reaching a nadir in the early adult life, and again rising in elderly. The International League against Epilepsy (ILAE) in 1981 has given clinical classification of seizure types based on the electroencephalographic (EEG) after discharges (AD).

Seizures are characterized by excessive discharges of neurons in the CNS. There are different neurotransmitters and neuromodulators in the brain that have been speculated to be involved in the neuronal

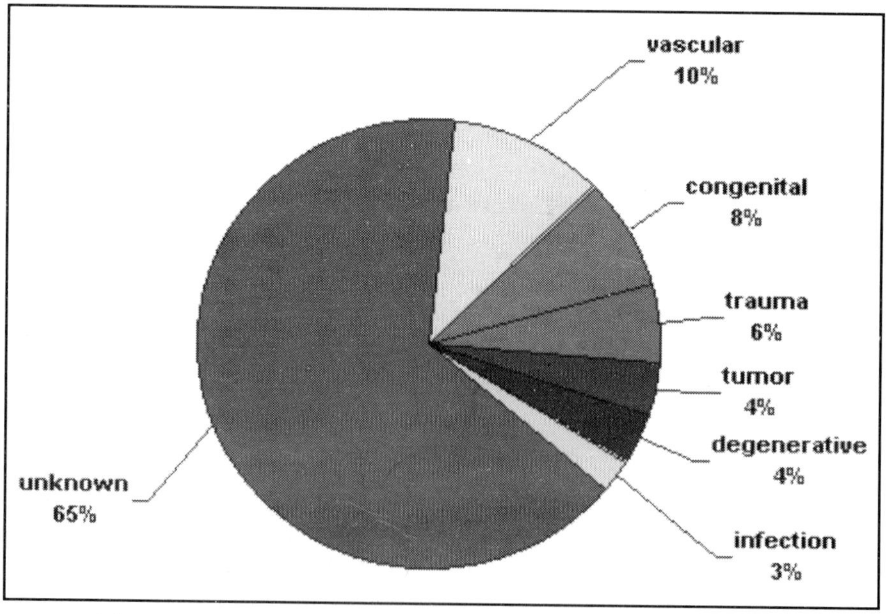

Fig. 1. Pie-chart illustrating the different causes of epilepsy

excitation. These predominantly include γ-amino butyric acid (GABA), glutamate, dopamine, and acetylcholine[3]. These neurotransmitters are broadly divided into inhibitory and excitatory types. Their receptor interplay have been recognized in the expression of complex behavioral and electrographic patterns seen in epilepsy. Fine tuning of various neurotransmitters is essential for the maintenance of homeostasis, particularly in brain structures which regulate emotion, behavior and cognitive function[4].

Three principal factors are thought to contribute to the initiation of epileptic discharges. Firstly, the population of excitatory neurons with the ability to generate so-called intrinsic bursts, namely, barrage of action potentials. The second is an increase in glutamatergic (excitatory) synaptic transmission particularly via recurrent connections; and the third is a decrease in the efficacy of GABA-mediated (inhibitory) connections[5,6]. Attenuation of seizures is frequently achieved with drugs that increase neuronal inhibition or decreases the excitatory neurotransmitter(s). Consequently, the inhibitory neurotransmitter GABA has been suggested to play an important role in regulating neuronal excitability, seizure production and its control. A loss or reduction (as little as 10-15 %) in GABAergic inhibition significantly facilitates seizure spread in cortical tissues[7].

GABA is known to produce its inhibitory response by increasing the conductance to chloride (Cl^-) ions. Activation of $GABA_A$ receptors, which are coupled directly to an ion-channel, results in an increase in chloride conductance, inducing early, short duration inhibitory post-synaptic potentials. $GABA_B$ receptors present in most brain structures are located in the post-synaptic membrane and on presynaptic axon terminals[8]. They are coupled to their effector via G-protein. Activation of postsynaptic $GABA_B$ receptor mediates a late long-lasting postsynaptic potential, while presynaptic $GABA_B$ receptors regulate the release of several neurotransmitters and neuropeptides from nerve terminals[9]. Blockade of presynaptic receptor increases the release of glutamate and GABA from cortical slices[10]. During the high frequency transmission at the glutamatergic system, the NMDA receptors in particular are activated as there is a simultaneously depression in GABA-mediated synaptic inhibition through $GABA_B$ autoreceptors. Thus, NMDA receptors remain in active state (increased efficiency) and calcium ions enter the cell through NMDA receptor channel to induce long-term potentiation (LTP). The LTP formation is considered as one of the mechanisms for learning and memory and also for excitotoxicity as in the case of epilepsy (Fig 2).

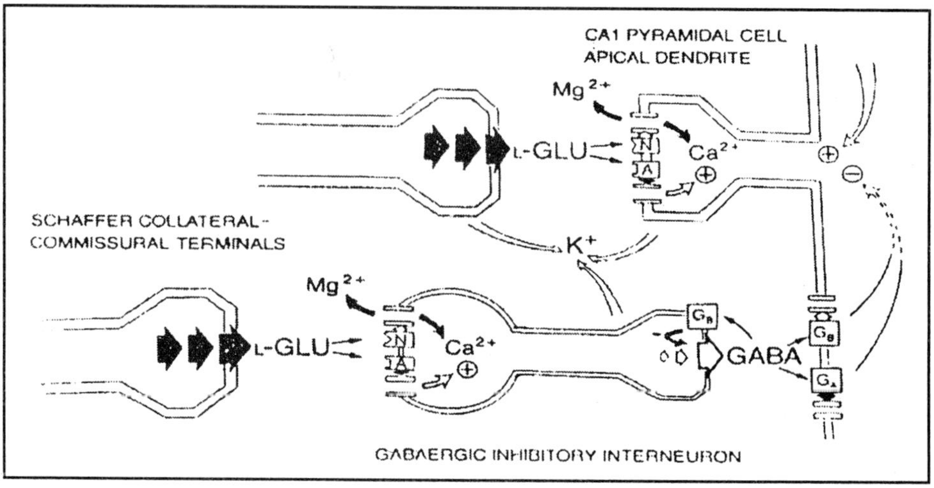

Fig. 2. Scheme for the induction of Long term potentiation (LTP) in the Schaffer collateral-commissural pathway. GABAergic system provides powerful synaptic inhibition; when activated it hyperpolarizes cells in the region where NMDA receptor-gated ion channel are subjected to substantial blockade by Mg^{2+} (present in the synaptic cleft). During high frequency transmission, synaptic inhibition fatigues and extracellular K^{+} elevates. Under these conditions cells stay depolarized for longer, the Mg^{2+} block of NMDA channel is reduced and NMDA receptors mediate a slow Excitatory Post Synaptic Potential (EPSP). Ca^{2+} enters the cell via the NMDA channels where it may activate local processes that sustain the enhanced response.

After release into the synapse, free GABA that does not bind to either the GABA-A or GABA-B receptor complexes can be taken up by neurons and glial cells by different transporters in the brain. Four membrane transporter proteins, known as GAT-1, GAT-2, GAT-3, and BGT-1, which differ in their distribution in the CNS, are believed to mediate the uptake of synaptic GABA into neurons and glial cells[11].

The highest concentrations of GABAergic neurons are found in the substantia nigra, basal ganglia, hypothalamus, periacqueductal grey and dentate nuclei[3]. There is also a high concentration of GABA in cortical grey matter and cortical interneurons. Understanding of the GABA/benzodiazepine (BZ) receptors has been greatly, enhanced by molecular biological approaches in the last 10 years[12,13] (*For details see earlier section).*

Numerous natural and synthetic compounds interact with the $GABA_A$ receptor at distinct, yet incompletely defined, sites. These compounds include barbiturates, benzodiazepines, neurosteroids, alcohol, anaesthetics and picrotoxin[14,15]. The benzodiazepine receptors complied to $GABA_A$ receptors are modulated by three distinct class of ligands, agonists, inverse agonists and neutral ligands. $GABA_A$ receptor agonists as well as drugs, which allosterically modulate the $GABA_A$ receptor channel complex, are therapeutically effective against convulsive seizures[16]. On the other hand, $GABA_A$ receptor antagonists like bicuculline, picrotoxin (*For details see Dhir, Naidu, and Kulkarni, 2005*) produce convulsions in animals. These convulsants are widely used as tool to screen the antiepileptic potential of different molecules.

Enhancement of GABA function can theoretically be effected through several mechanisms. These include direct receptor agonism which is the mode of action of the benzodiazepines, inhibition of the extraneuronal enzymatic breakdown of GABA, which is the mechanism of vigabatrin, modulation of GABA-coupled ion channels, which is the primary mode of action of topiramate, and inhibition of the reuptake of synaptic GABA by neurons and glial cells, which is the mechanism of tiagabine. Some drugs like gabapentin whose mechanism is still debatable, is hypothesized to act through GABAergic modulation[17]. The mechanism of action of these drugs which are used as antiepileptic agents are shown in the following Fig.3. and Table 1.

Electroconvulsive shock (ECS) treatment has been extensively employed for many years to treat psychiatric illness. Repeated ECS is known to cause an increase in GABA function in several brain regions[18]. Several experimental studies have supported the involvement of GABAergic tone in ECS mechanism[19]. Electroconvulsive shock (ECS) was given acutely as well as chronically. Neither acute nor chronic ECS had any significant effect on bicuculline-induced convulsions, whereas the latency for picrotoxin (PTX)-induced convulsions was delayed by both acute and chronic ECS.

Baclofen, a $GABA_B$ agonists treatment delayed significantly the latency for PTX-induced convulsions in animals which were subjected to both acute and chronic ECS, whereas in bicuculline-induced convulsions, it shortened the latency of convulsions 24 hr after acute ECS. Progabide, both $GABA_A$ and $GABA_B$ agonist delayed the bicuculline-induced convulsions. Fengabine, an agonist at $GABA_A$ receptor showed no significant effect on bicuculline-induced convulsions. However, on PTX-induced convulsions, the latency was delayed in animals not subjected to ECS and in those subjected to chronic ECS[20]. There is a possible alteration in receptor sensitivity, number or alterations in the levels of endogenous neurotransmitter following acute or chronic ECS, which is responsible for these observations (*For more details refer to Aley and Kulkarni, 1991).*

Kindling is a model of epilepsy and epileptogenesis. Daily electrical stimulation of the amygdaloid complex through low-intensity electric current has been shown to produce kindled seizures in animals. Repeated application of subconvulsive doses of CNS stimulants like pentylenetetrazol (PTZ), cocaine, picrotoxin, strychnine and bicuculline once every 24 or 48 hr over a period of time is also known to induce a permanent change in the epileptogenic sensitivity of forebrain structures, such that initial subconvulsive stimuli become capable of evoking fully developed seizures[21].

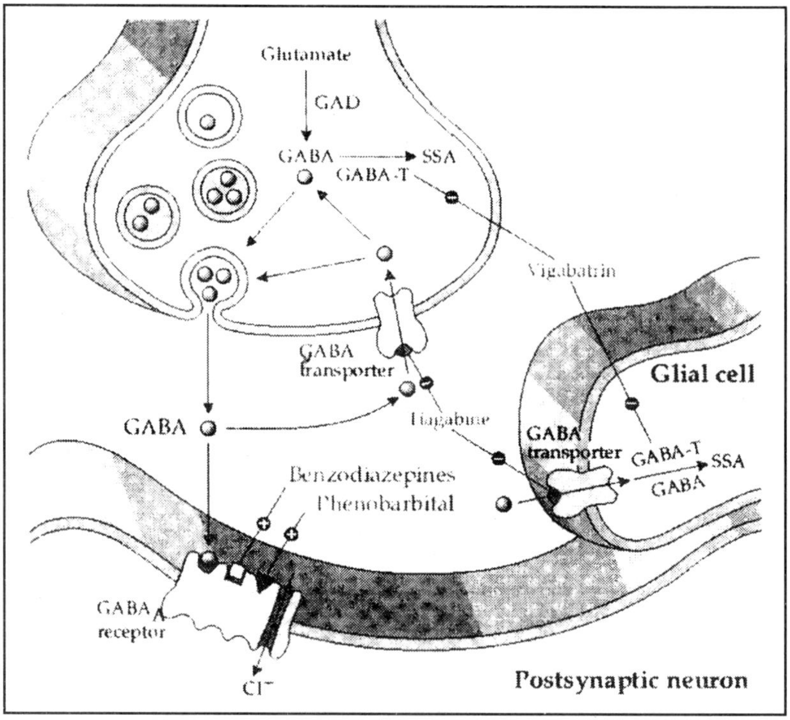

Fig. 3. Possible sites of interaction of antiepileptic drugs on GABA-mediated transmission. GABA is formed from glutamate by the action of glutamic acid decarboxylase (GAD), and metabolized by GABA aminotransaminase (GABA-T) to form succinic acid semialdehyde (SSA). The GABA$_A$ receptor is associated within ion channel permeable to Cl^-. GABA$_A$ receptor activation increases Cl^- conductance by opening the channel and hyperpolarization. Barbiturates and benzodiazepines act via associated modulatory sites to potentiate the effect of GABA on Cl^- conductance.

PTZ-induced kindling is related to the down regulation of $GABA_A$ergic transmission in the CNS[22]. PTZ is reported to inhibit $GABA_A$-induced chloride conductance in cultured mouse spinal-cord neurons, and also ^{35}[S] TBPS binding in rat brain homogenates in a concentration dependent manner. The drugs that protect from kindling in animals are said to be antiepileptic and acting via $GABA_A$ergic transmission.

Table 1. Pharmacological profiles of selective GABAergic drugs used as antiepileptic (*Adapted from Ketter et al., 1999*)[17].

Drug	GABAergic Potency	GABAergic effects	Profile
Tiagabine	Strong	GABA- reuptake inhibition	Sedating
Gabapentin	Strong	Increase glial GABA release	Sedating
Vigabatrin	Strong	GABA transaminase inhibition	Sedating
Valproate	Strong	Increase cerebral GABA concentration	Sedating

Status Epilepticus (SE) is a condition in which the seizure last or recur over a period of at least 30 minute without a return to normal baseline activity[23]. It is recognized as both a major neurological problem and an intriguing neurobiological phenomenon. SE may occur as a part of an acute illness or may be part of an existing seizure disorder[24]. In Lithium-pilocarpine model of status epilepticus there is marked reduction of $GABA_A$ receptor currents in the CA1 pyramidal neurons leading to loss of GABA-mediated inhibition. It is likely that $GABA_A$ receptor protein is modified during status epilepticus, thus producing the loss of affinity and activity of the receptor[25].

GABA/BZ Inverse agonist concept and convulsions

Benzodiazepine (BZ) receptor is the site of action for three classes of pharmacologically distinct agents. They are agonists, inverse agonists and competitive antagonists[26]. Evidences have indicated that certain benzodiazepine receptor ligands designated as inverse agonists such as β-carboline derivatives act by reducing GABA-ergic inhibition via an allosteric interaction with the $GABA_A$ receptor, thus produce anxiogenic, proconvulsant or convulsant effects. DMCM (6, 7 dimethoxy-4-ethyl-beta carboline-3-carboxylic acid methyl ester) is a benzodiazepine inverse agonist with anxiogenic and proconvulsant profile[27]. Ro 5-4864 (p-chlorodiazepam) is another BZ receptor ligand preferring the peripheral type of BZ receptors with anxiogenic and convulsant properties[26]. In another study, the difference in the mechanism of action of the benzodiazepine (BZ) inverse agonist DMCM and peripheral type BZ receptor agonist Ro 5-4864 were elucidated in mice. Both of them produced tonic-clonic convulsions in mice. Activation of central alpha$_2$ adrenoceptors by clonidine significantly delayed the onset of Ro 5-4864-induced convulsions while no significant effect was seen in DMCM-induced convulsions. Pretreatment of Ro15-1788 (flumazenil), a benzodiazepine receptor antagonist failed to antagonize the convulsant effect of Ro 5-4864. On the other hand it reversed the DMCM-induced convulsions. Ro 5-4864 is a selective ligand for GABA-independent peripheral and micromolecular binding site. PK 11195, the peripheral BZ antagonist, reversed the anxiogenic and convulsant profile of Ro 5-4864. It was suggested that Ro 5-4864 has been shown to interact with GABA-benzodiazepine receptor complex in the CNS, possibly, due to its ability to bind at high concentration to the picrotoxin domain on this complex[28]. The study also demonstrated that alpha$_2$ adrenoceptors can modulate picrotoxin site mediated GABAergic effects while BZ inverse agonists mediated GABAergic effects remain unclear (*For details see Kunchandy and Kulkarni, 1988*).

Flumazenil (Ro 15-1788), an imidazodiazepine, antagonizes a wide spectrum of behavioral effects of benzodiazepines. This molecule is also known to antagonize the effect of inverse agonists such as β-carbolines. But some studies have proved that flumazenil also possessed some intrinsic activity at GABA-BZ receptor channel[29] (*For details see Aley, Kulkarni, Mathur, and Nayar, 1990*). Benzodiazepine and inverse agonist sites are supposed to be up-regulated in rat cerebral cortex and hippocampus following chronic treatment with Ro15-1788 and its withdrawal. If this compound is supposed to have intrinsic activity, one may expect both behavioral and EEG changes in different brain areas. In one of the study[30], we have seen the effect of chronic treatment and its withdrawal due to Ro 15-1788 on cortical and hippocampal EEG discharges in conscious rat brains. Chronic treatment with Ro 15-1788 and its withdrawal reduced the cortical and hippocampal EEG amplitude as compared to control group (Fig.4.).

In animals chronically treated with the Ro15-1788, GABA reversed the effect of chronic Ro15-1788 treatment, while, baclofen a GABA$_B$ agonist and FG 7142, a benzodiazepine inverse agonist enhanced the effect. This may be due to allosteric interactions at GABA/BZ receptor complex. Also, biochemical studies have demonstrated that various sites on the macromolecular GABA receptor complex bear a relationship with each other in an allosteric manner[31]. Therefore, it may be suggested that the conformational changes produced on the GABA/BZ receptor complex by Ro 15-1788 treatment has a facilitatory effect on the action of other drugs which act on GABA/BZ receptor complex and the direction (positive or negative) of this enhancement depended on the nature of the drug (*For details see Aley, Kulkarni, Mathur, and Nayar, 1990*).

It has also been suggested that β-carbolines may share some of the pharmacological properties of adenosine antagonists such as caffeine and theophylline in addition to any action at the GABA-benzodioazepine receptor complex[32]. At cellular level, adenosine and its stable analogues have been shown to inhibit spontaneously evoked neuronal firing through activation of specific receptors at pre-and post-synaptic domains throughout the CNS[33]. Adenosine has been reported to be an endogenous anticonvulsant and neuroprotective agent[34]. Adenosinergic agents such as adenosine, 2-chloroadenosine, N^6-cyclohexyladenosine produced dose-dependent protective effect against DMCM- and Ro 5-4864-induced convulsions and mortality. N^6-cyclohexyladenosine produced most significant protective effect against Ro 5-4864-induced convulsions whereas 2-chloroadenosine was more effective than N^6-cyclohexyladenosine in antagonizing DMCM-induced convulsions. Pretreatment of animals with subprotective doses of adenosine and dipyridamole significantly prolonged the latencies for the onset of myoclonic jerks and convulsions due to both DMCM and Ro 5-4864. DMCM and Ro 5-4864-induced mortality rate was also significantly reduced by pretreatment with subprotective doses of adenosine and dipyridamole. Similarly, subprotective doses of adenosine and diazepam further delayed the latencies for myoclonic jerks and convulsions due to DMCM and Ro 5-4864 treatment. The results suggested that adenosine and adenosine receptor agonists, 2-chloroadenosine and N^6-cyclohexyladenosine are protective against both DMCM- and Ro 5-4864-induced convulsions. Throat and Kulkarni have suggested that adenosinergic agents via activation of central A_1 adenosine receptors may modulate the convulsant effects mediated by DMCM and Ro 5-4864[35]. These observations further supported the notion that adenosinergic mechanisms mediate neuroprotective effects in the central nervous system (*For details see Thorat and Kulkarni., 1990*).

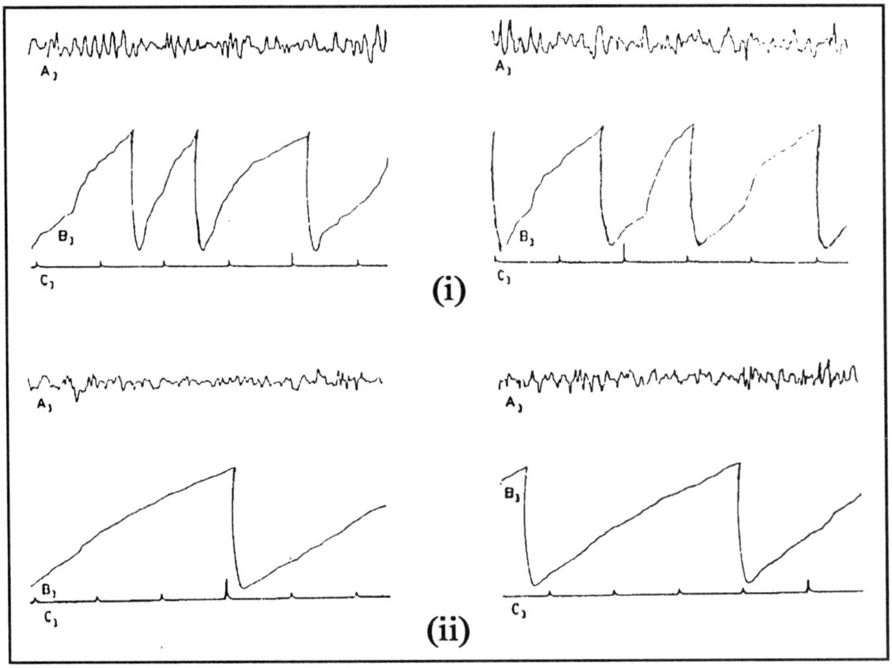

Fig. 4. Cortical and hippocampal EEG of rats chronically treated with **(i)** vehicle (control) **(ii)** Ro 15-1788 on the basal EEG, B: integrated voltage, C: time calibration, 48 hr after 14th dose of Ro 15-1788.

Inflammatory process and epilepsy: possible GABAergic mechanism

In recent years, increasing evidence has indicated that immune and inflammatory reactions occur in brain in various central nervous system diseases. Furthermore, inflammatory processes, such as the production of proinflammatory cytokines (IL-1α, IL-1β) and related molecules like cyclooxygenases, have been described in brain after seizures induced in experimental models of epilepsy. Although little is known about the role of inflammation in epilepsy, it has been hypothesized that activation of the innate immune system and associated inflammatory reactions in brain may mediate some of the molecular and structural changes occurring during and after seizure activity. Whether the innate immune response that takes place in epileptic tissue is beneficial or noxious to the CNS is still an open and intriguing question.

Arachidonic acid which is converted into prostaglandins by the action of cyclooxygenase, has been proposed to be a diffusible second messenger in the CNS with a pathophysiological role in epilepsy. This is possibly due to the ability of arachidonic acid to enhance extra-neuronal glutamate concentration[36]. Therefore, we examined the effects of combining COX-inhibitors with subprotective dose of muscimol, a $GABA_A$ agonists against bicuculline and picrotoxin-induced convulsions.

Convulsions were induced with bicuculline, picrotoxin (both GABA receptor antagonists) or electroshock. Various COX-inhibitors were administered 45 minutes prior to an epileptic challenge. Onset, duration of clonus and percentage mortality/recovery were recorded. Bicuculline, picrotoxin or electroshock significantly induced convulsions. Nimesulide or rofecoxib prolonged mean onset time of convulsions, decreased duration of clonus and decreased % mortality rate against bicuculline- and picrotoxin- induced convulsions in mice. COX-2 inhibitors were ineffective towards maximal electroshock-induced convulsions. Nimesulide and rofecoxib in lower doses also enhanced the effect of subprotective dose of muscimol against picrotoxin-induced convulsions[37] (Fig.5.).

The study carried out by Dhir, Naidu and Kulkarni strongly suggested the possible role of cyclooxygenase isoenzymes particularly COX-2, in the pathophysiology of epilepsy and they may modulate GABAergic mechanisms in the treatment of epilepsy *(For details see Dhir, Naidu and Kulkarni, 2006).*

There may be other possibility that cyclooxygenase enzyme induction leads to increase in prostaglandin levels particularly PGE_2, which facilitates glutamate release from the nerve terminal and astrocytes[38]. In one study PGE_2 increased the mean size of evoked excitatory postsynaptic currents (EPSC) in a proportion of rat nucleus tractus solitarii neurons and increased the frequency of miniature EPSCs mediated by non-NMDA glutamate receptors[39]. Third possibility is that activation of cyclooxygenases cause an increase in the free radical production leading to oxidative stress, thus leading to apoptosis of GABAergic neurons, thus, causing epileptic discharges. COX-2 enzyme may also have a role to play in excitatory synapse as excitatory amino acid agonists such as NMDA induce strong COX-2 immunostaining in many regions of the limbic cortex, isocortex, hippocampus and amygdala[40].

Role of other neurotransmitters in epilepsy

The amino acid glutamate is widely distributed in mammalian brain and is considered as the primary excitatory neurotransmitter in

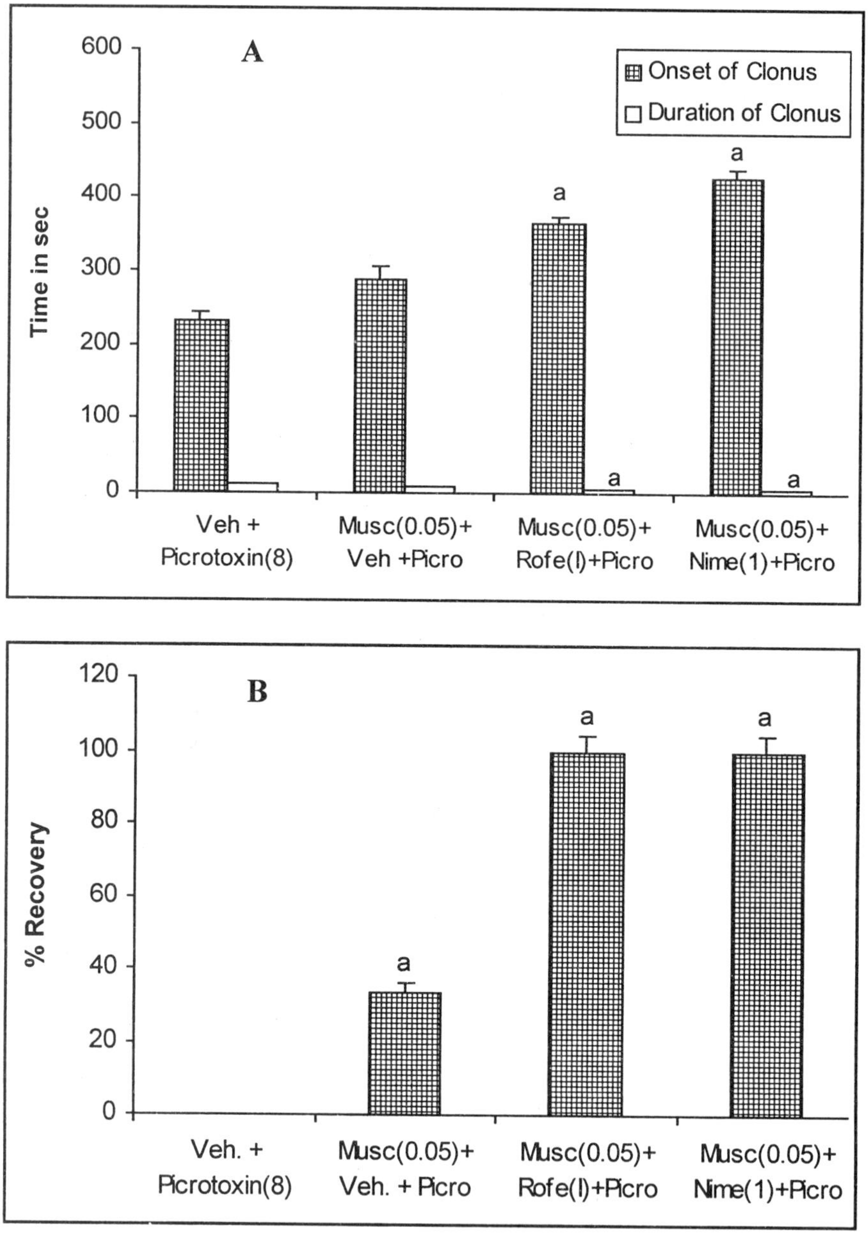

Fig. 5. Effect of subprotective dose of muscimol (0.05 mg/kg) and its combination with rofecoxib (1 mg/kg) or nimesulide (1 mg/kg) on (A) onset time of convulsions and duration of clonus (B) percentage recovery against picrotoxin-induced convulsions in mice (n=6-18). [a]$P<0.05$ as compared to picrotoxin treated group (ANOVA followed by Dunnett's test) (*For details see Dhir, Naidu and Kulkarni, 2006*).

the CNS. But only a small part of intracerebral glutamate is involved in synaptic transmission. There are at least five types of excitatory amino acids (EAA) receptors have been recognized, all of which bind to glutamate with high affinity[41]. These are the N-methyl-D-aspartate (NMDA), α- amino-3-hydroxy-5-methyl-4-isoxazolepropionate (AMPA, also known as quisqualate), kainate, 1-2-amino-4-phosphonobutyrate (AP4, an inhibitory autoreceptor), and trans-l-amino-cyclopentane-1-3-dicarboxylic acid (ACPD), a metabotropic receptor that stimulates inositol phosphate metabolism, and is also activated by quisqualate). NMDA, kainate and AMPA receptors are coupled to ion channels having diverse conductance capacities that are regulated by various ionic- and voltage-dependent mechanisms. The NMDA receptor is the best defined of all glutamate receptors[42]. *In vitro* pharmacological studies suggest that lamotrigine modulates the release of excitatory amino acids such as glutamate and aspartate by inhibiting to voltage-sensitive sodium channels, thereby stabilizing neuronal membranes.

In one of the studies conducted, the combined effect of GABAergic agents and MK-801 was investigated against digoxin-induced pop-corn type convulsions to assess the relative role of GABAergic transmission and glutamate receptor antagonism in chemoconvulsions in rats. There was a GABAergic influence in digoxin-induced convulsions as pentobarbital and diazepam showed significant protection against digoxin-induced neurotoxicity. Muscimol, a $GABA_A$ agonist and baclofen, a $GABA_B$ agonist showed only partial protection against digoxin-induced convulsions suggesting that another neurotransmitter is also involved in its pathophysiology. The NMDA receptor antagonist MK-801 showed significant protection against digoxin-induced convulsions. Furthermore, MK-801 (0.5 mg/kg) when combined with various GABAergic agonists, it provided significant protection against digoxin-induced convulsions. MK-801 has been reported to inhibit NMDA receptor subtypes via Ca^{2+} gated ion channels[43]. The study suggested the possible interaction of glutamate receptors, particularly, NMDA receptor subtypes and GABA-receptor ionophore complex in digoxin-induced convulsions (*For details see Gautam and Kulkarni, 1991*).

Dopaminergic (DAergic) system in various parts of the brain is involved in the control of motor activity, autonomic processes and emotional behavior. The agents which alter the synthesis, release, reuptake or catabolism of DA are useful therapeutically in Parkinson's disease. Drugs acting on DA receptors influence biochemical, electrophysiological and behavioral functioning of the DAergic system. DA may play an important role in the modulation of neuronal activity in the hippocampus. DA has been traditionally regarded as being anticonvulsant, though experimental work has occasionally thrown up conflicting results, suggesting there might be an opposite side to dopamine's action. L-deprenyl (selegiline) is an irreversible inhibitor of MAO-B enzyme and being used in the therapy of Parkinson's disease. Besides inhibition of MAO type B, it also inhibits reuptake of dopamine and noradrenaline, increases the turnover of dopamine, enhances striatal enzymes which include superoxide dysmutase (SOD), catalase and is reported to be involved in the detoxification of free radicals. The study conducted in our laboratory, demonstrated to possess anticonvulsant actions against PTZ-induced convulsions. It is well known that DA - Acetylcholine - GABA system is mutually dependent and regulate brain homeostasis in neurotoxic insults. The possible GABAergic mechanism of L-deprenyl was explored by combining it with sub-protective dose of diazepam[44]. The combination of sub-protective doses of L-deprenyl (10 mg/kg) and diazepam (1 mg/kg) showed potentiation of its anticonvulsant effect. Anticonvulsant activity of deprenyl was also checked against maximal electroshock-induced convulsions or Li-pilocarpine-induced status epilepticus. L-deprenyl significantly delayed the onset and decreased the duration of extensor phase against maximal electroshock-induced convulsions. Its combination with lower dose of phenytoin showed potentiation of the protective effect. Deprenyl however, was not effective against status epilepticus. The above observation suggested that in epilepsy, L-deprenyl may be acting partially by influencing the $GABA_A$-benzodiazepine mechanism in brain and may also affect dopamine-GABA balance in the critical areas of brain (*For details see Gupta and Kulkarni., 2000*).

Brain serotonin (5-HT) has been shown to participate in the mechanisms regulating various types of experimentally induced seizures[45,46], However, very little is known about the role of 5- HT receptor subtypes in the modulation of seizure activation. The activation of 5-HT_{1A} receptors leads to an inhibition of seizure activity, whereas 5-HT_2 receptors play an excitatory role in this model[47]. 5-HT_3 receptor agonist (m-CPBG) has been found to increase the duration of fully kindled seizures and facilitate the development of seizure process, suggesting an excitatory role of 5-HT_3 receptors in the kindling model of epilepsy.

Calcium channels and its glutamatergic modulation in epilepsy

Accumulating evidences suggest that abnormalities in calcium-regulated ion channels or enzymatic processes may underlie alterations in neuronal excitability and result in seizure activity. Increased Ca^{2+} influx in epileptogenesis is well established and it is assumed that both receptor-operated and voltage sensitive Ca^{2+} channels take active part in this processes. Desmedt *et al*, demonstrated that two piperazine derivatives, flunarazine and cinnarizine antagonized PTZ and electroshock-induced seizures[48]. The development and evaluation of drugs which block Ca^{2+} channels have therefore, been an important rational strategy for anticonvulsant drug design. In one study, the effect of various calcium channel blockers has been studied in lithium-pilocarpine model of status epilepticus. Status epilepticus was induced by administration of lithium chloride (3meq/kg) followed 21 hr later by a higher dose of pilocarpine. Diltiazem was not effective in delaying onset of convulsions. Verapamil showed protection against lithium-pilocarpine-induced convulsions. Amlodipine was partially protective (Fig 6). Flunarizine delayed the onset of forelimb clonus and rearing and only 60% of the rats underwent status in this group. Pre-treatment of MK-801, a NMDA antagonist led to a potentiation of the antiseizure activity of calcium channel inhibitors. The percent increase in amplitude at various time points with amlodipine pretreatment was significant only at the 30th min recording and at the rest of the time frames it was practically similar as the controls. It was concluded that the anticonvulsant action of MK-801 could be enhanced by centrally acting calcium channel inhibitors. Ca^{2+} ions also play a pivotal role in EAA-mediated events. In this study, MK-801 was administered before the subeffective doses of Ca^{2+} channel inhibitors (diltiazem, verapamil, nifedipine, amlodipine, and flunarizine) in Li-pilocarpine model led to a potentiation of the antiseizure activity. The exact nature of the interaction between voltage-dependent calcium channels and EAA receptors remains to be determined. NMDA and non-NMDA receptors differ substantially in ion selectivity. It is known that the NMDA receptor-mediated effects are calcium dependent due to the high permeability of the NMDA receptor to Ca^{2+} ions. Calcium channel inhibitors, therefore, may synergistically increase the protective action of competitive NMDA receptor antagonists against convulsions[49]. It was concluded that the anticonvulsant action of MK-801 could be enhanced by centrally acting calcium channel inhibitors (*For details see George and Kulkarni, 2000*).

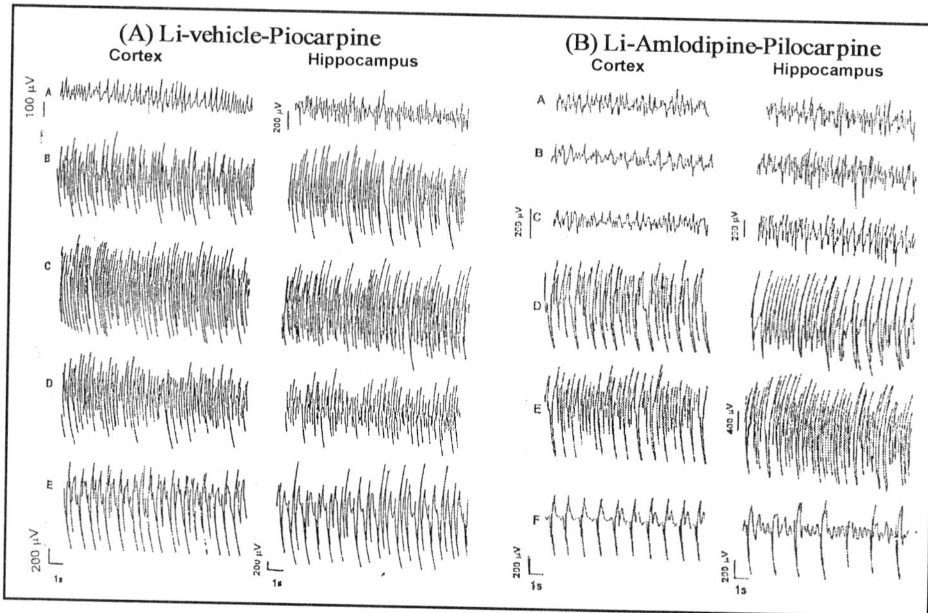

Fig. 6. Representative cortical and dorsal hippocampal EEG showing the development of status epilepticus in amlodipine (10 mg/kg) pretreated rats at different time intervals. A: Basal recording; B, C, D, E: 0.5, 1, 1.5 and 4 hr post pilocarpine (30 mg/kg) challenge. The cortical amplitude corresponding to A$\rightarrow$C (200mV), D$\rightarrow$E (400mV), F (200mV), respectively are indicated (*For details see George and Kulkarni, 2000*).

GABA and Anxiety

There are a variety of explanations for the cause of panic disorder which increasingly define it as a physiological condition, rather than a purely psychological one as was previously believed. Several theories exist that attempt to discuss the causes of panic disorder in terms of biochemical imbalances. One proposed explanation links levels of the monoamine neurotransmitters in the central nervous system (dopamine, norepinephrine, and serotonin) to the pathology of anxiety. Individuals with panic disorder may produce insufficient amounts of serotonin that results in a high level of anxious behavior, (and) a low level of norepinephrine (that) results in a hyperactive alarm system and sensitization to novel stimuli. Similarly, GABA is another neurotransmitter that has been implicated in panic disorder[50]. GABA is the main inhibitory neurotransmitter in the central nervous system (CNS). GABAergic inhibition is seen at all levels of the CNS, including the hypothalamus, hippocampus, cerebral cortex and cerebellar cortex. The activity of GABAergic neurones is decreased in generalized anxiety disorder[51]. Benzodiazepines are widely used to treat a variety of disorders, including anxiety, panic attacks, insomnia and muscle spasm.

Table 2. Various neurotransmitter, neuromodulators and receptor systems involved in anxiety (*Adapted from Kulkarni, 1999a*)[52]

GABA-A/benzodiazepine chloride ionophore (GABA/BZD)
5-HT_{1A}, 5-HT_2, 5-HT_3
N-Methyl-D-aspartate (NMDA)
Neurosteroids (NS)
Neuropeptide Y
Norepinephrine (NE)
Cholecystokinin (CCK)
Corticotropin-releasing factor
Adenosine/ purinoceptors

GABA is associated with other neurotransmitters system also. Benzodiazepines potentiate the GABA system, which then exerts inhibitory effects on other neurotransmitter systems which may account for the behavioral effects of anxiolytics (Fig. 7).

Exposure of animals (rats and mice) to elevated plus-maze is known to evoke approach-avoidance conflict behavior and anxiety related movements. The test has been validated behaviorally, biochemically and pharmacologically. This test is usually based on the observations of Montgomery in which the authors showed that exposure of animals to an elevated (open) maze alley evoked an approach-avoidance conflict that was considerably stronger than that evoked by exposure to an enclosed maze alley and animals preferred enclosed alley and explored it considerably more than those exposed to open maze alley.

Montgomery suggested that exposure of rats to novel stimuli (in the form of maze alley) can evoke both exploratory drive and fear drive and generate approach-avoidance conflict response. The elevation of maze further adds greater strength of fear and more avoidance conflict[53]. These observations then led Handley and Mithani to describe plus-maze apparatus consisting of two open and two closed arms, facing each other, to measure anxiety response[54]. The procedure was further validated physiologically, pharmacologically and behaviorally by Pellow et al., for rats[55] and Lister[56] for mice. The

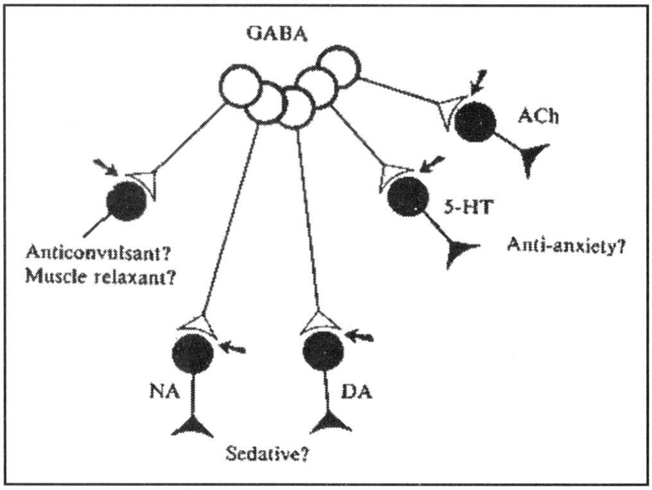

Fig. 7. Possible interaction of GABA with other neurotransmitter systems

pictorial view of plus-maze is shown below (Fig 8) in which plus maze consisted of two open (16 X 5 X 12 cm in case of mice and 50 X 10 X 40 cm in case of rats) with an open roof and elevated at a height of 25cm for mice and 50 cm for rats, respectively[52].

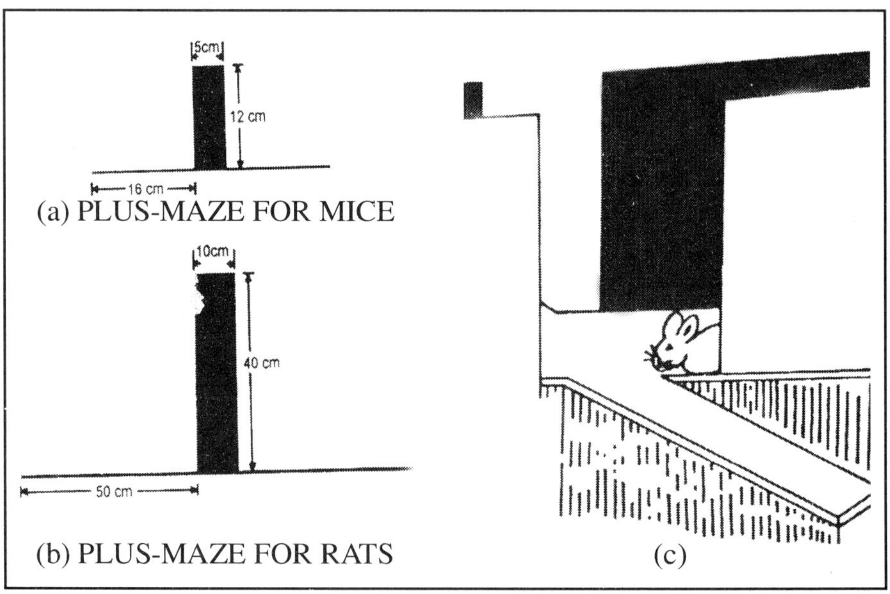

Fig. 8. Picture of elevated plus maze-showing open and closed (dark shaded) arms for (a) mice, (b) rats, and (c) a three dimensional view of elevated plus-maze depicting the animal in enclosed arm.

Elevated plus-maze is a fast and reliable procedure to detect anxiety related behaviors and to test antianxiety agents. Anxiogenic drugs like PTZ, amphetamine, caffeine, DMCM, FG 7142 enhances and anxiolytic drugs (diazepam, chlordiazepoxide) reduce anxiety response[57]. The antianxiety response of diazepam is shown in Table 3:

Table 3. Effect of diazepam on anxiety-related parameters on elevated plus-maze apparatus in mice[a]

Treatment (mg/kg; ip)	% preference to open arm	Closed arm: Number of entries (M ± SEM)	Closed arm: Average time spent (M ± SEM)	Open arm: Number of entries (M ± SEM)	Open arm: Average time spent (M ± SEM)	Total number of entries (M ± SEM)
Control	13.3	6.2± 0.75	46.21± 7.83	2.46 ± 0.52	5.60 ± 2.03	7.91 ± 1.51
Diazepam (1)	50.00	7.0 ± 0.80	19.43± 2.81**	5.1± 0.79**	5.42 ± 1.00	12.66± 1.28
Diazepam (2)	83.3	9.40± 1.75	17.58 ± 6.23**	8.10 ± 0.86**	5.70± 1.52*	17.6± 2.50**
Diazepam (2) +	0	6.5± 0.55	34.44 ± 2.9*	1.5 ± 0.93**[b]	1.08± 0.57**[b]	8.0± 1.38

[a] Abstracted from Kulkarni & Sharma, 1993[58]

*P<0.05; **P< 0.01 as compared to control ,[b]as compared to the effect of diazepam (2 mg/kg)

Alprazolam, a benzodiazepine produced dose dependant increase in antianxiety response, 100% first preference to open arm, increase in open arm entries and exploratory behaviour. Further, alprazolam like diazepam, affected both learning and acquisition behaviour. When tested for transfer latency, a parameter for learning and memory, both diazepam and alprazolam interfered with cognitive behaviour. Besides these actions, alprazolam also possessed anti-depressant property[58]. The antidepressant effect was sensitive to reversal by flumazenil; thereby, substantiating the GABA/benzodiazepine receptor involvement in the pathogenesis of anxiety associated depression (*For details see Kulkarni and Sharma, 1993*).

Several studies have suggested for an interaction of NMDA receptor and GABA/BZ receptor complex in the manifestation of behavioral patterns and drug action[59]. MK 801 is the most potent and selective noncompetitive NMDA receptor antagonist known so far, which appears to act within the ion channel coupled to NMDA receptors now known as phencyclidine (PCP) receptors[60]. MK 801 and related drugs have been reported to be useful in progressive neurodegenerative disorders including epilepsy[61]. It also produces amnesic, locomotor and anticonflict activities[62]. As GABA acting through GABA/BZ chloride ionophore complex, plays a predominant role in the neurochemistry of anxiety and stress, and therefore, the study was designed to investigate the role of BZ receptor ligands namely, diazepam (agonist), FG-7142 (partial inverse agonist) and flumazenil (Ro 15-1788, antagonist) in elevated plus-maze behavioural paradigm, a model of anxiety in rodents and the interaction of NMDA receptor antagonist MK 801. MK 801 produced anxiolytic effect at all the doses studied in rats. Effect was potentiated by diazepam. Both, FG-7142 and Ro 15-1788 reversed the effects of MK 801 and diazepam, when these agents were concomitantly administered. The study revealed anxiolytic profile of MK 801 and indicated that NMDA receptors could modulate the benzodiazepine receptor activity in rodents in elevated plus-maze apparatus. The present study also revealed that MK-801[63] when administered concurrently with diazepam further increased the percent preference and number of entries in the open arm suggesting the potentiating influence of MK-801 on the anxiolytic profile of diazepam (*For details see Sharma and Kulkarni, 1993*).

GABA and Memory

Elucidation of the biochemical and molecular mechanisms underlying learning and memory remains perhaps one of the greatest challenges for neuroscientists. A number of neurotransmitters and neuromodulators are involved in the learning and memory process. Various studies have reported the cholinergic involvement in the learning and memory process. Decline in the cognitive function in dementia is associated with decrease in cholinergic neurotransmission. The cholinergic muscarinic antagonist scopolamine has been most widely used to induce amnesia in experimental animals. L-glutamate is an excitatory neurotransmitter and is involved in learning and memory processes. Activation of N-methyl-D-aspartate (NMDA) receptor, a subtype of the glutamate receptors has been proposed for memory-producing process[64]. Also, stimulation of serotonergic neurotransmission disrupts behavioral performance while inhibition enhances the performance in experimental animals. 5-HT_3 receptor antagonists such as ondansetron and zacopride have shown promise in enhancing cognitive performances.

The different neurotransmitter and neuromodulators involved in the memory process are summarized in the Table 4:

Table 4- Different neurotransmitter and neuromodulators involved in the memory process *(Adapted from Kulkarni, 1999)*[64]

Neurotransmitter/Neuromodulator	Receptor system(s)
Glutamate	NMDA, AMPA receptors
Acetylcholine	Muscarinic, nicotinic
Dopamine	D_1, D_2 receptors
Serotonin	5-HT_3, 5-HT_{1A} receptors
Noradrenaline	α, β receptors
Neuropeptides	G-protein coupled peptidergic receptors
GABA-β-carbolines	GABA-A/BZD receptor complex
Neurosteroids	NMDA/GABA-A receptors

Considerable evidence has been provided for last few years for the involvement of the $GABA_A$ receptor complex in memory processes. Compounds that enhance the action of GABA, such as benzodiazepines, impair memory processing. On the contrary, compounds that reduce the action of GABA, such as β-CCM, pentylenetetrazol or picrotoxin, have the opposite action, that is they enhance memory processing. All these actions seem to focus mainly on the acquisition (learning) processes. Mainly, two subtypes of GABA receptors, $GABA_A$ and $GABA_B$ having selective agonists and antagonists have been characterized in CNS. A possible link between $GABA_B$ receptor activation and consolidation of memory is known[65]. N-methyl-D-aspartate receptor activation for induction of long-term potentiation has been found to be facilitated by $GABA_B$ receptors[66]. Interaction of cholinergic and GABA/benzodiazepine receptor system in the brain is also hypothesized. In one of the studies conducted in our laboratory, the modulation of cholinergic neurotransmission by $GABA_A$ and $GABA_B$ ligands in information storage mechanisms was investigated using scopolamine-induced short-term memory deficit on step-down task paradigm in mice. Atropine or scopolamine (anticholinergics) and GABA showed retention enhancing effects in scopolamine-treated and untreated animals but GABA agonist progabide did not affect any of the parameter significantly. $GABA_A$ agonist, muscimol and $GABA_B$ agonist, baclofen and (-) baclofen also displayed memory enhancing action. Whereas, $GABA_A$ antagonist, bicuculline produced hind limb rigidity, $GABA_B$ antagonist, CGP 35348 did not show any effect *per se,* but reversed the baclofen-induced delay in latency, without affecting retention enhancing action of baclofen. Combined administration of sub-effective dose of GABA and baclofen, showed a significant improvement in acquisition and retention[65]. However, the effect of GABA on acquisition was reversed by bicuculline and by CGP 35348 while improving retention. The study extended the support to the cholinergic concept in cognitive performance and provided an evidence for the influence of GABAergic (particularly $GABA_B$) modulation in scopolamine-induced learning and memory deficits in mice (*For details see Sharma and Kulkarni, 1993*).

Melatonin and GABAergic system

The pineal hormone, melatonin, can exert sedative/hypnotic, anxiolytic and other neuropharmacological effects in experimental animals. Melatonin has an overall central nervous system depressant activity. These effects of melatonin are generally produced by large pharmacological doses of melatonin, which are known to interact with benzodiazepine (BZ) receptors in the central nervous system (CNS). There is evidence that flumazenil, a specific central-type BZ antagonist, can block some of these effects of melatonin. Therefore, it is thought that activation of central-type BZ receptors on the BZ-$GABA_A$ receptor complex, with consequent allosteric enhancement of GABAergic activity, is the primary mechanism underlying the neuropharmacological effects of melatonin[67,68]. The interaction of melatonin with different neurotransmitter system particularly GABAergic system in producing hypothermia, sedation, hypolocomotion, anticonvulsant, antidopaminergic, anticonvulsant and analgesia actions are depicted in the following Fig. 9.

In an extensive study carried out in our laboratory, melatonin potentiated pentobarbitone (45 mg/kg)-induced hypnosis (Fig.10.). Melatonin in higher doses decreased both total and ambulatory activity, produced hypothermia and possessed significant analgesic property both in tail-flick and acetic acid-induced writhing tests. Melatonin in low dose significantly reduced the forced-swimming-induced immobility period *per se* and also reserpine-induced immobility. It also potentiated the effect of desipramine. Higher doses of melatonin significantly enhanced the reserpine-induced immobility time[69]. These studies suggested that GABA is an essential modulator of dopamine related functions in the striatal and limbic system and melatonin through its complex interactions with cerebral adrenergic system

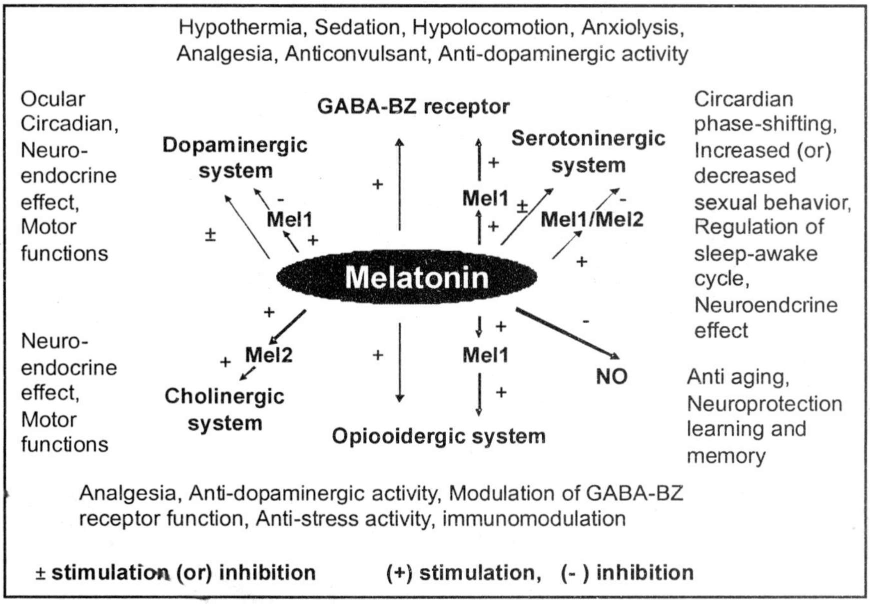

Fig. 9. Melatonin interaction with different neurotransmitter system of the body

brings about antidepressant action (*For details see Shaji and Kulkarni, 1998*).

Possible GABAergic mechanism of Herbal drugs in epilepsy

The use of herbal remedies and dietary supplements has become increasingly popular. These preparations are used for a wide range of perceived benefits in enhancing learning and memory, treatment of other specific conditions. Anecdotal accounts suggest that some herbal preparations may have anticonvulsant effect, however, randomized double-blind controlled trails of modern concept are lacking. *Withania somnifera* or Aswagandha (Winter Cherry) is a popular herb that finds its wide utility in epilepsy. It has been shown to possess anticonvulsant properties in acute and chronic models of epilepsy[70,71]. The root extract has been demonstrated to have antiepileptic activity against pentylenetetrazol (PTZ)-induced kindling in mice[72], amygdaloid kindling in rats[73], and in status epilepticus[74]. The protective effect of *Withania somnifera* in epilepsy is proposed to be through its GABAergic modulation.

The extensive studies carried out in our laboratory have shown the GABAergic modulatory activity of Aswagandha and its usefulness in epilepsy. Herbal formulation containing aswagandha (Siotone

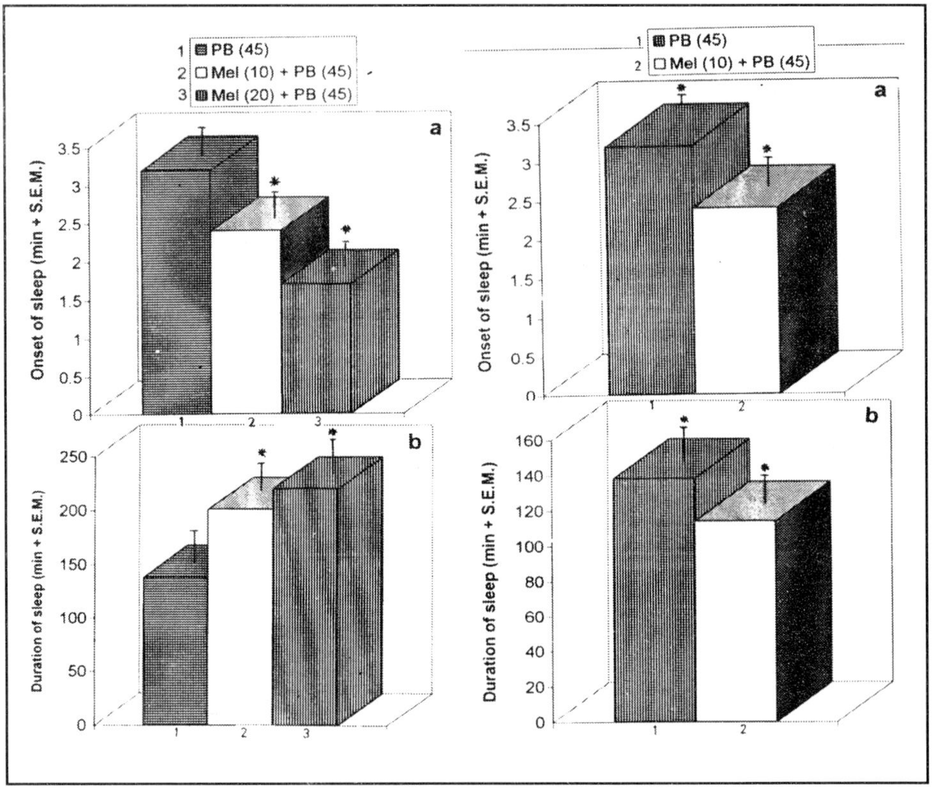

Fig. 10. Effect of (A) acute and (B) chronic treatment (X 8 days) of melatonin (10 or 20 mg/kg) on pentobarbitone (PB 45 mg/kg)-induced (a) onset of sleep (b) duration of sleep in mice (n=5). *P< 0.05 as compared to acute pentobarbitone treated group (*For details see Shaji and Kulkarni, 1998*).

granules)[75] was found to be protective against PTZ, maximal electroshock and strychnine-induced convulsions. When combined with sub-protective dose of diazepam, a GABA facilitator or MK-801, a NMDA receptor antagonist, the formulation showed enhanced anti-epileptic activity. The anti-convulsant action was also blocked by flumazenil, a benzodiazepine antagonist, suggesting the involvement of GABA-BZ receptor mechanism in its protective action (Fig. 11) (*For details see Kulkarni and Joseph, 1998*).

Another herbal psychotropic preparation BR-16A (Mentat ®), that contains various ingredients reputed in the ancient system of Ayurvedic medicine to be useful in the management of nervous disorders. These include: brahmi *(Hydrocotyl asiatica)*, shatavari *(Asparagus racemosus)*, buchh *(Acorus calamus)*, jatamansi

(Nardostachys jastamansi), aswagandha *(Withania somnifera)*, shankpushpi *(Evolvulus alsinoides)*, kuth *(Sausurea lappa)* and triphala *(Terminalia chebula)*. Some of the CNS activities of BR-16A has been related to its modulatory action on $GABA_A$ergic transmission. BR-16A has been recently tried as an adjuvant to the commonly used antiepileptic drugs in clinical trials and was found to significantly reduce seizure frequency.

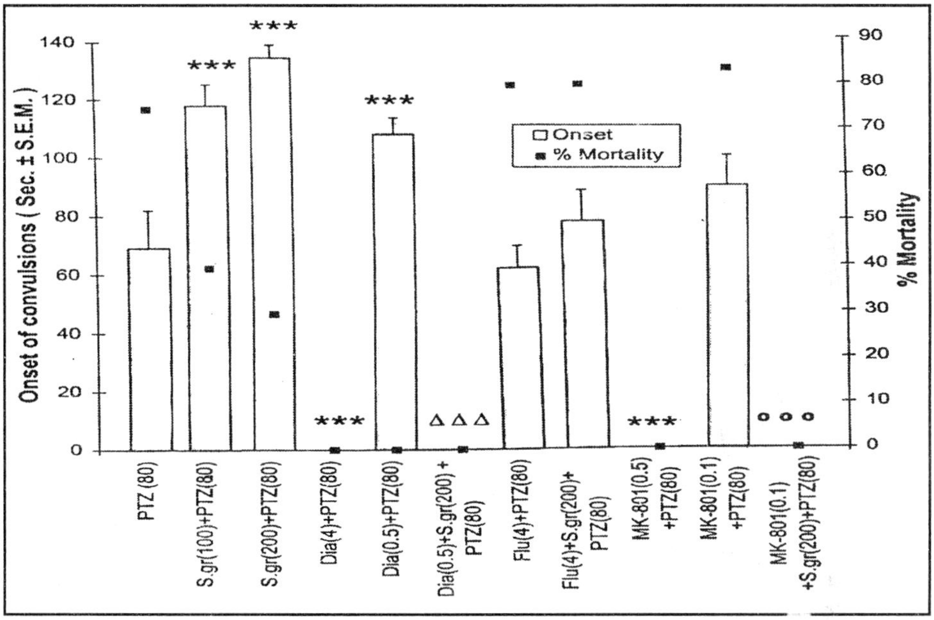

Fig. 11. Effect of Siotone granules on pentylenetertazol-induced convulsions in mice. ***P< 0.001 compared to PTZ (80) ΔΔΔ P< 0.001 as compared to sub-protective dose of diazepam (0.5); °°°P < 0.001 as compared to sub-protective dose of MK-801 (0.1). S.gr-Siotone granules; Dia- Diazepam; Flu-Flumazenil (For details see Kulkarni and Joseph, 1998).

Repeated administration of pentylenetetrazol (PTZ, 30 mg/kg, thrice a week) to mice for 9 weeks and subsequent challenge of the animals with the same dose of PTZ on the last chronic dose produced chemical kindling. The mice showed myoclonic jerks, clonus, Straub's tail, falling back response and full blown convulsion. The anticonvulsant profile of chronic administration of BR-16A was studied in this model of epilepsy. BR-16A offered protection against PTZ-induced chemical kindling. The percent animals showing myoclonic jerks and clonus was reduced to 40 and 34 with lower and 54 and 27 with higher doses of BR-16A, respectively. The protective effect was compared with diazepam (Table 5)[76]. The results demonstrated $GABA_A$ receptor mediated PTZ-induced kindling and protective effect of BR-16A therein (*For details see Kulkarni and George, 1995).*

Similarly, BR-16 A also showed protective effect on alcohol abstinence-induced anxiety and convulsions. Ethanol withdrawal sensitized the animals to convulsogenic reaction to pentylenetetrazol. A non-convulsive dose (40 or 60 mg/kg) of PTZ produced full blown convulsions in ethanol-withdrawn rats or mice[77]. Both acute and chronic administration of BR-16A (100 mg/kg) exhibited significant protection against ethanol withdrawal-induced reduction in PTZ threshold in rats and mice (*For details see Kulkarni and Verma, 1993*).

Table 5. Protective effect of BR-16A on pentylenetetrazol (PTZ)-induced kindling in mice on 10th day of last PTZ challenge dose (*For more details refer to Kulkarni and George., 1995*).

Treatment (mg/kg, i.p/p.o)	N	Onset (sec ± SEM)		Severity of clonus
		jerks	clonus	
Control PTZ 30 (i.p)	14	194.1 ± 96.68 (14)	324.8 ± 177.84 (9)	++
BR 16A 100 (p.o)	15	295.6 ± 122.18 (8)	275 (1)	+
BR 16A 500 (p.o)	14	235.3 ± 47.71 (8)	266.7 ± 20.19 (3)	+
Diazepam 1 (i.p)	8	-	-	-

GABA, BR-16A and de-addiction

Chronic use of opiates is known to produce tolerance to their analgesic effect and produce dependence. The management of drug dependence/addiction, particularly the withdrawal reactions to substances of abuse is a serious medical and social problem. Among the pharmacological approach of management many anticraving drugs have been recently tried with varying success rates. Since, BR-16A mediated many behavioral paradigms, we examined the role of BR-16A in the prevention of tolerance and dependence to opiates in animals. BR-16A when administered to animals prevented the development of tolerance and dependence to opiates in mice. Repeated administration of BR-16A (20-500 mg/kg) for 9 days attenuated the development of tolerance to the analgesic effect of morphine (10 mg/

kg)[78]. BR-16A (20-500 mg/kg) also suppressed the development of morphine dependence as assessed by naloxone (2 mg/kg) precipitated withdrawal jumps on day 10 of testing (*For details see Kulkarni and Verma, 1992*) as pretreatment with different doses of BR-16A decreased the number of withdrawal jumps induced by naloxone injection to the morphine dependent animals (Fig.12). The results speculated that the GABAergic system may be down-regulated during opiate withdrawal, leading to hyperexcitability and, further, BR-16A brings about its effect by modulating GABAergic tone.

Like other hypnotics and narcotics, benzodiazepines have the pharmacological potential to produce dependence and thereby, withdrawal symptoms in experimental animals and human beings. Biochemical studies have revealed that chronic diazepam treatment caused a selective supersensitivity to GABA in serotonergic dorsal raphe nucleus in rats which can be correlated with the abstinence syndrome. Similarly, abrupt cessation of chronic treatment of diazepam (20 mg/kg/day for 21 days) produced withdrawal reactions. BR-16A earlier shown to reverse the withdrawal reactions to opiates was studied against diazepam-induced withdrawal reactions in mice. Acute dose of diazepam (20 mg/kg) produced a decrease in the ambulatory and total activity. However, chronic administration for 21 days produced tolerance and no significant change in the ambulatory and total activity. On abrupt termination of diazepam treatment after 21 days, the animals showed anxiety and excitement as there was an increase in ambulatory and total activity. The withdrawal excitement was highest at 72 hr of the last dose of diazepam. Concomittant administration of BR 16-A reversed the acute effect of diazepam in a dose dependent manner. Similarly, chronic administration of BR 16-A (for 21 days) with diazepam also reversed the withdrawal induced hyperambulation and total activity. BR-16A with its CNS profile of activity could be a useful in the management of withdrawal reactions to substances of abuse[79] (*For details see Kulkarni and Sharma, 1994*).

Besides GABAergic mechanism in the development of tolerance and dependence to drugs, the possibility of non-GABAergic mechanism has also been suggested. The change in other brain monoamines during chronic diazepam treatment and diazepam withdrawal reaction is tabulated below (Table 6).

As shown in the table chronic diazepam treatment resulted in reduction of norepinephrine, 5-hydroxytryptamine and its metabolite

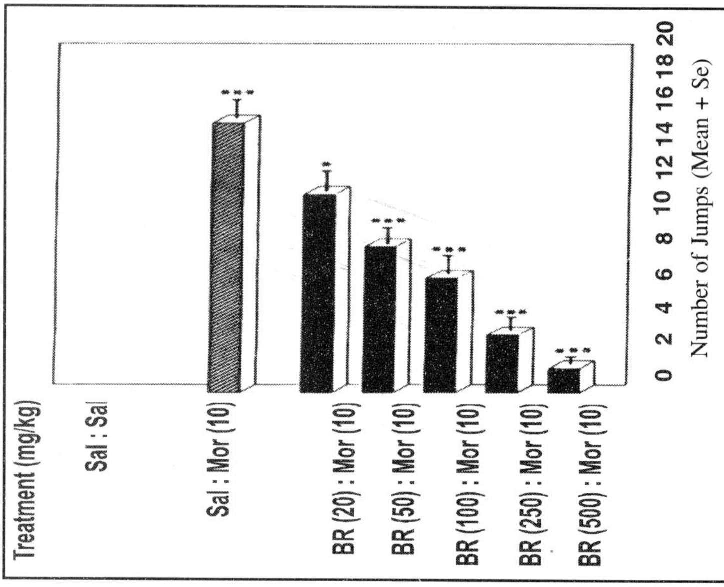

Fig. 12. Effect of various doses of BR-16A on naloxone precipitated jumps in morphine-withdrawn mice. *P< 0.05, *** P< 0.001 as compared with the sal-Mor-treated control. (*For details see Kulkarni and Verma, 1992*)

5-hydroxy indole acetic acid (5-HIAA) contents in the whole brain while and an increase in dopamine contents was noted. On abrupt termination of chronic diazepam, noradrenaline, 5-hydroxytryptamine, 5-hydroxyindoleacetic acid (5-HIAA) levels increased while DA levels were reduced. An increase in NA and 5-HT brain levels was seen in diazepam withdrawn rats when compared with control and with rats on chronic diazepam treatment indicating higher levels of central autonomic function. An adrenergic hyperactivity is documented in diazepam abstinence since $alpha_2$ adrenoceptor agonists such as clonidine, guanfacine and B-HT 920 were shown to be effective in such situations[80] (*For details see Kunchandy and Kulkarni, 1987*).

Physiology of Stress

Stress is defined as a state of threatened homeostasis or dysharmony and is counteracted by a complex range of physiologic, biochemical and behavioral responses that reestablish homeostasis. Hans Selye[81] first popularized the concept of "stress" in the 1950s. Selye theorized that all individuals respond to all types of threatening situations in the same manner, and he called this the *General Adaptation*

Table 6- Brain monoamines during chronic diazepam treatment and diazepam withdrawal reaction

S.No.	Treatment (Dose)	No. of animals	Brain tissue ηg/g			
			NA	DA	5-HT	5-HIAA
1	Control	8	522.3 ± 6.00	1203.2 ± 55.8	1293.7 ± 107.4	601.6 ± 12.9
2	On chronic diazepam (20 mg/kg, ip)	6	389.9 ± 24.6[a]	2018.0 ± 280[c]	796.3 ± 95.0[b]	485.3 ± 18.6[a]
3	Diazepam withdrawn (third day)	6	687.03 ± 27.8[b]	1080.0 ± 92.3	1338.8 ± 113.3	644.4 ± 35.3
4	Diazepam withdrawn + Clonidine (100 μg/kg, ip twice daily)	6	606.5 ± 9.85	1378.5 ± 184	2155.75 ± 93.5[a]	337.2 ± 55.5[a]

NA; Noradrenaline, DA; Dopamine, 5-HT; 5-hydroxytryptamine; 5-HIAA; 5-hydroxy indole acetic acid. [a]P<0.001 when compared with 2:1, 4:1; [b]P<0.01 when compared with 2:1,3:1; [c]P<0.02 when compared with 2:1

Syndrome (GAS). He claimed that, in addition to Sympathetic Nervous System (SNS) arousal, other bodily systems such as the adrenal cortex and pituitary gland may be involved in a response to threat. For example, chemicals such as epinephrine (adrenaline) may serve to focus the body's attention just on immediate self-preservation by inhibiting such functions as digestion, reproduction, tissue repair, and immune responses. Ultimately, as the threat wanes, Selye suggested, body functions return to normal, allowing the body to focus on healing and growth again. But if the threat is prolonged and chronic, the SNS arousal never gets "turned off," and health can be impaired. With a continuously suppressed immune system, for example, a person would be more vulnerable than usual to infection—which is one explanation of why some individuals get sick so often. And, regardless of whether Selye was right or not, psychology, as well as medicine and popular culture, have accepted the concept of "stress" as an unpleasant fact of life. The stress response is subserved by a complex neuroendocrine, cellular and molecular infrastructure, the stress system, which is located in both the central nervous system and the periphery.

Hypothalamic-pituitary-adrenal (HPA) axis and stress

Any stress lasting longer than a few minutes results in increased levels of cortisol being released from the adrenal cortex. Cortisol is the anti-stress hormone. The release of cortisol is controlled by the paraventricular nucleus of the hypothalamus, where corticotropin-releasing hormone (CRH) is released in response to the stress. CRH then acts on the pituitary gland, causing it to release adrenocorticotrophic hormone (ACTH), which in turn causes the adrenal cortex to release corticosteroids out of which cortisol is the major hormone released[82]. CRH and ACTH are released in short pulses, each of which causes a (roughly) 15 minute sustained release of cortisol from the adrenal cortex, which then has a half-life of 100 minutes in the blood. Prolonged release of ACTH causes the adrenal cortex to increase in size (presumably to cope with a greater need for cortisol production), whereas long-term ACTH deficiency causes it to shrink. The combined system of CRH-ACTH-cortisol release is referred to as the hypothalamic-pituitary-adrenal axis (or HPA axis). Positive and negative feedback occurs at various sites in the brain to ensure that cortisol production stays within certain bounds, depending on current requirements and stress levels (Fig. 13).

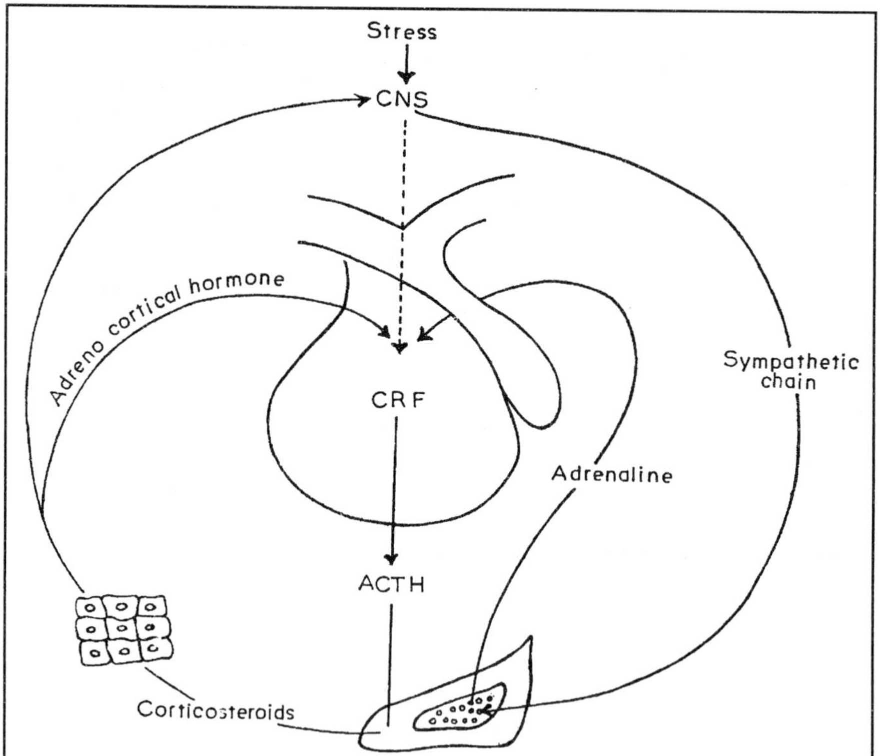

Fig. 13. Overview of the HPA axis

The circadian pattern of cortisol release is controlled by the suprachiasmatic nucleus (SCN) of the hypothalamus, also known as the body clock. Nerve signals from the SCN cause the paraventricular nucleus of the hypothalamus to release pulses of CRH roughly once per hour, resulting in HPA axis activation and cortisol release. There are also direct links between the SCN and the adrenal gland itself (bypassing the HPA axis) through sympathetic nerve fibres, causing the adrenal gland to become more sensitive to ACTH stimulation during the morning, further adding to the circadian pattern of cortisol release throughout the day[83].

The endocrine response to stress also involves increased sympathetic stimulation of the adrenal medulla. Increased sympathetic stimulation of the adrenal medulla increases adrenaline secretion. Physiological stressors are known to enhance urinary excretion of 3-methoxy 4-hydroxy mandelic acid, an end product of catecholamines[84] (*For details see Kulkarni, Dandiya and Khuketa, 1973*). Adrenaline normally helps the body adjust to sudden stress[85]. When a person becomes angry or frightened, the adrenal glands release large amounts of adrenaline into the blood. The hormone causes changes in the body to make it more efficient for "fight or flight."

Together adrenaline and cortisol increase blood glucose levels and the release of fatty acids from adipose tissue and the liver. Sympathetic innervation of the pancreas decreases insulin secretion. Consequently, most tissues do not readily take up and use glucose. Thus glucose is available primarily to the nervous system; and fatty acids are used by skeletal muscle, cardiac muscle, and other tissues. Adrenaline and sympathetic stimulation also increase cardiac output, increase blood pressure, and act on the central nervous system to increase alertness and aggressiveness. Cortisol also decreases the initial inflammatory response.

The HPA axis, which has traditionally been seen as the body's "stress system", and which ultimately controls levels of cortisol and other important stress related hormones, is generally underactive in people suffering from chronic fatigue syndrome (CFS) and burnout. New research is beginning to show that the HPA axis should instead be thought of as the body's energy regulator, as it is ultimately responsible for controlling virtually all of the hormones, nervous system activity and energy expenditure in the human body, as well as modulating the immune system. In CFS the HPA axis becomes suppressed, resulting in the various physical and mental symptoms associated with these conditions.

Stress induces various neurochemical and behavioral deficits that result in depressant like behavioral effects. It is well known that many of the effects of chronic stress are thought to be mediated by stress-induced increases in circulating levels of glucocorticoids, the major stress hormone. In fact, chronic elevation of circulating glucocorticoids has been shown to produce a variety of cognitive deficits. For instance, chronic administration of corticosterone demonstrated impaired acquisition of a passive avoidance and T maze tasks. Indeed, chronic stress procedures weaken working memory functions. In humans and animals, adrenal cortex contains a higher concentration of ascorbic acid than other tissues and the acute administration of ACTH caused decrease in ascorbic acid levels.

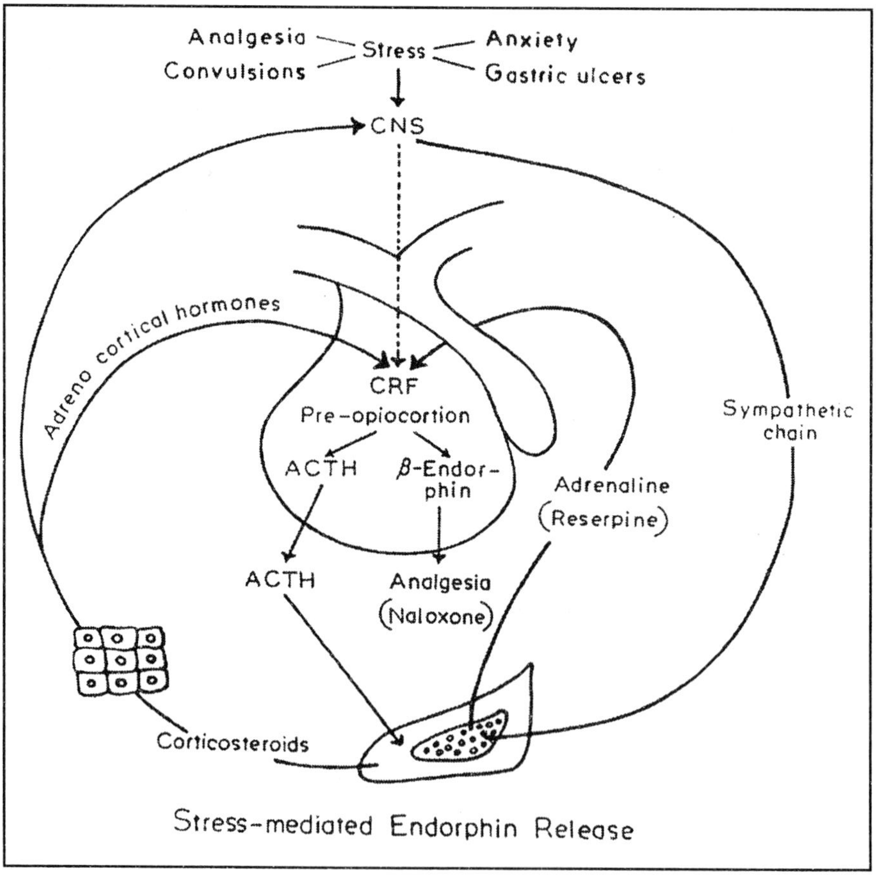

Fig. 14. Stress mediated endorphin release

Another important hormone released by the pituitary along with ACTH is beta-endorphin, a morphine-like hormone[86]. Both ACTH and beta-endorphin are similar in structure, and are released together during acute stress in response to CRH stimulation by the hypothalamus (Fig. 14). Endorphins are pain regulatory hormones and released in acute stressful situation exhibiting analgesic response[87]. Furthermore, stress also leads to decrease in seizure threshold and producing convulsions.

In addition to cortisol, the adrenal cortex also releases dehydroepiandrosterone (DHEA), a precursor to the sex hormones testosterone and oestrogen, and aldosterone, a mineralocorticoid that maintains blood volume and pressure by controlling the sodium/ potassium balance of the blood. Both DHEA and cortisol are released in response to ACTH stimulation, but aldosterone is relatively independent of HPA axis stimulation.

The ratio of cortisol to DHEA depends on a number of factors. During acute stress and illness, the balance shifts towards cortisol and away from DHEA. Interestingly, mental attitude has been shown to influence the DHEA/cortisol ratio, with high DHEA-to-cortisol ratios corresponding to feelings of warm-heartedness, and low ratios corresponding to feelings of being stressed.

REFERENCES

1. Fong GCY & Fong JKY, Recent advances in the diagnosis and management of epilepsy. *Hong Kong Med J* 7(2001) 73

2. Hauser WA, Annegers JF & Kurland LT, Incidence of epilepsy and unprovoked seizures in Rochester, Minnesota: 1935-1984. *Epilepsia* 34 (1993)453.

3. Fisher RS & Coyle JT, (1991) In Summary: Neurotransmitters and epilepsy Fisher, RS, Coyle JT (Eds.) Wiley-Liss: NY, pp 247-252

4. Kohling R, GABA Becomes Exciting. *Science* 298 (2002)1350.

5. Traub RD, Borck C, Colling SB & Jefferys JG, On the structure of ictal events in vitro. *Epilepsia* 1996 Sep; 37(9):879-91.

6. Dichter M A, In: *Epilepsy A Comprehensive Textbook*. Engel J, Pedley TA (Eds.) Lippincott-Raven: Philadelphia; 1997, Section 2.

7. Chagnac-Amitai Y & Connors BW, Synchronized excitation and inhibition driven by intrinsically bursting neurons in neocortex *J Neurophysiol* 62 (1989)1149.

8. Deisz RA, Billard JM & Zieglgansberger W, Pre- and postsynaptic GABAB receptors of rat neocortical neurons differ in their pharmacological properties *Neurosci Lett* 154 (1993)209.

9. Pende M, Lanza M, Bonanno G & Raiteri M, Release of endogenous glutamic and aspartic acids from cerebrocortex synaptosomes and its modulation through activation of a gamma-aminobutyric acid B (GABA-B) receptor subtype. *Brain Res* 604(1993)325.

10. Waldmeier PC, Wicki P, Feldtrauer JJ, Mickel SJ, Bittiger H & Baumann PA, GABA and glutamate release affected by GABA-B receptor antagonists with similar potency: no evidence for pharmacologically different presynaptic receptors. *Br J Pharmacol* 113(1994)1515.

11. Borden LA, GABA transporter heterogeneity: pharmacology and cellular localization. *Neurochem Int* 29 (1996)335.

12. Wisden W & Seeburg PH, GABAA receptor channels: from subunits to functional entities. *Curr Opin Neurobiol* 2(1992): 263.

13. Macdonald RL & Olsen RW, GABA-A receptor channels. *Annu Rev Neurosci*17(1994)569

14. Sieghart W, $GABA_A$ receptors: ligand-gated Cl^- ion channels modulated by multiple drug-binding sites. *Trends Pharmacol Sci* 13(1992)446.

15. Smith GB & Olsen RW, Functional domains of GABAA receptors. *Trends Pharmacol Sci* 16 (1995)162.

16. David M, GABAergic mechanism in epilepsy, *Epilepsia* 42 (2001) 8.

17. Ketter TA, Post RM & Theodore WH, Positive and negative psychiatric effects of antiepileptic drugs in patients with seizure disorders. *Neurology* 53 (1999) Suppl 2:S53-S67.

18. Green AR, Minchin MC & Vincent ND, Inhibition of GABA release from slices prepared from several brain regions of rats at various times following a convulsion. *Br J Pharmacol* 92 (1987)13.

19. Gray JA & Green AR, Increased $GABA_B$ receptor function in mouse frontal cortex after repeated administration of antidepressant drugs or electroconvulsive shocks. *Br J Pharmacol* 92 (1987)357.

20. Aley KO & Kulkarni SK, Altered response to GABAergic agents following electro and chemo convulsions in mice. *Ind J Exp Biol* 29 (1991) 241.

21. Goddard GV & Douglas RM, Does the engram of kindling model the engram of normal long term memory? *Can J Neurol Sci* 2 (1975) 385.

22. Barkai E, Grossman Y & Gutnick MJ, Long-term changes in neocortical activity after chemical kindling with systemic pentylenetetrazole: an in vitro study. *J Neurophysiol* 72 (1994) 72.

23. Delgado-Escueta AV, Wasterlain CG, Treiman D & Porter, RJ, Status epilepsticus: Summary In : *Advance in Neurology*. Delgado-Escueta, AV, Wasterlain, CG, Treiman D, Porter, RJ (Eds). Raven Press: NY; 1985. pp 539-541.

24. Dodson WE, DeLorenzo RJ & Pedley TA, The treatment of convulsive status epeilspticu: recommendations of the epeilpsy foundation of America's working group on status epilepticus. *JAMA*, 270(1993) 854.

25. Kapur J, Lothman EW & DeLorenzo RJ, Loss of $GABA_A$ receptors during partial status epilepticus. *Neurology* 44 (1994)2407.

26. Kulkarni SK, Development of and anti-alcohol pill: a myth or reality, *The Eastern Pharmacist* 1988 (1988) 51.

27. Braestrup C, Schmiechen R, Neef G, Nielsen M & Petersen EN, Interaction of convulsive ligands with benzodiazepine receptors. *Science* 216 (1982) 1241.

28. Kunchandy J & Kulkarni SK, On the convulsant action of DMCM and Ro 5-4864 in mice. *Ind J Exp Biol* 26(1988)625.

29. File SE & Pellow S, Intrinsic actions of the benzodiazepine receptor antagonist Ro 15-1788. *Psychopharmacology (Berl)* 88 (1986) 1.

30. Aley KO, Kulkarni SK, Mathur R, & Nayar U, Effect of chronic treatment of Ro 15-1788 and its withdrawal on cortical and hippocampal EEG activity in rats. *Ind J Exp Biol* 28 (1990) 1149.

31. Ticku MK, Benzodiazepine-GABA receptor-ionophore complex: Current concepts. *Neuropharmacology* 22(1983)1459.

32. Phillis JW & O'Regan MH, The role of adenosine in the central actions of the benzodiazepines. *Prog Neuropsychopharmacol Biol Psychiatry*12 (1988)389.

33. Phillis JW & Wu PH, The role of adenosine and its nucleotides in central synaptic transmission. *Prog Neurobiol* 16(1981)187.

34. Dragunow M & Faull R L M, Neuroprotective effects of adenosine. *Trends in Pharmacol Sci* 9 (1988)193.

35. Thorat SN & Kulkarni SK, Benzodiazepine inverse agonist, DMCM- and peripheral agonist, Ro 5-4864-induced convulsions in mice: Effect of adenosinergic agents. *Ind J Exp Biol* 28(1990)1160

36. Dickie BG, Annals SJ & Davies JA, Effect of cyclooxygenase inhibition upon glutamate release from rat cerebellum. *Neuroreport* 5 (1994) 393-396

37. Dhir A, Naidu PS & Kulkarni SK, Effect of cyclooxygenase-2 (COX-2) inhibitors in various animal models (bicuculline, picrotoxin, maximal electroshock-induced convulsions) of epilepsy with possible mechanism of action. *Ind J Exp Biol* 44 (2006) 286.

38. Takemiya T, Suzuki K, Sugiura H, Yasuda S, Yamagata K Kawakami Y & Maru E, Inducible brain COX-2 facilitates the recurrence of hippocampal seizures in mouse rapid kindling. *Prostaglandins & Other Lipid Meadiators* 71 (2003) 205

39. Sekiyama N, Mizuta S, Hori A, & Kobayashi S, Prostaglandin E2 facilitates excitatory synaptic transmission in the nucleus tractus solitarii of rats. *Neuro Sci Lett* 188(1995)101.

40. Knapp DJ & Crews FT, Induction of cyclooxygenase - 2 in brain during acute and chronic ethanol treatment and ethanol withdrawal. *Alcohol: Clin and Experim Res* 23 (1999) 633.

41. Watkins JC, Krogsgaard-Larsen P & Honore T, Structure-activity relationships in the development of excitatory amino acid receptor agonists and competitive antagonists. *Trends Pharmacol Sci* 11(1990)25.

42. Monaghan DT & Cotman CW, Identification and properties of N-methyl-D-aspartate receptors in rat brain synaptic plasma membranes. *Proc Natl Acad Sci USA* 83(1986)7532.

43. Gautam SK & Kulkarni SK, GABA/BZ-and NMDA-receptor interaction in digoxin-induced convulsions in rats. *Ind J Exp Biol* 29 (1991)636.

44. Gupta M & Kulkarni SK, Studies on anticonvulsant actions of L-deprenyl. *Ind J Exp Biol* 38 (2000) 332.

45. Wada Y, Hasegawa H, Nakamura M & Yamaguchi N, Behavioral and electroencephalographic effects of a serotonin receptor agonist (5-methoxy-N,N-dimethyltryptamine) in a feline model of photosensitive epilepsy. *Neurosci Lett* 138(1992)115.

46. Wada Y, Shiraishi J, Nakamura M & Hasegawa H, Prolonged but acute fluoxetine administration produces its inhibitory effect on hippocampal seizures in rats. *Psychopharmacology* 118 (1995) 305.

47. Wada Y, Shiraishi J, Nakamura M & Koshino Y, Effects of the 5-HT3 receptor agonist 1-(m-chlorophenyl)-biguanide in the rat kindling model of epilepsy. *Brain Res* 759(1997)313.

48. Desmedt LKC, Niemegeers CJE & Janssen PAJ, Anticonvulsant proprerties of cinnarizine and flunarazine in rats and mice. *Drug Res* 25 (1976) 1408.

49. George B, Kulkarni SK & Mathur R, Motor and electrographic response of refractory experimental status epilepticus in rats and effect of calcium channel blockers. *Ind J Exp Biol* 38 (2000)105.

50. Zivkovic B, Perrault G & Sanget DJ, In: Target receptors for anxiolytics and hypnotics: From molecular pharmacology to therapeutics, J Mendlewicz & G Racagni (Eds) Karger: Basel; 1992

51. Rago L, Kiivet RA, Harro J & Pold M, Behavioral differences in an elevated plus-maze: correlation between anxiety and decreased number of GABA and benzodiazepine receptors in mouse cerebral cortex. *Naunyn Schmiedebergs Arch Pharmacol* 337 (1988) 675.

52. Kulkarni SK, Animal models for testing antianxiety drugs. In: Handbook of Experimental Pharmacology, Vallabh Prakashan: New Delhi; 1999a. p 27-42

53. Montgomery KC, The relation between fear induced by novel stimulation and exploratory behaviour. *J Comp Physiol Psychol* 48 (1958) 254

54. Handley SL & Mithani S, Effects of alpha-adrenoceptor agonists and antagonists on maze-exploration model of fear-motivated behavior. *Naunyn-Schimed Arch Pharmacol* 327 (1984)1.

55. Pellow S, Chopin P, File SE & Briley M, Validation of open/closed arm entries in an elevated plus-maze as a measure of anxiety in the rat. *J Neurosci Meth* 14 (1985)149.

56. Lister RG, The use of a plus-maze to measure anxiety in the mouse. *Psychopharmacology* 92 (1987) 180.

57. Kulkarni SK, Sharma AC & Verma A, Strain difference and bidirectional activity of benzodiazepine ligands in rodents subjected to elevated plus-maze. *Ann Natl Acad Med Sci* 27 (1991) 61.

58. Kulkarni SK & Sharma K, Alprazolam modifies animal behaviour on elevated plus-maze. *Ind J Exp Biol* 31(1993)908.

59. Kulkarni SK & Ticku MK, Interaction between GABAergic anticonvulsants and the NMDA receptor antagonist MK 801 against MES- and picrotoxin-induced convulsions in rats. *Life Sci* 44(1989)1317.

60. Lodge D & Johnson KM, Noncompetitive excitatory amino acid receptor antagonists. *Trends Pharmacol Sci* 11 (1990)81.

61. Woodruff GN, Foster Ac, Wong EHF, Gill R, Kemp JA & Iversen LL, Excitatory amino acids in health and disease, Lodge D (Eds). Wiley: New York; 1988. P- 379.

62. Whishaw IQ & Auer RN, Immediate and long-lasting effects of MK-801 on motor activity, spatial navigation in a swimming pool and EEG in the rat. *Psychopharmacology (Berl)* 98(1989)500.

63. Sharma AC & Kulkarni SK, Evidence for benzodiazepine receptor interaction with MK 801 in anxiety related behaviour in rats. *Ind J Exp Biol* 31(1993)191.

64. Kulkarni SK, Preclinical and clinical behavioural paradigms for testing drugs that affect learning and memory In: Handbook of Experimental Pharmacology, Vallabh Prakashan: New Delhi; 1999. p 43-84.

65. Sharma AC & Kulkarni SK, (+/-) Baclofen sensitive scopolamine-induced short-term memory deficits in mice. *Ind J Exp Biol* 31(1993)348.

66. Collingridge GL & Singer W, Excitatory amino acid receptors and synaptic plasticity. *Trends Pharmacol Sci* 11 (1990)290.

67. Holmes SW & Sugden D, Effects of melatonin on sleep and neurochemistry in the rat. *Br J Pharmacol* 76 (1982)95.

68. Coloma FM & Niles LP, Melatonin enhancement of [3H]-gamma-aminobutyric acid and [3H] muscimol binding in rat brain. *Biochem Pharmacol* 37 (1988) 1271.

69. Shaji AV & Kulkarni SK, Central nervous system depressant activities of melatonin in rats and mice. *Ind J Exp Biol* 36(1998)257.

70. Kulkarni SK & Verma A, Protective effect of BR-16A (Mentat), a herbal preparation on alcohol abstinence-induced anxiety and convulsions. *Ind J Exp Biol* 31(1993) 435.

71. Kulkarni SK, Sharma A, Verma A, & Ticku MK, GABA receptor mediated anticonvulsant action of *Withania somnifera* root extract. *Indian Drugs* 30 (1993) 305.

72. Kulkarni, SK & George B, Anticonvulsant action of *Withania somnifera* (Aswagandha) root extract against pentylenetetrazol-induced kindling in mice. *Phytother Res* 10 (1996) 447.

73. Kulkarni SK & George B, Amygdaloid kindling in rats, Protective effect of *Withania somnifera* (Aswagandha) root extract. *Indian Drugs* 32 (1995) 37.

74. Kulkarni SK, George B & Mathur R, Neuroprotection by *Withania somnifera* root extract against Lithium-pilocarpine-induced seizures. *Indian Drugs* 35 (1998) 208.

75. Kulkarni SK & Joseph P, Anticonvulsant profile of Siotone granules, a herbal preparation. *Ind J Exp Biol* 36 (1998) 658.

76. Kulkarni SK & George B, Pentylenetetrazol-induced kindling in animals: protective effect of BR-16A. *Ind J Exp Biol* 33 (1995) 424.

77. Kulkarni SK & Verma, AV, GABA receptor mediated anticonvulsant action of *Withania somnifera* root extract. *Indian Drugs* 30 (1993) 305

78. Kulkarni SK & Verma A, Prevention of development of tolerance and dependence to opiate in mice by BR-16A (Mentat), a herbal psychotropic preparation. *Ind J Exp Biol* 30 (1992) 885.

79. Kulkarni SK & Sharma A, Reversal of diazepam withdrawal induced hyperactivity in mice by BR 16-A (Mentat), a herbal preparation. *Ind J Exp Biol* 32 (1994) 886.

80. Kunchandy J, Kulkarni SK & Shukla VK, Autonomic hyperactivity on diazepam withdrawal in rats. *Ind J Exp Biol* 25 (1987)115.

81. Selye H, The Stress of Life New York: McGraw-Hill, 1956, Rev. ed. 1976.

82. Gianoulakis C, Alcohol-seeking behavior: The roles of the hypothalamic-pituitary-adrenal axis and the endogenous opioid system. *Alcohol Health & Research World* 22 (1998)202.

83. Jameson D, Hypothalamic-Pituitary-Adrenal (HPA) Axis. In: Mind-body Health and Stress Tolerance 2003 p 1-178.

84. Kulkarni SK, Dandiya PC & Khuteta KP, Effect of reserpine, chlorpromazine and meprobamate on stress induced metabolic alterations in urinary excretion of 3-methoxy, 4-hydroxymandelic acid. *Ind J Exp Biol* 11(1973)229.

85. Atkinson R L, Glossary: Epinephrine, Endocrine system, Fight or Flight, Hormone, Stress. In *Hilgard's introduction to psychology* 1996 Eds. Asaf Rolef Ben-Shahar; Ch 2.

86. Stocker S, Studies link stress and drug addiction *NIDA Notes* 14(1999)12.

87. Kulkarni SK, Heat and other physiological stress-induced analgesia: catecholamine mediated and naloxone reversible response. *Life Sci* 27 (1980) 185.

3

On the GABAergic actions of *Withania somnifera*: An Indian Ginseng

S.K.KULKARNI
Pharmacology Division, University Institute of Pharmaceutical Sciences, Panjab University, Chandigarh - 160014

Introduction

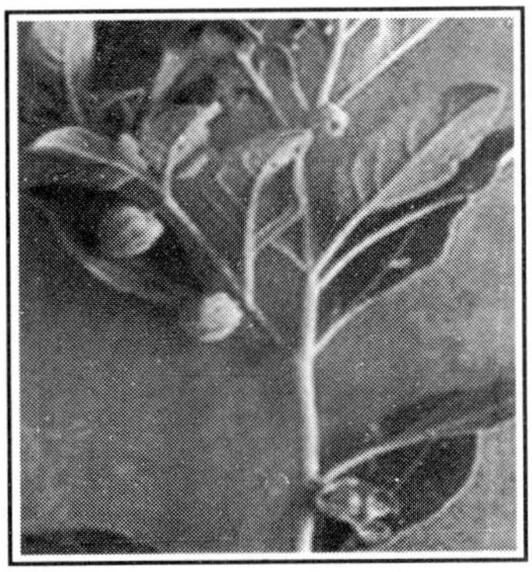

Withania somnifera is popularly known as Aswagandha or Winter Cherry[1]. It is an evergreen shrub belonging to family Solanaceae[2]. The plant is found through out the drier parts of India, Baluchistan, Pakistan, Afghanistan, Sri Lanka, Congo, South Africa, Egypt, Morocco and Jordan. In India, it is widely grown in the provinces of Madhya Pradesh (MP), Uttar Pradesh (UP), plains of Punjab and northwestern parts of Gujarat and Rajasthan[3]. The practitioners of the traditional Indian system of medicine regard *Withania somnifera* as the "Indian Ginseng"[4].

Many pharmacological studies have been conducted to investigate the properties of Aswagandha in an attempt to authenticate its use as a multi-purpose medicinal agent[5]. The extensive pharmacological studies carried out on the plant indicated Aswagandha to have beneficial effects in almost every disorder of the body system like inflammatory arthritis[6], cancer[7, 8], stress[9-11], disorders of immune system[12], nervous system[13, 14-18], endocrine system[19] and cardiovascular system[5, 20]. Besides, it is also known to possess adaptogenic activity and modulate neurotransmitters like the GABAergic [(γ-amino-butyric acid (GABA)][21,22] or cholinergic systems[23]. Some of its beneficial effects have been correlated to its antioxidant potentials. The present review attempts discuss the pharmacological basis of the use of Aswagandha in epilepsy and related CNS disorders based on its GABAergic actions.

Constituents: The major biochemical constituents of Aswagandha are steroidal alkaloids and steroidal lactones, a class of constituents together known as withanolides (steroidal lactones with ergostane skeleton)[24]. At present 12 alkaloids, 35 withanoloids and several sitoindosides have been isolated and their structures have been elucidated.

The structures of important constituents [(withaferin A, withanolide G or sitoindoside (IX, X)] of *Withania somnifera* root extract are given in Fig. 1.

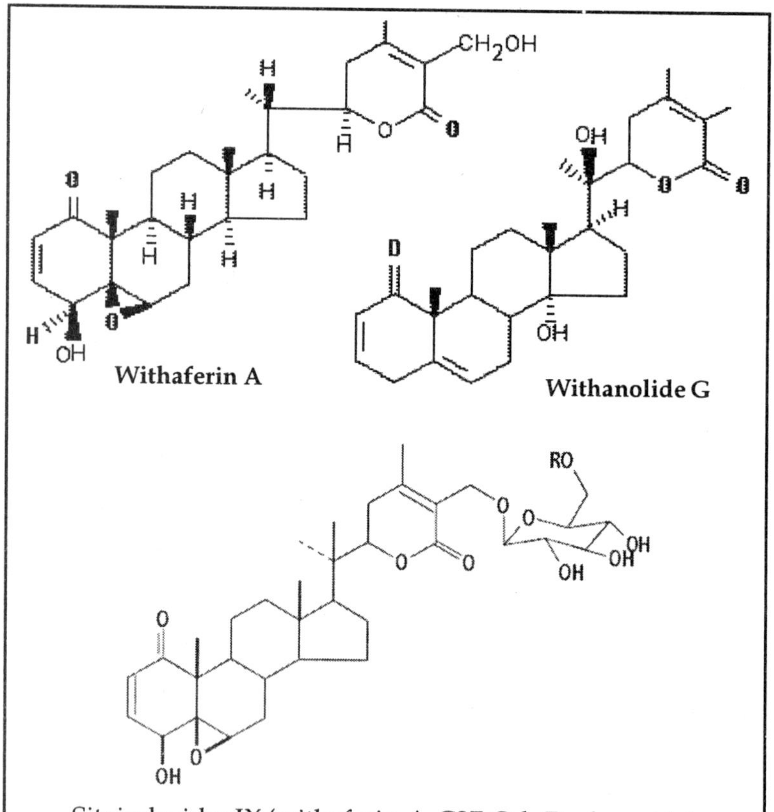

Sitoindosides IX (withaferin-A-C27-O-b-D-glucoside)
Sitoindosides X (6′-O-palmitoyl-A-C27-O-b-D-glucoside)

Fig. 1. Active constituents of *Withania somnifera*[5]

Epilepsy

Withania somnifera has profound CNS depressant actions. It has been shown to possess anticonvulsant properties in acute and chronic models of epilepsy[25,26]. The root extract has antiepileptic activity against pentylenetetrazol (PTZ)-induced kindling in mice[22], amygdaloid kindling in rats[27], and in status epilepticus in rats[13]. The protective effect of *Withania somnifera* in epilepsy is considered to be through GABAergic modulation.

Withania somnifera possessed protective activity against pentylenetetrazol (PTZ) (80 mg/kg i.p.) -induced convulsions in mice. PTZ when injected intraperitoneally produced severe tonic-clonic convulsions in mice. *Withania somnifera* dose dependently offered significant protection against convulsions as shown by an increase in the onset time of extensor and protection against mortality due to PTZ (Fig 2)[26]. Pretreatment with Aswagandha extract at 200 mg/kg completely abolished the extensor phase in mice due to PTZ.

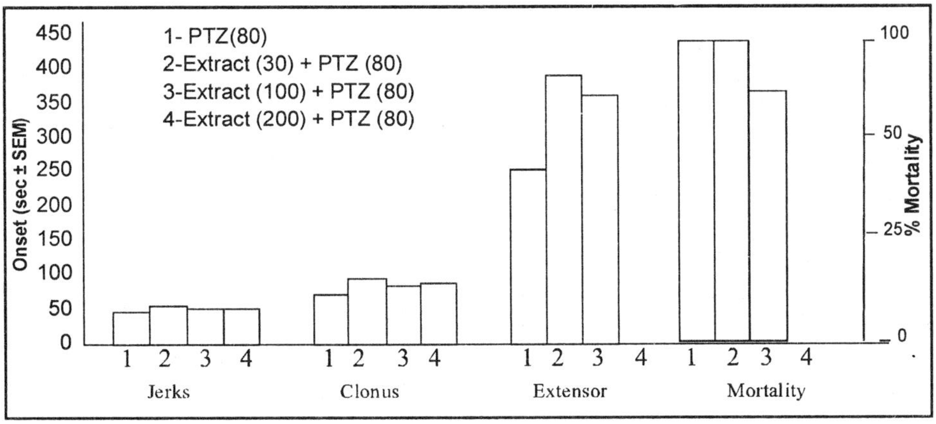

Fig. 2. Effect *of Withania somnifera* (30-200 mg/kg) against PTZ-induced convulsions.

Pretreatment of the animals with GABA (100 mg/kg) produced no significant delay in the onset of clonus and extensor phase, but a significant delay in the onset of jerks, and reduction of mortality rate to 87.5 % was observed. When GABA (200 mg/kg) was administered similarly, a significant delay in the onset of jerks and extensor phase was observed. The mortality rate was reduced to 57.2%. Concomittant administration of GABA (100 mg/kg) with the subprotective dose of the extract (30 mg/kg) produced a significant delay in the onset of the extensor phase and a significant reduction of the mortality to 80 %. Concomittant administration of a higher dose of GABA (200 mg/kg) with the extract (30 mg/kg) produced a significant delay in the onset of clonus and a significant reduction of mortality to 50 %. On increasing the dose of the extract to 100 mg/kg there was no significant delay in the onset of the three stages or the mortality rate[26]. These observations tend to suggest that the effect of the extract and GABA when given together did not show any potentiation or additive response (Fig 3). Similarly, when the *Withania* extract was combined with diazepam there was no significant interaction (not reported here).

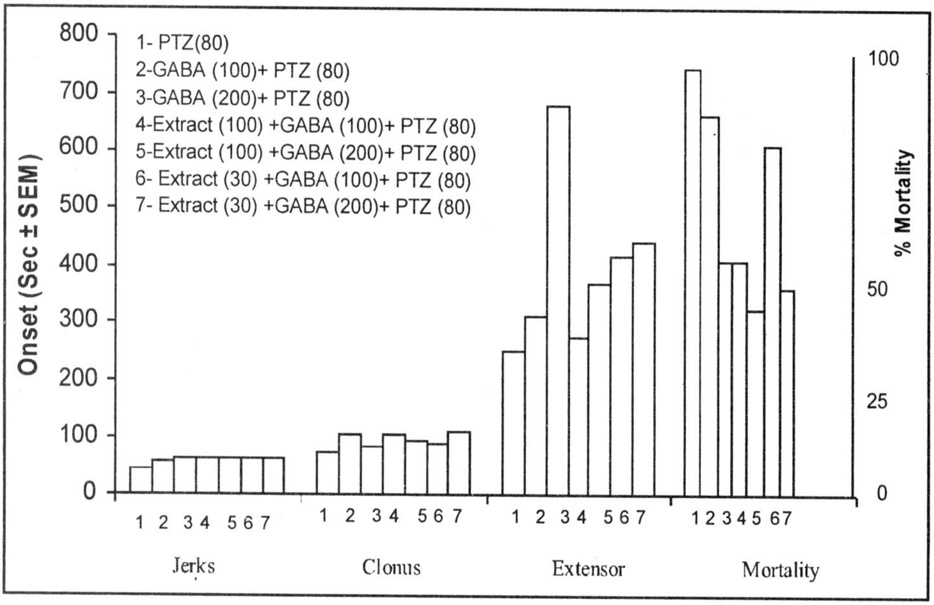

Fig 3. Effect of GABA (100 or 200 mg/kg) and its combination with *Withania somnifera* (30 or 100 mg/kg) against PTZ- induced convulsions.

However, when *Withania somnifera* was combined with different doses of pentobarbitone it enhanced the protective effect of pentobarbitone (5 and 10 mg/kg). The combination of *Withania somnifera* (100 mg/kg) with pentobarbitone (10 mg/kg) completely abolished the extensor phase against PTZ-induced convulsions[26] (Fig 4) thereby suggesting that extract may act at the barbiturate modulatory centre on the $GABA_A$ receptor to show the protective effect.

To further study the GABAergic mechanism of action of *Withania somnifera,* when the root extract was co-administered with

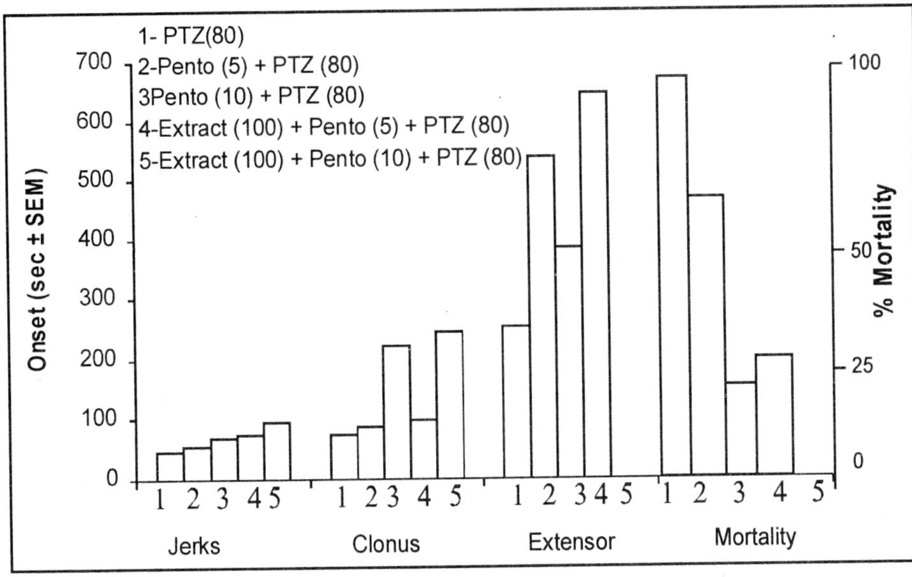

Fig 4. Effect of pentobarbitone (Pento) (5 and 10 mg/kg) and its combination with *Withania somnifera* (100 mg/kg) on against PTZ- induced convulsions.

γ-aminobutyric acid (GABA) (100 and 200 mg/kg), it (30 and 100 mg/kg) enhanced the protective action of GABA against bicuculline-induced ($GABA_A$ receptor antagonist) convulsions, supporting the GABAergic mechanism of action of *Withania somnifera*[26].

Kindling is a chronic model of epilepsy and epileptogenesis. In PTZ or electrical kindling, the repeated application of convulsants (PTZ or electrical stimulation) applied once a day or alternate days, which initially has no effect on behavior but slowly culminating into full blown convulsions. PTZ-induced kindling is one such type of model in which subconvulsant dose of PTZ (40 mg/kg) on alternate days for 15 days lead to full blown convulsions and the animals go into a continuous state of convulsions (kindling) and become seizure prone.

Withania somnifera protected the animals against PTZ-induced kindling, although, the effect was less potent as compared to diazepam treatment[28] (Table 1A, 1B).

Amygdala-pyriform cortex is the most responsive within the limbic system in the rate of kindling development as compared to hippocampus and cortex. The regularity and predictability of amygdaloid kindling under a given set of stimulus conditions makes this model ideal for study of neuronal mechanisms that may underlie seizure development. In one of the studies reported from our laboratory, an attempt was made to study the protective effect of *Withania somnifera* root extract in amygdaloid kindled rats. The electrical stimulation was given for total of 15 days and animals showed persistent kindling. EEG recording showed epileptic changes in both the amplitude and frequency of wave patterns. Treatment with *Withania somnifera* (100 mg/kg, p.o.) given acutely, 30 minutes prior to stimulus, showed significant reduction in severity of motor seizures as was evident from the amplitude and frequency of wave pattern.

Table 1. Effect of *Withania somnifera* (100 mg/kg) on onset time of clonus, jerks, severity of clonus and % animals showing jerks or clonus against PTZ-induced kindling **(A)** on 3rd day of last challenge day of PTZ **(B)** on 10th day of last challenge day of PTZ[28]

A

Treatment (mg/kg)	N	Onset (sec ± SE)		Severity of clonus	% Showing	
		Jerks	Clonus		Jerks	Clonus
Control PTZ i.p.	14	173.1 ± 26.97 (14/14)	331.2 ± 31.8 (9/14)	++	100	64.3
W.S. (100) p.o.	12	346.7 ± 50.44 (3/12)	-	-	25	0
Diazepam (1.0) i.p.	9	435 (1/9)	-	-	11.1	0

B

Treatment (mg/kg)	N	Onset (sec ± SE)		Severity of clonus	% Showing	
		Jerks	Clonus		Jerks	Clonus
Control PTZ i.p.	14	194.1 ± 25.84 (14/14)	324.8 ± 59.28 (9/14)	++	100	64.3
W.S. 100 p.o.	10	352.2 ± 67.77 (7/10)	448 (1/10)	+	70	10
Diazepam 1.0 i.p.	8	-	-	-	0	0

In another experimental model of status epilepticus, *Withania somnifera* was given acutely and it delayed the onset of forelimb clonus and rearing but the drug was not able to reduce the mortality rate against lithium-pilocarpine-induced status epilepticus in rats. When the root extract of *Withania somnifera* (50, 100, 200 mg/kg. p.o.) was given chronically for 7 days followed by lithium-pilocarpine challenge, it protected the animal from mortality to 60 % but did not reduce the latency of forelimb clonus with rearing (results were not significant). Furthermore, *Withania somnifera* was also combined with the standard anti-epileptic drugs. All the anticonvulsant drugs namely, diazepam (1, 2.5 and 5 mg/kg), clonazepam (0.25, 0.5 and 1 mg/kg), sodium valproate (100, 300 mg/kg) and phenytoin (50, 100 mg/kg) produced a dose dependent protection. When *Withania somnifera* was combined with these standards agents, the combination was able to reduce significantly the effective dose of diazepam and clonazepam to offer full protection with no mortality[29] (Table 2).

Table 2. Effect of *Withania somnifera* alone and in combination with known anticonvulsants against lithium-pilocarpine-induced status epilepticus (SE) in rats. Each value represents mean ± SD. n=6-9 in each group. $^{a}p< 0.05$, $^{b}p< 0.01$ (Kruskal-wallis test followed by student's t-test)[8]. *F.C + R, forelimb clonus with rearing, NS-Not significant*[29].

Treatment (mg/kg)	Onset of F.C + R	Mortality (%)
Control (Lithium + Pilocarpine)	25.4 ± 0.97	100
Acute study		
W.s (100)	56 ± 2.12^{NS}	100
Diazepam (2.5)	60.4 ± 15.73 ^{NS}	50
W.s (100) + Diazepam (2.5)	85 ± 5.01^{a}	20
Sodium Valproate (100)	38.2 ± 5.2^{a}	80
Sodium valproate (300)	74.83 ± 9.09^{a}	66
W.s (100) + Sodium valproate (300)	75.8 ± 5.94^{a}	66
Clonazepam (0.25)	72 ± 11.09^{a}	40
W.s (100) + Clonazepam (0.25)	100 ± 0^{b}	0
Phenytoin (100)	79 ± 7.16^{a}	40
W.s (100) + Phenytoin (100)	78.2 ± 7.45^{a}	40
Chronic study		
W.s (50) X 7d	45 ± 9.6 ^{NS}	83
W.s (100) X 7d	50.2 ± 5.87 ^{NS}	60
W.s (200) X 7d	57.2 ± 11.3 ^{NS}	66.6

When checked for EEG recordings the cortical amplitude showed reduced amplitude (Fig. 5) with *Withania somnifera* pretreatment until 60 minutes compared with the control groups. The results were comparable with the effect of clonazepam (1 mg/kg)[8].

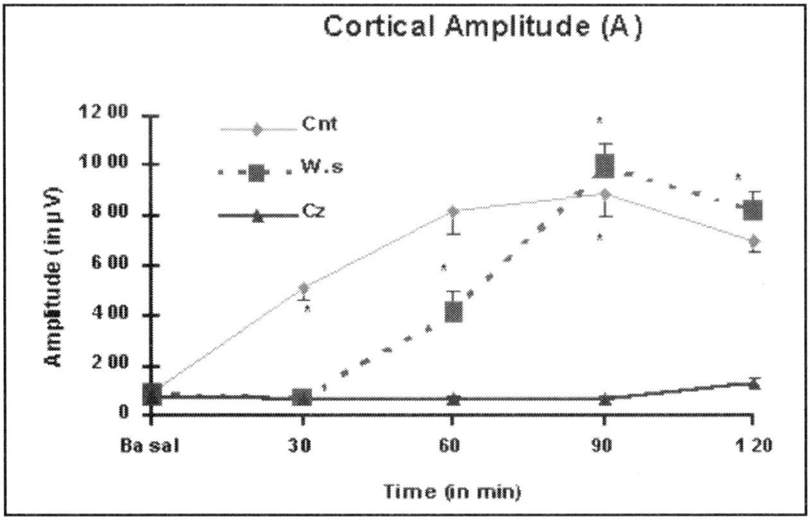

Fig. 5. Time course change in the cortical amplitude in (µV) in Li-pilocarpine model of status epilepticus following different drug pretreatment [control, clonazepam (1 mg), *W. somnifera* (100 mg) groups] in rats. $^{*}p < 0.05$ (significance with respect to basal values, Friedman's test). Overall significant difference exists between the area under the curves of Cnt and Cz; Cz and *Ws* (in A); and between Cnt and Cz (in b) at $^{*}p < 0.01$ (Kruskal-Wallis test followed by multiple range test)[13].

The profound anticonvulsant activity of *Withania* root extract as reported in various animal models is hypothesized to be through $GABA_A$ receptors[21]. As discussed in the previous chapters, the $GABA_A$-benzodiazepine receptor-ionophore complex is a major site of drug action for a variety of centrally acting drugs including benzodiazepines and barbiturates[30,31]. Barbiturates and benzodiazepines facilitate the effect of GABA mediated Cl^- conductance. *Withania somnifera* root extract is reported to have anxiolytic[32] and CNS inhibitory effects[33]. To test this hypothesis. Mehta *et al*[21] conducted functional assays using neuronal membranes to determine the modulatory effect of a methanol extract of *Withania somnifera* on the binding of $[^3H]$ GABA, $[^{35}S]$ t-butylbicyclophosphorothionate (TBPS) and $[^3H]$ flunitrazepam to their respective sites in the brain.

The extract was more potent in inhibiting $[^3H]$ GABA and $[^{35}S]$ (TBPS) binding. The methanol extract of *W. somnifera* increased the specific binding of $[^3H]$ flunitrazepam in cerebral cortex. Also the effect of extract on $[^3H]$ flunitrazepam binding was additive with that of pentobarbital. When the extract and GABA were tested, in combination on [^{3}H] flunitrazepam binding the effect was not additive. The effect of combination treatment indicated that the extract decreased the enhancing effect of GABA. Similar results were obtained when the effect of two GABA agonists (GABA and muscimol) was examined in combination with [^{3}H] flunitrazepam binding. These functional studies indicated that *Withania somnifera* possessed its anticonvulsant activities through $GABA_A$ receptor system.

Anxiety

Anxiety disorders have a lifetime prevalence that exceeds 15 % in the general population[34]. In India, Aswagandha (*Withania somnifera*) has been widely used for centuries in Ayurvedic medical practice to reduce symptoms of anxiety and stress[35]. As demonstrated earlier *Withania somnifera* possessed GABA-mimetic properties[21, 26]. Since GABA agonism has been linked to anxiolysis[36], the extracts of Aswagandha may be expected to have beneficial effect in anxiety and related disorders. A double blind placebo control study conducted by other investigators, in patients with ICD-10 anxiety disorders, 6 weeks of treatment with ethanolic extract of Aswagandha, the patients met with priori response criteria in the drug group (88.2 %) as compared with the placebo group (50%). The extract was well tolerated and did not cause more adverse effects than placebo. So, it was concluded that the ethanolic extract of *Withania somnifera* has useful anxiolytic potential[37]. Also, in one study carried out by Bhattacharya et al., (2000)[38] regarding the anxiolytic action of *W. somnifera* root extract in rats, it (20 and 50 mg/kg) was administered orally once daily for 5 days and the results were compared with lorazepam (0.5 mg/kg, i.p.). *Withania somnifera* extract induced an anxiolytic effect, in the elevated plus-maze, and social interactions studies in rats, an effect comparable to that produced by lorazepam [38]

Shaligram and colleagues carried out a clinical study with Aswagandha tablets on the psychomotor performance. The study was carried out in a double blind cross over manner. The volunteers were required to state their position along the three 100 mm scales for anxious-calm mode, relaxed tense mode and the drowsy alert mode. It was concluded that Aswagandha tablets had a beneficial effect in the tense and anxious state but this was not accompanied by sedation or drowsiness. The effect was compared with diazepam where diazepam reported to produce sedation besides producing the anxiolytic action (unpublished data).

Summary

From the above observations, it may be concluded that *Withania somnifera* could be a useful protective therapy in epilepsy, possibly through its GABAergic mechanism. The drug is without having any serious toxicity or side effects known till date and thus safe to be used in human disorders particularly of central nervous system disorders.

REFERENCES

1. Andallu B & Radhika B, Hypoglycemic diuretic and hypocholesterolemic effect of winter cherry (*Withania somnifera* Dunal) root. *Indian J Exp. Biol* 38 (2000) 607.
2. Dafni A & Yaniv Z. Solanaceae as medicinal plants in Israel. *J Ethnopharmacol.* 44 (1994) 11.
3. Bhatia P, Rattan SIS, Cavallius J & Clark BFC, *Withania somnifera* (Aswagandha) a so-called rejuvenator inhibits growth and macromolecular snthesis of human cells. *Med Sci Res* 15 (1987)515.
4. Singh B, Saxena AK, Chandan BK, Gupta DK, Bhutani KK & Anand KK, Adaptogenic activity of a novel withanolide-free aqueous fraction from the roots of *Withania somnifera* Dun. *Phytother Res* 15(2001) 311.
5. Mishra LC, Singh BB & Dagenais S, Scientific basis for the therapeutic use of *Withania somnifera* (ashwagandha) a review. *Altern Med Rev* 5(2000) 334.
6. Bhattacharya SK, Satyan KS & Ghosal S, Antioxidant activity of glycowithanolides from *Withania somnifera*. *Indian J Exp Biol* 35(1997) 236.
7. Devi PU, Sharada AC, Solomon FE & Kamath MS, In vivo growth inhibitory effect of *Withania somnifera* (Ashwagandha) on a transplantable mouse tumor Sarcoma 180. *Indian J Exp Biol* 30(1992) 169.
8. Mohan R, Hammers HJ, Bargagna-Mohan P, Zhan XH, Herbstritt CJ, Ruiz A, Zhang L, Hanson A.D, Conner BP, Rougas J & Pribluda VS, Withaferin A is a potent inhibitor of angiogenesis. *Angiogenesis* 7(2004) 115.
9. Dhuley JN, Effect of ashwagandha on lipid peroxidation in stress-induced animals. *J Ethnopharmacol* 60(1998) 173.
10. Rai D, Bhatia G, Sen T & Palit G, Anti-stress effects of *Ginkgo biloba* and *Panax ginseng* a comparative study. *J Pharmacol Sci* 93(2003) 458.
11. Archana R & Namasivayam A, Antistressor effect of *Withania somnifera*. *J. Ethnopharmacol* 64 (1999) 91.
12. Ziauddin M, Phansalkar N, Patki P, Diwanay S & Patwardhan B, Studies on the immunomodulatory effects of Ashwagandha. *J Ethnopharmacol* 50 (1996) 69.

13. Kulkarni SK, George B & Mathur R, Neuroprotection by *Withania somnifera* root extract against Lithium-pilocarpine-induced seizures. *Indian Drugs* 35 (1998) 208.

14. Naidu PS, Singh A, & Kulkarni SK, Effect of *Withania somnifera* root extract on haloperidol-induced orofacial dyskinesia possible mechanisms of action. *J Med Food* 6(2003) 107.

15. Ahmad M, Saleem S, Ahmad AS, Ansari MA, Yousuf S & Hoda MN, Islam F, Neuroprotective effects of *Withania somnifera* on 6-hydroxydopamine induced Parkinsonism in rats. *Hum Exp Toxicol* 24(2005) 137.

16. Dhuley JN, Nootropic-like effect of ashwagandha (*Withania somnifera* L.) in mice. *Phytother Res.* 15(2001)524.

17. Chaudhary G, Sharma U, Jagannathan NR, & Gupta YK, Evaluation of *Withania somnifera* in a middle cerebral artery occlusion model of stroke in rats. *Clin Exp Pharmacol Physiol* 30 (2003) 399.

18. Jain S, Shukla SD, Sharma K & Bhatnagar M, Neuroprotective effects of *Withania somnifera* Dunn. in hippocampal sub-regions of female albino rat. *Phytother Res* 15(2001) 544.

19. Panda S & Kar A, Changes in thyroid hormone concentrations after administration of ashwagandha root extract to adult male mice. *J Pharm Pharmacol* 50 (1998) 1065-1068.

20. Mohanty I, Arya DS, Dinda A, Talwar KK, Joshi S & Gupta SK, Mechanisms of cardioprotective effect of *Withania somnifera* in experimentally induced myocardial infarction. *Basic Clin Pharmacol Toxicol* 94(2004) 184.

21. Mehta AK, Binkley P, Gandhi SS & Ticku MK, Pharmacological effects of *Withania somnifera* root extract on $GABA_A$ receptor complex. *Indian J Med Res* 94 (1991) 312.

22. Kulkarni SK. & George B, Anticonvulsant action of *Withania somnifera* (Aswagandha) root extract against pentylenetetrazol-induced kindling in mice. *Phytother Res* 10(1996) 447.

23. Schliebs R, Liebmann A, Bhattacharya SK, Kumar A, Ghosal S & Bigl V, Systemic administration of defined extracts from *Withania somnifera* (Indian Ginseng) and Shilajit differentially affects cholinergic but not glutamatergic and GABAergic markers in rat brain. *Neurochem Int* 30(1997) 181.

24. Elsakka M, Grigorescu E, Stanescu U, Stanescu U & Dorneanu V, New data referring to chemistry of *Withania somnifera* species. *Rev Med Chir Soc Med Nat Iasi* 94(1990) 385.

25. Kulkarni SK & Verma AV, GABA receptor mediated anticonvulsant action of *Withania somnifera* root extract. *Indian Drugs* 30 (1993) 305.

26. Kulkarni SK, Sharma A, Verma A & Ticku MK, GABA receptor mediated anticonvulsant action of *Withania somnifera* root extract. *Indian Drugs* 30 (1993) 305-312

27. Kulkarni SK & George B, Amygdaloid kindling in rats Protective effect of *Withania somnifera* (Aswagandha) root extract. *Indian Drugs* 32 (1995) 37.

28. Kulkarni SK & George B, Anticonvulsant action of Withania somnifera (aswagandha) root extract against pentylenetetraol-induced kindling in mice. *Phytother Research* 10 (1996)447-449.

29. Kulkarni SK, George B & Mathur R, Protective effect of Withania somnifera root extract on electrographic activity in a Lithium-pipcarpine model of status epilepticus. *Phytother Research* 12 (1998) 451-453.

30. Olsen RW, The GABA postsynaptic membrane receptor-ionophore complex. Site of action of convulsant and anticonvulsant drugs. *Mol Cell Biochem* 39(1981) 261-279.

31. Ticku MK, (1983) Benzodiazepine-GABA receptor-ionophore complex. Current concepts. *Neuropharmacology*. 22 1459-1470.

32. Bhattacharya SK, Goel RK, Kaur R & Ghoshal S, Anti-stress activity of sitoindosides VII and VIII New acylsterylglycosides from *W.somnifera*. *Phytother Res* 1 (1987) 32.

33. Malhotra CL, Mehta VL, Das PK & Dhalla NS Studies on Withania-ashwagandha Kaul. V. The effect of total alkaloids (ashwagandholine) on the central nervous system. *Indian J Physiol Pharmacol* 9(1965) 127.

34. Kessler RC, McGonagle KA, Zhao S, Nelson CB, Hughes M, Eshleman S, Wittchen HU & Kendler KS, Lifetime and 12-month prevalence of DSM-III-R psychiatric disorders in the United States. Results from the National Comorbidity Survey. *Arch Gen Psychiatry* 5(1994) 18.

35. Handa SS, Plants and plant products for mental health. In: Koslow S.H. Murthy R.S. Coelho G.V (Eds.) Decade of the Brain Rockville MD U.S. Department of Health and Human Service pp. (1995) 163-171.

36. Stahl SM, Essential Psychopharmacology. New Delhi. Cambridge University Press 1998.

37. Andrade C, Aswath A, Chaturvedi SK, Srinivasa M & Raguram R, A double-blind placebo-controlled evaluation of anxiolytic efficacy of an ethanolic extract of *Withania somnifera*. *Indian J of Psychiatry* 42 (2000) 295.

38. Bhattacharya SK, Bhattacharya A & Chakrabarti A, Adaptogenic activity of Siotone a polyherbal formulation of Ayurvedic rasayanas. *Indian J Exp Biol* 38(2000) 119.

4

Effect of cyclooxygenase-2 (COX-2) inhibitors in various animal models (bicuculline, picrotoxin, maximal electroshock-induced convulsions) of epilepsy with possible mechanism of action

ASHISH DHIR, PATTIPATI S NAIDU & SHRINIVAS K KULKARNI
Pharmacology Division, University Institute of Pharmaceutical Sciences,
Panjab University, Chandigarh 160 014, India

Enzyme cyclooxygenase (COX) is reported to play a significant role in neurodegeneration and may play a significant role in the pathogenesis of epilepsy. Bicuculline (4 mg/kg; ip), picrotoxin (8 mg/kg; ip) and electroshock (60 mA for 0.2 sec) significantly induced convulsions in male Laka mice. COX-inhibitors viz. nimesulide (2.5 mg/kg; ip) and rofecoxib (2 mg/kg; ip) administered 45 minutes prior to an epileptic challenge prolonged mean onset time of convulsions, decreased duration of clonus and decreased % mortality rate against bicuculline- and picrotoxin-induced convulsions in mice. COX-2 inhibitors were ineffective towards maximal electroshock-induced convulsions. Nimesulide (1 mg/kg) and rofecoxib (1 mg/kg) also enhanced the effect of subprotective dose of muscimol against picrotoxin-induced convulsions. The result of the present study strongly suggests for a possible role of cyclooxygenase isoenzymes particularly, COX-2 in the pathophysiology of epilepsy and its GABAergic modulation.

Keywords: Bicuculline, Convulsions, Cyclooxygenases, Epilepsy, Nimesulide, Picrotoxin, Rofecoxib

Introduction

Epilepsy is a common neurological disorder affecting about 0.5-1% of the world's population[1]. Clinical signs of epilepsy arise from the intermittent, excessively synchronized activity of group of neurons.

Different neurotransmitters and neuromodulators are known to play a significant role in the system of excitation[2]. Therefore, there is always a continuous research being done to unravel the pathophysiology of epilepsy and the development of newer therapeutic strategies. Cyclooxygenase is the key enzyme that converts arachidonic acid, derived from membrane phospholipids to prostaglandins (PGs) which have important signaling and house keeping functions particularly in platelets, gastrointestinal tract, lungs and kidneys[3]. The neuromodulation by prostaglandins and their possible role in epileptogenesis has been reported[4]. The involvement of COX-2 in acute and chronic neurodegenerative syndromes has promoted the development of neuroprotective treatment strategies involving COX-inhibitors, such as non-steroidal antiinflammatory drugs (NSAIDs). Although studies suggest that NSAIDs may be protective in chronic neurodegenerative conditions, little is known of their clinical efficacy in treating acute neurodegeneration.

It has been reported that COX-2 mRNA and protein are specifically and rapidly increased in brain by electroconvulsive seizure activity[5]. There are recent reports regarding the up-regulation of cyclooxygenase enzyme particularly COX-2 isoform following seizures activity[6]. But there are some contradictory results on the role of cyclooxygenase in epilepsy as there was lowering of the convulsive threshold by non-steroidal anti-inflammatory drugs[7] like aspirin and paracetamol. In one report, COX-2 selective inhibitor as well as non-selective COX-inhibitor such as indomethacin, aggravated kainic acid-induced seizure activity and the following hippocampal neuronal death[8] and there is no mentioning regarding the mechanism of action of COX-inhibitors in epilepsy. With this background, the present study has been undertaken to elucidate the effect of cyclooxygenase inhibitors in various animal models of epilepsy and the possible mechanism of action.

Materials and Methods

Animals- Male Albino mice (Laka strain) weighing 22-30 g and bred in Central Animal House (CAH) facility of Panjab University, Chandigarh were used. The animals were housed under standard laboratory conditions, maintained on a natural light and dark cycle and had free access to food and water. Animals were acclimatized to laboratory conditions before the experiment. All the experiments were carried out between 0900 and 1500 hrs. The experimental protocols were approved by Institutional Animal Ethics Committee (IAEC) and conducted according to the Indian National Science Academy Guidelines [icmr.nic.in/bioethics/INSA_Guidelines.pdf] for the use and care of experimental animals.

Drugs and treatment schedule

The following drugs were used: picrotoxin (Sigma, USA), bicuculline (Sigma, USA), nimesulide and rofecoxib (Panacea Biotec, India). The drugs doses were selected according to the previous studies[9]. Picrotoxin was dissolved in normal saline. Bicuculline was dissolved in saline with the aid of 0.1 N HCl and the COX-inhibitors were suspended in 0.25% carboxymethylcellulose (CMC). Different COX-inhibitors were administered 1 hr before bicuculline or picrotoxin challenge. To see the mechanism of action, COX-inhibitors were given 30 min before subprotective dose of muscimol and after 30 min challenged with picrotoxin.

The experiment protocol comprises the following groups, each constitutes 6-18 animals:

Bicuculline-induced convulsions-Following groups were used: -

Group-1 control i.e. treated with vehicle (0.25% CMC, ip); Group-2 treated with rofecoxib (2 mg/kg; ip) or nimesulide (2.5 mg/kg; ip).

Picrotoxin-induced convulsions– Group-1 control treated with vehicle (0.25% CMC, ip); Group-2 treated rofecoxib (1 and 2 mg/kg; ip) or nimesulide (1 and 2.5 mg/kg; ip); Group-3 given sub-protective dose of muscimol (0.05 mg/kg; i.p.); Group-4 given a combination of sub-protective dose of muscimol and sub-protective dose of rofecoxib (1 mg/kg; ip) or nimesulide (1 mg/kg; ip) against picrotoxin-induced convulsions.

Maximal electro-shock induced seizures-The following groups were used: Group-1 control treated with vehicle (0.25% CMC, ip); Group-2 treated rofecoxib (2 mg/kg; ip) or nimesulide (2.5 mg/kg; ip).

Experimental Models

Bicuculline- and picrotoxin- induced convulsions–Bicuculline (4 mg/kg; ip) and picrotoxin (8 mg/kg; ip) were used to induce chemoconvulsions in mice. Different parameters of chemoconvulsions were noted like onset time of convulsions, duration of convulsions and recovery/death. Each animal was observed individually for the presence or absence of above phases of convulsions up to 2 hr and thereafter at 24 hr for mortality. Bicuculline and picrotoxin produced severe tonic-clonic convulsions followed by 100% mortality at respective doses[10].

Maximal electro-shock induced seizures (MES)–The mice were subjected to maximal electroshock (MES) using an electroconvulsometer. A current of 60 mA for 0.2 sec was used to induce convulsions. The parameters observed were tonic hind limb extension of mice and percentage mortality of animals[11].

Statistical analysis–One specific group of mice was assigned to one specific drug treatment condition and each group comprised 6-18 mice (n=6-18). All the values are expressed as mean ± SE. The data were analyzed by using analysis of variance followed by Dunnett's test. In all tests, the criterion for statistical significance was $P < 0.05$.

Results

Effect of selective COX-2 inhibitors on bicuculline-induced convulsions–Bicuculline (4 mg/kg; ip) produced severe tonic-clonic convulsions followed by 100% mortality. Pretreatment with rofecoxib (2 mg/kg; ip) or nimesulide (2.5 mg/kg; ip) significantly decreased the severity of bicuculline-induced seizures as these drugs prolonged the mean onset time of convulsions and decreased the duration of clonus (Fig. 1A). Pretreatment with rofecoxib (2 mg/kg; ip) or nimesulide (2.5 mg/kg; ip) decreased the % mortality (Fig. 1B) after bicuculline challenge.

Effect of selective COX-2 inhibitors on picrotoxin-induced convulsions–Pretreatment with rofecoxib (2 mg/kg; ip) or nimesulide (2.5 mg/kg; ip) significantly decreased the severity of picrotoxin-induced convulsions (Fig. 2A). Rofecoxib (1 mg/kg; ip) or nimesulide (1 mg/kg; ip) was not effective against picrotoxin-induced convulsions, as rofecoxib and nimesulide at 1 mg/kg did not prolonged the mean onset time of convulsions. Pretreatment with either rofecoxib or nimesulide decreased the % mortality in mice. (Fig. 2B).

Effect of combination of sub-effective dose of selective COX-2 inhibitors and sub-effective dose of muscimol against picrotoxin-induced convulsions–Muscimol (0.05 mg/kg) *per se* was not effective in preventing seizures against picrotoxin-induced convulsions. Pretreatment with rofecoxib (1 mg/kg) or nimesulide (1 mg/kg; ip) potentiated the effect of subprotective dose of muscimol (0.05 mg/kg) against picrotoxin-induced convulsions (Fig. 3) and the combination showed 100% recovery against picrotoxin-induced convulsions (Fig. 4).

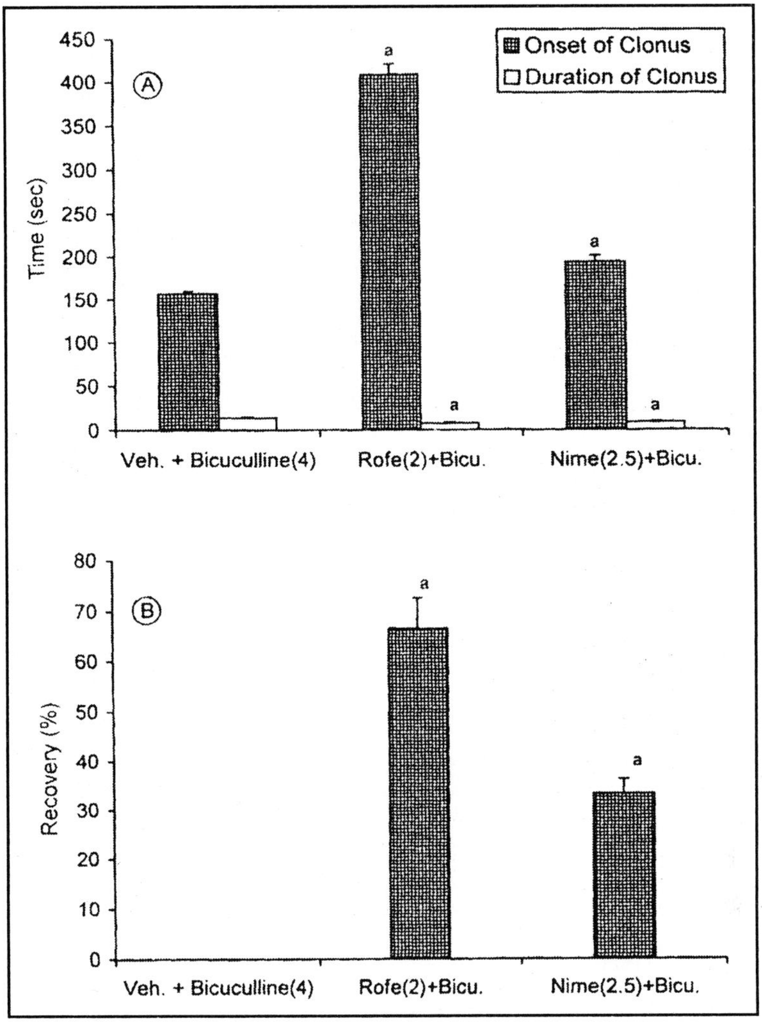

Fig. 1. Effect of COX-2 inhibitors on **(A)** onset of convulsions or duration of clonus and **(B)** recovery (%) against bicuculline-induced convulsions (n=6-18). [a]$P<0.05$ as compared to bicuculline treated group (ANOVA followed by Dunnett's test).

Effect of selective COX-2 inhibitors on maximal electroshock-induced convulsions–Rofecoxib (2 mg/ kg) or nimesulide (2.5 mg/kg) were selected as these doses were effective against bicuculline or picrotoxin induced convulsions. Pretreatment with rofecoxib (2.0 mg/kg) or nimesulide (2.5 mg/kg) did not affect the mean onset time of convulsions in maximal electroshock-induced convulsions. These drugs did not decrease the duration of extensor phase (Fig. 5) and also did not decrease the % mortality in mice.

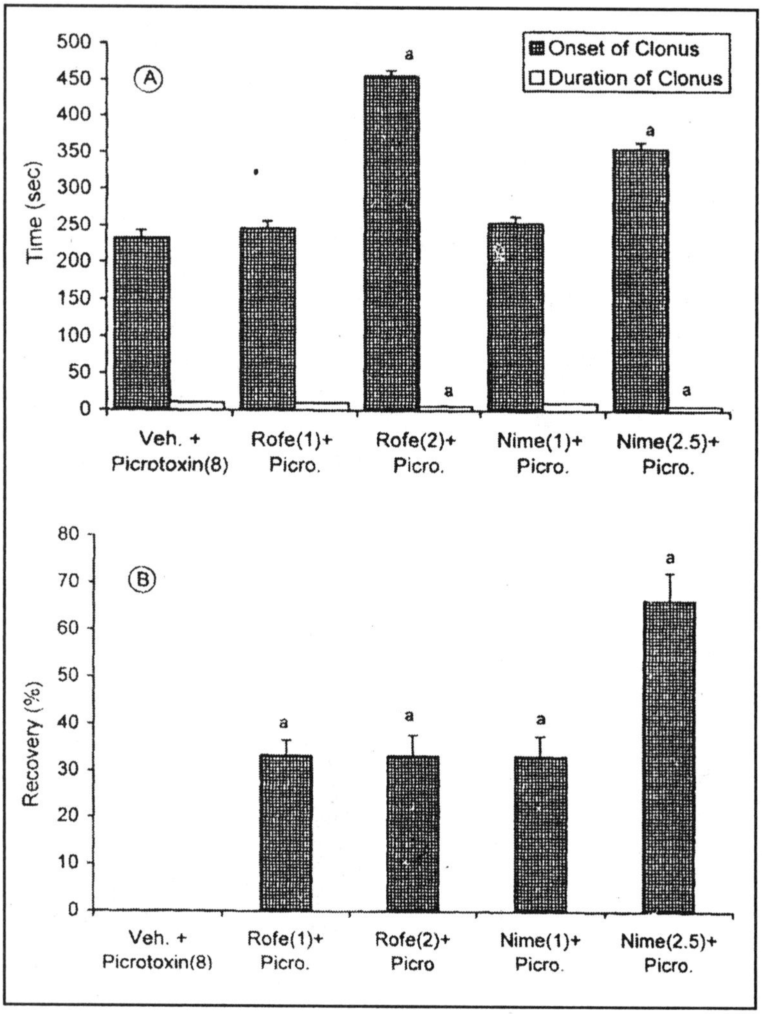

Fig. 2. Effect of COX-2 inhibitors on (A) onset time of convulsions and duration of clonus and (B) recovery (%) against picrotoxin-induced convulsions (n=6-18). [a]P<0.05 as compared to picrotoxin treated group (ANOVA followed by Dunnett's test).

Discussion

The presence of prostaglandins in the mammalian brain is well-documented[12] and prostaglandins are either directly or indirectly involved with neuronal activity[13]. The role of prostaglandins in seizures is known, as there are increased levels of PGD_2 and PGE_2 following PTZ-induced seizures. PGE_1 and PGE_2 have excitatory action on cerebral cortex[14]. Prostaglandins and cyclooxygenases, levels tend to

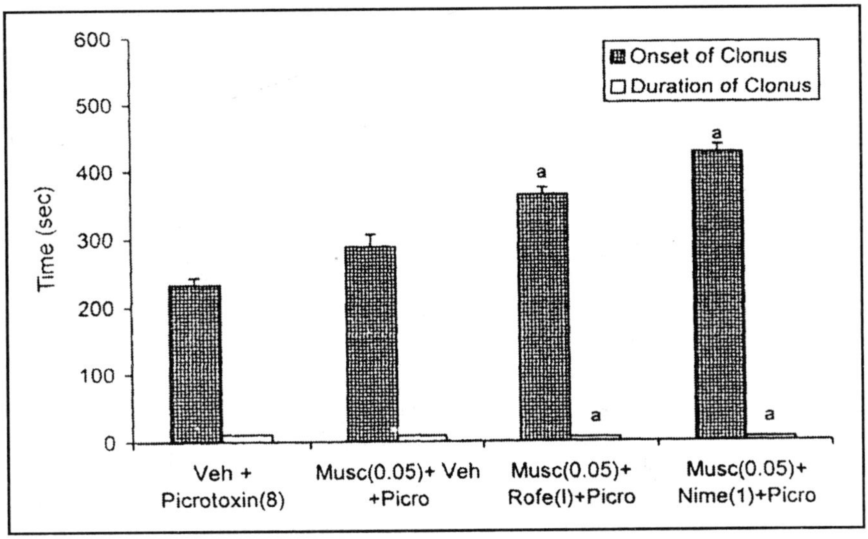

Fig. 3. Effect of subprotective dose of muscimol (0.05 mg/kg) and its combination with rofecoxib (1 mg/kg) or nimesulide (1 mg/kg) inhibitors on onset time of convulsions and duration of clonus against picrotoxin-induced convulsions (n=6-18). [a]P<0.05 as compared to picrotoxin treated group (ANOVA followed by Dunnett's test).

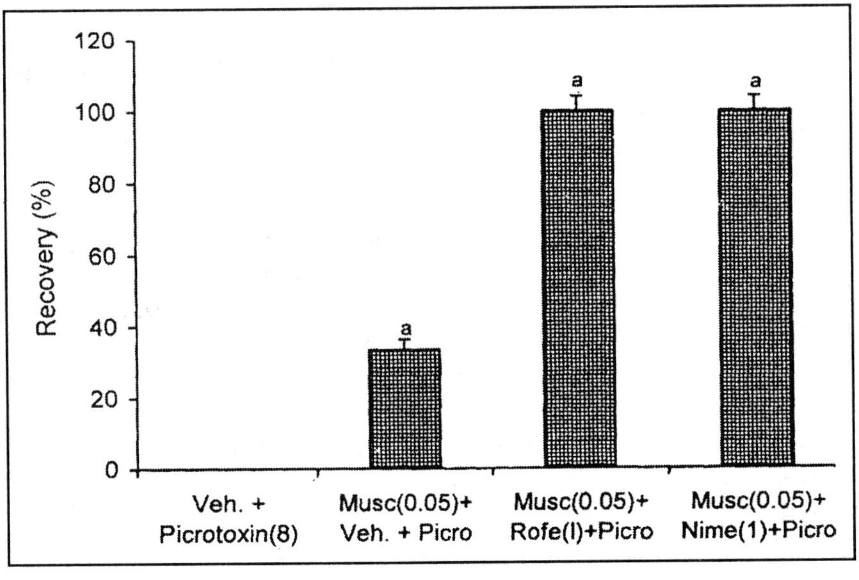

Fig. 4. Effect of subprotective dose of muscimol and its combination with COX-2 inhibitors on recovery (%) against picrotoxin-induced convulsions (n=6-18). [a]P<0.05 as compared to picrotoxin treated group (ANOVA followed by Dunnett's test).

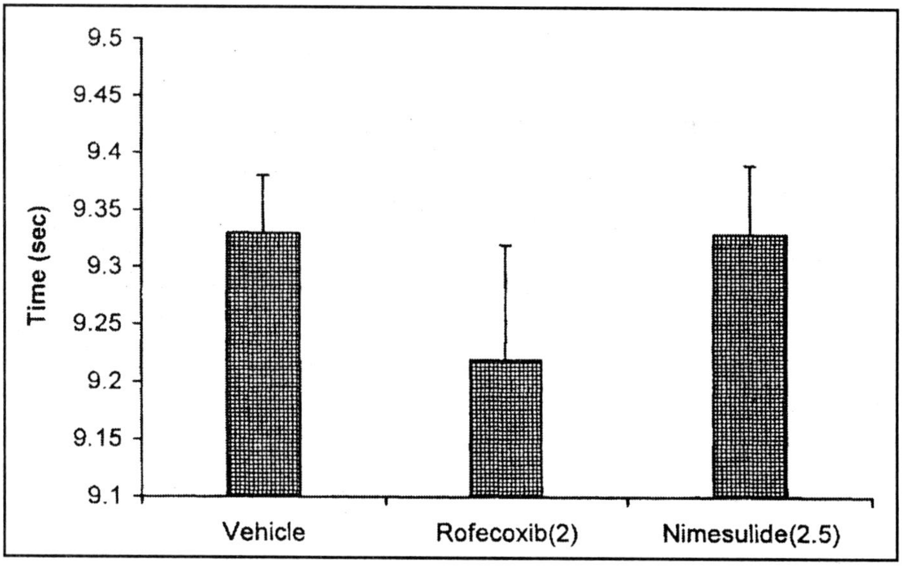

Fig. 5. Effect of COX-2 inhibitors on duration of extensor phase against maximal electroshock-induced convulsions (n=6-18).

rise in both chemically and electrically induced seizures[15]. PGE_1 and PGE_2 have excitatory effects on the cerebral cortex, the area that plays an important role in the onset of seizure activity. PGF_2 is the predominant prostaglandin identified in the experimentally induced as well as spontaneous seizure activity[16]. It was hypothetized that COX-inhibitors reduce seizures by inhibiting the synthesis of prostaglandins. Also PGE_2 which is preferentially formed during the activity of COX-2 rather than COX-1, could participate in through several mechanisms, including modulation of glutamatergic neurotransmission[17]. There was increased expression of COX-2 in the genetically epilepsy susceptible E_1 mice[18]. In one model of lithium chloride and tacrine (5 mg/kg; ip) induced status epilepticus seizures, there was also an expression of COX-2 enzyme protein particularly in dorsal hippocampus and elevated brain PGE_2 levels[19]. Cyclooxygenase-2 expression is markedly and transiently up regulated in neurons in response to excitatory stimuli such as seizures and kainic acid[20]. COX-2 induction appears to be the characteristic of forebrain seizures since COX-2 was not induced in mid-brain seizures, but was dramatically up regulated in ipsilateral cortex following seizure generalization[5]. Takemiya et a[16], studied the expression of cyclooxygenase-2 isoenzyme in the mouse brain after rapid kindling.

Evidences support the involvement of GABA in seizures paradigm. $GABA_A$ receptor agonist as well as drugs, which allosterically modulate the receptor channel complex, is therapeutically active against convulsive seizures[21]. Both picrotoxin and bicuculline affect GABA neurotransmission. Picrotoxin appears to interfere indirectly with the tonic presynaptic inhibition action of GABA, thus induced convulsions through rapid summation of synaptic activity[22]. Bicuculline is a pure GABA receptor antagonist, as assessed by ligand binding studies[23]. Zath and Roth[24] observed that electroconvulsive stimuli increase PGF in rat cerebral cortex. In the present study, rofecoxib (2 mg/kg) or nimesulide (2.5 mg/kg) significantly decreased the incidence of bicuculline-induced convulsions. γ-amino butyric acid (GABA), the principal inhibitory neurotransmitter in the cerebral cortex maintained the inhibitory tone that counterbalances neurons excitation. When this balance is disturbed, seizures ensue. Reduction in GABAmediated inhibitory activity of glutamate decarboxylase has been reported in studies of human epileptic brain tissues[25]. Glutamate concentration increased before seizure onset and found to be highest in the epileptic hippocampus than non-epileptic hippocampus while GABA levels increased during seizures was greater in non-epileptic hippocampus than in epileptic hippocampus showing decreased levels of GABA in epilepsy[26]. The $GABA_A$ receptor is responsible for most fast inhibitory neurotransmission in the central nervous system. Consequently, this receptor has been targeted for the pharmacological control of anxiety, sleep, and epilepsy. Numerous natural and synthetic compounds interact with the $GABA_A$ receptor at distinct, yet incompletely defined, sites. These compounds include barbiturates, benzodiazepines, neurosteroids, and picrotoxin[27,28]. The drugs, which enhance the anti-epileptic activity of $GABA_A$ agonist such as muscimol, are thought to act through $GABA_A$ receptors. In the present study, pretreatment with rofecoxib (2 mg/kg) or nimesulide (2.5 mg/kg) significantly decreased the incidence of picrotoxin-induced convulsions while rofecoxib (1 mg/kg) and nimesulide (1 mg/kg) were not effective against picrotoxin-induced convulsions. Rofecoxib (1 mg/kg) or nimesulide (1 mg/kg) potentiated the effect of sub-effective dose of muscimol (0.05 mg/kg) against picrotoxin-induced convulsions. These combinations also decreased the duration of clonus and combining rofecoxib (1 mg/kg) and nimesulide (1 mg/kg) with sub-effective dose of muscimol (0.05 mg/kg) showed 100% recovery in animals against picrotoxin-induced convulsions. This further proves the GABAergic mechanism of action of COX-inhibitors. Arachidonic acid which by cyclooxygenases action formed prostaglandins has been proposed a diffusible second messenger in CNS with a pathophysiological role in epilepsy. This is possibly due to ability of arachidonic acid to enhance extraneuronal glutamate concentration[29]. Also arachidonic acid cannot be only considered as a facilitatory neuromodulator in the hippocampus as the arachidonic acid facilitation of the release of the main inhibitory neurotransmitter GABA. Also majority of cyclooxygenases are excitatory and express in glutamatergic neurons[30]. Increased in glutamate levels may leads to decrease in GABAergic output, which may be responsible for increased seizures susceptibility. In the present study, COX-inhibitors proved to be ineffective against maximal-electroshock induced convulsions. Further studies are needed at higher doses to see the effect of COX-inhibitors against maximal electroshock induced seizures paradigm. Finally, the result of the present study suggested that COX-2 have significant protection against the bicuculline- and picrotoxin-induced convulsions via GABA/ Benzodiazepine receptor mechanism.

REFERENCES

1. Hackinski V, New antiepileptic drugs, the cost of innovation, Arch Neurol, 55 (1998) 1142.
2. Fisher R S & Coyle J T, In summary: Neurotransmitters and epilepsy, (Wiley-Liss: New york) 1991, 247.
3. Griffin M R, Epidemology of nonsteroidal anti-inflammatory drug associated gastrointestinal injury, Am J Med, 104 (1999) 155.
4. Foko G C, Longiava D & Bosisco E, Relation between prostaglandins E2, F2 and cyclic nucleotides levels in rat brain and induction of convulsions, Prostaglandins, 13 (1977) 893.
5. McCown T J, Knapp D J & Crews F T, Inferior collicular seizure generalization produces site-selective cortical induction of cyclooxygenase-2 (COX-2), Brain Res, 767 (1997) 370.
6. Takemiya T, Suzuki K, Sugiura H, Yasuda S, Yamagata K Kawakami Y & Maru E, Inducible brain COX-2 facilitates the recurrence of hippocampal seizures in mouse rapid kindling, Prostaglandin & Other Lipid Mediators, 71 (2003) 205.
7. Hjalmar B S & George H, Lowering of the convulsive threshold by non-steroidal anti-inflammatory drugs, European Journal of Pharmacology. 69 (1981) 199.
8. Bark EJ, Kein EK Lee S H & Moon C, COX-2 selectins inhibitors aggravate kainic acid induced seizures and neuronal cell death in the hippocampus, Brain Res, 843 (1999) 118.

9. Dhir A, Naidu P S & Kulkarni S K, Protective effect of cyclooxygenase-2 (COX-2) inhibitors but not non-selective cyclooxygenase (COX)-inhibitors on ethanol withdrawal-induced behavioural changes, Addict Biol, 10 (2005) 329.

10. Kulkarni S K & Ticku M K, RO15-4513 but not FG-7142 reverses anticonvulsant effects of ethanol against bicuculline- and picrotoxin-induced convulsions in rats, Pharmacol Biochem Behavi, 32 (1989) 232.

11. Kulkarni S K, Handbook of experimental pharmacology (Vallabh Prakashan, Delhi) 3 (1999) 117.

12. Wolfe L S, Possible role of prostaglandins in the nervous system, Adv. Neurochem, 1 (1975) 1.

13. Haris R H & Ramwell P W, Cellular mechanism of prostaglandin action, Ann. Rev. Physiol, 41 (1979) 653.

14. Bradley P B, Synaptic transmission in the CNS and its relevance for drug action, edited by CC Pfeiffer & JR symthies in The international review of neurobiology. edited by CC Pfeiffer & JR symthies London. (Academic Press, London) 1968, 2.

15. Wallenstein M C & Mauss E A, Effect of prostaglandin synthetase inhibitors on experimentally induced convulsions in rats, Pharmacology, 29 (1984) 85.

16. Tandon M, Anuradha K & Pandhi, P, Evaluation of antiepileptic activity of aspirin in combination with newer antiepileptic lamotrigine in mice, Method Find Ex. Clin Pharmacol, 25 (2003) 607.

17. Bazan N G, Synaptic lipid signaling: significance of polyunsaturated fatty acids and platelet-activationg factor, J. Lipid Res, 44(2003) 2221.

18. Okada K, Yuhi T, Tsuji S & Yamashita U, Cyclooxygenase-2 expression in the hippocampus of genetically epilepsy susceptible E1 mice was increased after seizure, Brain Res, 894 (2001), 332.

19. Paoletti A M, Piccirilli S, Costa N, Rotiroti D, Bagetta G & Nistico G, Systemic administration of N-nitro-L-arginine methyl ester and indomethacin reduces the elevation of brain PGE2 content and prevents seizures and hippocampal damage evoked by Licl and tacrine in rat, Experimental Neurology, 149 (1998) 349.

20. Yamagata K, Andreasson K I, Kaufmann W E, Barnes C A & Worley P F, Expression of a mitogen inducible cyclooxygenase in brain neurons: regulation by synaptic activity and glucocorticoids, Neuron, 11 (1993) 371.

21. Mohler H, Benke D, Benson J, Luscher B, Rudolph U & Fritschy J M, Diversity in structure, pharmacology and regulation of $GABA_A$ receptors.

The GABA receptors, edited by S J Enna & N.G Bowery (Humana Press, Totowa, N.J) 11.

22. Barker J L & MacDonald J F, Picrotoxin convulsions involve synaptic and nonsynaptic mechanisms on cultured mouse spinal neurons, Science, 208 (1980) 1054.

23. Snodgras S R, Use of 3H-muscimol for GABA receptor studies, Nature, 273 (1978) 392.

24. Zath M & Roth R H, Electroshock raises prostaglandins F in rat cerebral cortex, Biochem Pharmacol 24 (1975) 2101.

25. David M, GABAergic mechanism in epilepsy, Epilepsia 42 (2001) 8.

26. During M J & Spancer D D, Extracellular hippocampal glutamate and spontaneous seizures in the conscious human brain, Lancet, 341 (1993) 1607.

27. Sieghart W, $GABA_A$ receptors: ligand-gated Cl ion channels modulated by multiple drug-binding sites, Trends Pharmacol Sci, 13 (1992) 446.

28. Smith GB & Olsen CE, Functional domains of GABAA receptors, Trends Pharmacol Sci, 16 (1995) 162.

29. Dickie B G, Annals S J & Davies J A, Effect of cyclooxygenase inhibition upon glutamate release from rat cerebellum, Neuroreport, 5 (1994) 393.

30. Kaufman W E, Worley P F, Bremer, P J & Isakson P, COX 2 a synaptically induced enzyme is expressed by excitatory neurons at post synaptic sites in rat cerebral cortex, Proc Natl Acad Sci, USA, 93 (1996) 2317.

Paper Published In:
I.J.E.B (Vol. 44, April 2006, pp 286-291)

5

Motor and electrographic response of refractory experimental status epilepticus in rats and effect of calcium channel blockers

B. GEORGE & S.K. KULKARNI
Pharmacology Division, University Institute of Pharmaceutical Sciences, Panjab University, Chandigarh 160 014, India
and **R. MATHUR**
Department of Physiology, All India Institute of Medical Sciences, New Delhi 110 029, India

Effects of various calcium channel inhibitors have been studied in lithium-pilocarpine model of status epilepticus. Status epilepticus (SE) was induced by administration of lithium chloride (3 meq/kg) followed 21 hr later by pilocarpine (30 mg/kg). Diltiazem (5 and 10 mg/kg) was not effective in delaying onset of convulsions. Verapamil (20 mg/kg) showed protection against lithium-pilocarpine-induced convulsions. The dihydropyridine nifidepine (2.5 and 5 mg/kg) did not show any protection in this model. Amlodipine (5 and 10 mg/kg) is partially protective. Flunarizine (10 and 20 mg/kg) delayed the onset of forelimb clonus and rearing and only 60% of the rats underwent status in the 20 mg/kg group. Pre-treatment of MK-801 led to a potentiation of the antiseizure activity of calcium channel inhibitors. The percent increase in amplitude at various time points with amlodipine pretreatment was significant only at the 30th min recording, and at the rest of the time frames was practically similar as the controls. It can be concluded that the anticonvulsant action of MK-801 can be enhanced by centrally acting calcium channel inhibitors.

Accumulating experimental evidence suggest that abnormalities in calcium-regulated ion channels or enzymatic processes may underlie alterations in neuronal excitability and result in seizure activity.

Increased Ca^{2+} influx in epileptogenesis is well established, and it is assumed that both receptor operated and voltage-sensitive Ca^{2+} channels take active part in these processes. Desmedt *et at.*[1] demonstrated that two piperazine derivatives, flunarazine and cinnarizine antagonized PTZ and electroshock-induced seizures. These observations were confirmed and extended for calcium channel inhibitors (CCIs) from two other classes, dihydropyridine and benzothiazepines. Consistent with these findings, BAY K 8644, an L-type Ca^{2+} channel agonist, can elicit seizures by itself and potentiate audiogenic, PTZ- or NMDA-induced convulsions. CCIs are the only effective drugs for BAY K 8644-induced seizures. Representatives of the class I CCIs (verapamil, gallopamil) do not appear to exhibit significant anticonvulsant activity in any of the above mentioned models, with the notable exception of BAY K 8644-induced seizures[2]. BAY K 8644 augments NMDA-induced seizures whereas CCIs such as diltiazem, nifidepine or verapamil antagonize NMDA- and kainate-induced convulsions in mice. Convulsions elicited with intrahippocampal injections of quinolinic acid, an endogenous agonist acting preferentially at NMDA-type, receptors are suppressed by flunarizine or verapamil, but not by nifedipine[3].

The development and evaluation of drugs which block Ca^{2+} channels has therefore been an important rational strategy for anticonvulsant drug design[4]. Most selective CCIs which have been evaluated for anticonvulsant effects primarily block the L-type channel. Evidence suggest that dihydropyridines (nifidepine) may act on T-type channels at higher doses, and some CCIs may act at other non-calcium binding sites as well[5]. Flunarizine is able to block T-type as well as L-type Ca^{2+} channels in several tissues including brain membranes. Nifedipine and flunarizine, partially protects the kindled rats from subsequent kindling stimuli[3]. CCI nimodipine, has been shown to block amygdalar and hippocampal kindling[6].

The metabolic demands and physiological changes associated with SE indicate a major role of Ca^{2+} in modulating continued excitability and cytotoxicity[7] and this high $[Ca^{2+}]$ has been repeatedly shown to cause cell death[8]. Griffiths *et al.*[9] were the first to suggest this to be the mechanism of status-induced cellular damage. They showed that during 2 hr of status epilepticus induced by bicuculline or L-allylglycine in rats, Ca^{2+} accumulates in the swollen and disrupted mitochondria in basal dendrites and selected neuronal cell bodies within the hippocampus. *In vitro* studies indicate that hippocampal bursting activity is Ca^{2+} dependent and dihydropyridine channels are localized in regions such as the hippocampus which are related to epileptogenesis, CCIs acting at CNS sites may be useful in treating epilepsy.

Materials and Methods

Animals– Wistar rats of either sex, 200-250 g from Central Animal house facility, Punjab University were used. Animals were housed in cages and received standard laboratory chow and water. Animals were acclimatized to the laboratory conditions and all experiments were carried out between 9.00 and 17.00 hrs.

Drugs– The following drugs (with their respective source) were used during the entire study: lithium chloride (Merck, Germany), atropine sulphate, pilocarpine nitrate, (Boehringer Ingelheim, Germany), ketamine (Themis, India), MK-801 (Merck Sharp and Dohme, UK), nifedipine (Torrent Labs, Ahemedabad), diltiazem (Torrent Labs, Ahemedabad), verapamil (Torrent Labs, Ahemedabad), amlodipine (Systopic Laboratories Ltd., Faridabad, India), flunarizine (Torrent Pharmaceutical Ltd, Baroda, India). The doses used in the present study are based upon the previous studies carried out in our laboratory.

Experimental procedure– SE was induced by the method of Honchar and colleagues[10] by administering lithium chloride (3 meq/kg, ip) followed 21 hr later by pilocarpine (30 mg/kg, sc), following which rats were observed continuously for occurrence of behavioural and electroencephalographic (EEG) seizures (Fig. 1). In the interaction studies, the drugs were administered 30 min prior to pilocarpine challenge. The latency to attain forelimb clonus with rearing was noted and seizures were monitored till 90 min post pilocarpine behaviourally.

For electrophysiologic study, under ketamine anaesthesia (80 mg/kg, im) rats were stereotaxically[12] (David Kopff, Model-1404, USA) implanted with both cortical bilateral watch screw electrodes and unilateral unipolar electrode in the right dorsal hippocampus (-2.8 mm posterior, 2 mm lateral and 3.5 mm ventral). Prior to ketamine atropine sulphate (7 mg/kg, ip) was given to rats to reduce respiratory secretions. After 5 days recovery each animal was allowed atleast 30 min for habituation to the transparent recording cage (modified skinner box, 25x25x29 cm) permitting free movement with the experimental set up following which SE was induced[6]. Onset of seizures was

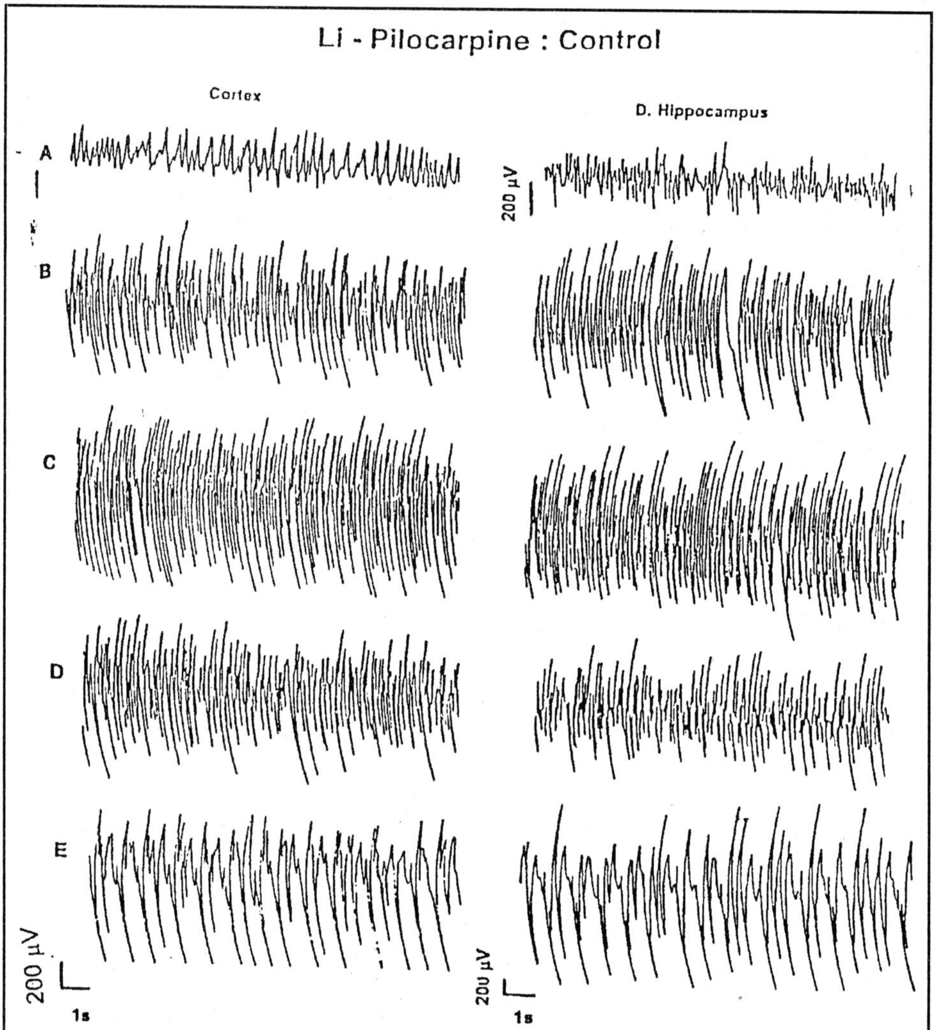

Fig. 1. Representative cortical and dorsal hippocampal (DHc) EEG in Li-pilocarpine control rats showing the development of SE at different time intervals. A: Basal recording; B, C, D, E: 0.5, 1, 1.5 and 4 hr post pilocarpine (30 mg) challenge (n=6). The cortical amplitude corresponding to A (100 mV); B→E (200 mV) and DHc amplitude corresponding to A (200 mV); B→E (200 mV) respectively are indicated.

characterised electrographically by the occurrence of generalized spikes and polyspikes for longer than 20s associated with sniffing, chewing, eye blinking and head nodding as reported by Hirsch *et al*[11]. SE was defined as continuous convulsions for a period longer than 30 min associated with continuous spikes of high amplitude. EEG signals were recorded on the chart paper of Grass Model 7D polygraph (Grass Instruments Co., Quincy, Mass, USA).

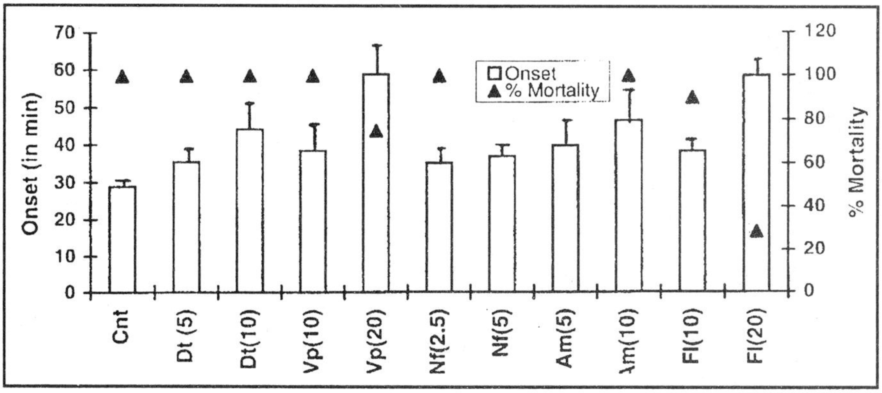

Fig. 2. Effect of different calcium channel blockers diltiazem (Dt: 5 and 10 mg/kg), verapamil (Vp: 10 and 20 mg/kg), nifedipine (Nf: 2.5 and 5 mg/kg), amlodipine (Amd: 5 and 10 mg/kg), and flunarizine (Fl: 10 and 20 mg/kg) administered 30 min before pilocarpine (30 mg/kg) challenge in Li-pretreated rats. Severity was assessed as onset of F.C+R and percent mortality. Each value represents mean+S.E. (n=7-9). ΔP<0.05 [compared w.r.t. control (Cnt), Kruskal Wallis test followed by Student's t-test].

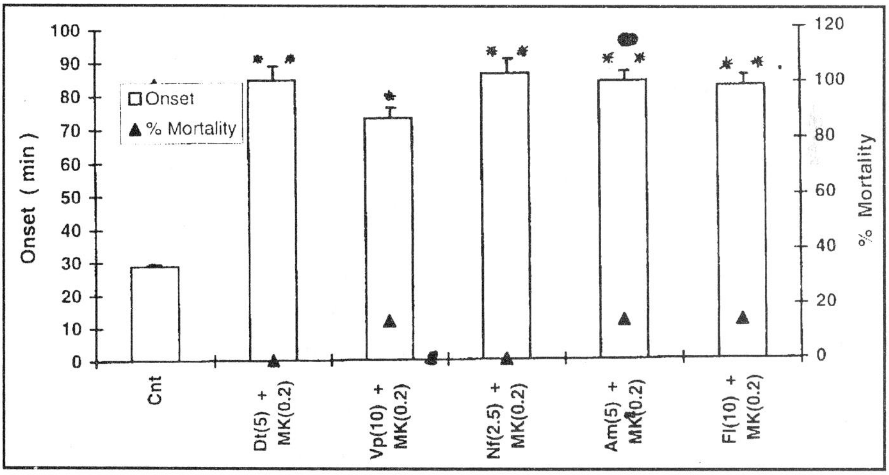

Fig. 3. Effect of combination of MK-801 (0.3 mg/kg) with different calcium channel blockers administered 45 and 30 min before pilocarpine (30 mg/kg), respectively in Li-pretreated rats. Diltiazem (Dt: 5 mg/kg), verapamil (Vp: 10 mg /kg), nifedipine (Nf: 2.5 mg/kg), amlodipine (Amd: 5 mg/kg), and flunarizine (Fl: 10 mg/kg). Severity was assessed as onset of F.C+R and percent mortality. Each value represents mean±S.E. (n=7-9). *P<0.05, **P<0.01 [compared w.r.t. control (Cnt), Kruskal Wallis test followed by Student's t-test].

Prior to recording, calibration of EEG signals was done by determining the height of signal having voltage of 50 μv. Frequency was determined by calculating the average number of peaks recurring per second taken up from three 5 s intervals, similarly for amplitude, determined by measuring peak to peak voltage manually. The changes in EEG were recorded alternately for cortex and hippocampus 30 min before lithium (basal), 30 min after amlodipine (20.5 hr post lithium), and after administering pilocarpine (21 hr post lithium) at 30 min intervals up to 90th min, and finally after 4 hr of pilocarpine.

Statistical analysis– In behavioural studies data on onset of forelimb clonus with rearing was subjected to Kruskal-Wallis one-way analysis of variance output test followed by Student's t-test. Descriptive statistics for amplitude and frequency in the cortex and hippocampus at various time points was calculated by mean and standard deviation for all the groups separately. Freidmans test (non-parametric test) was applied to find out at what time from the basal value changes become significant. This was done for both the parameters in the cortex and hippocampus group wise. Area under the curve (AUC) was compared among the groups by Kruskal Wallis test. In case of overall significance, multiple range test was applied. The data on the percent change in amplitude and frequency was analyzed by one way analysis of variance (ANOVA) amongst the groups. Further application of least significant difference procedure was performed for testing significance of each group. $P < 0.05$ was considered statistically significant.

Results

Behavioural studies– Among the CCIs, diltiazem (5 and 10 mg/kg) was not effective in delaying onset of status. Representatives of the class I CCIs, verapamil (10 and 20 mg/kg) which is effective against kindling was effective only at the higher dose. The dihydropyridine nifidepine (2.5 and 5 mg/kg) did not show any protection in this model. Amlodipine (5 and 10 mg/kg) was partially protective. Flunarizine (10 and 20 mg/kg, po), a diphenylalkylamine and a potent CCI, able to block T-type as well as L-type Ca^{2+} channels in several tissues including brain membranes was successful in delaying the onset of F.C+R, and only 60% of the rats underwent status in the 20 mg/kg group (Fig. 2).

MK-801 when given 15 min before the subeffective doses of CCIs studied [diltiazem (5 mg/kg), verapamil (10 mg/kg), nifedipine (5 mg/

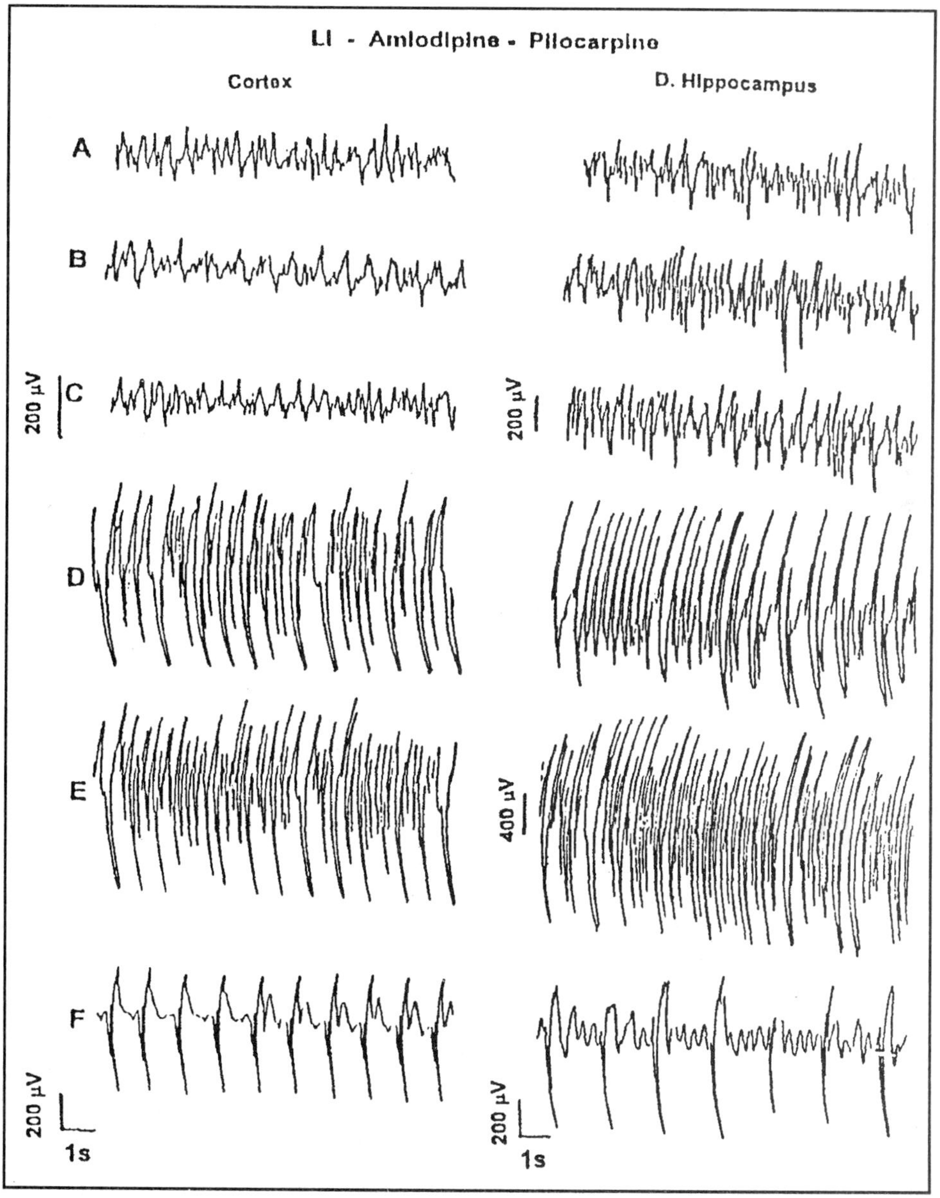

Fig. 4. Representative cortical and dorsal hippocampal (DHc) EEG, showing the development of SE in amlodipine (10 mg/kg) pretreated rats at different time intervals. A: Basal recording; B, C, D, E: 0.5, l, 1.5 and 4 hr post pilocarpine (30 mg/kg) challenge. The cortical amplitude corresponding to A→C (200 mV), D→E (400 mV), F (200 mV), respectively, are indicated.

kg), amlodipine (5 mg/kg), and flunarizine (10 mg/kg, po)] led to a potentiation of the antiseizure activity (Fig. 3).

EEG studies– However, amlodipine (10 mg/kg) neither reduced the severity of SE nor the subsequent mortality apart from the fact that it delayed the onset of status (Figs 4-6). The % increase in amplitude (with reference to the basal value) at various time points with amlodipine pretreatment was significant only at the 30th min recording, and at the rest of the time frames was practically similar as the controls (Fig. 7A). The hippocampal frequency in amlodipine group remained more or less at the basal value till 60th min. record, whereas in the control rats the DHc frequency increased right from the 30th min. record till the 90th min post pilocarpine. Recording taken at the 4th hr (240 min) showed a drop in frequency (Fig. 7B).

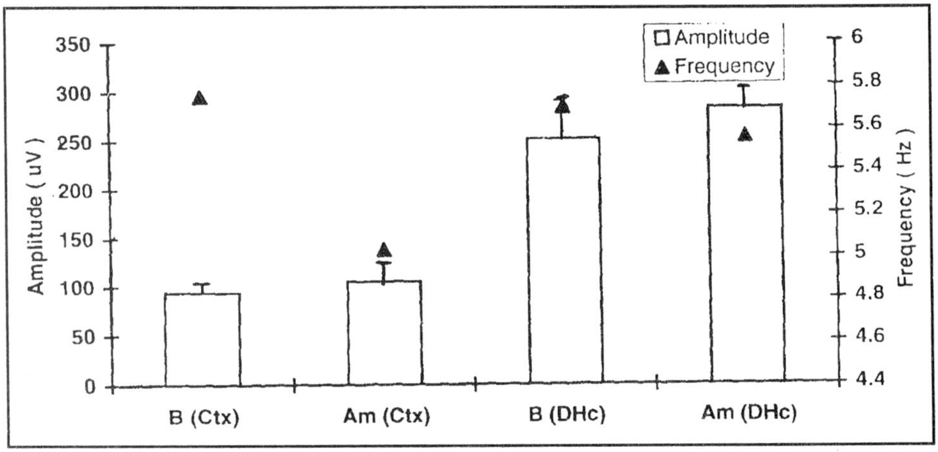

Fig. 5. Effect of amlodipine (Amd: 10 mg/kg) pretreatment in Li-pretreated rats on cortical (Ctx) and dorsal hippocampal (DHc) amplitude and frequency, compared with respect to basal (B) values. Each value represents mean±S.D. (n=4). (Friedmans test).

Discussion

Intracellular Ca^{2+} plays a crucial role in the initiation and regulation of a variety of physiological cellular processes, which include release of neurotransmitters and hormones, neuronal electrical activity, muscle contraction, gene expression, cell growth and differentiation and cell death[13].

This potentiation of the antiseizure activity could be the result of simultaneous blockade of excitatory events and voltage-dependent

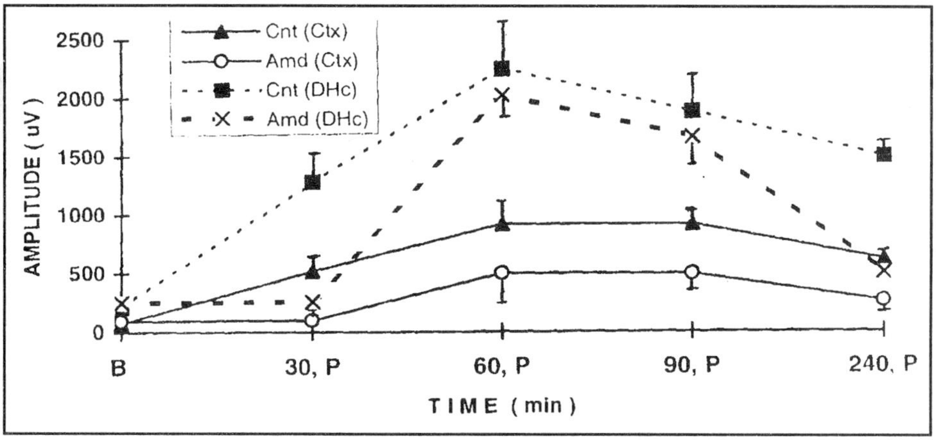

Fig. 6. Time course changes in the cortical (Ctx) and dorsal hippocampal (DHc) EEG amplitude in amlodipine (Amd: 10 mg/kg) pretreated rats as compared to the controls in Li-pilocarpine model. Each value represents mean±S.D. (n=4-6). The AUC of Cnt (Ctx) v/s Amd (Ctx) and Cnt (DHc) v/s Amd (DHc) showed no significant difference (Kruskal Wallis test).

calcium channels. Because of the reported role of neuronal Ca^{2+} channels in seizure disorders, various CCIs were examined for anticonvulsant activity in Li-pilocarpine model of SE.

The CCI, diltiazem (5 and 10 mg/kg), a potent coronary dilator, was not protective in the present model of SE. Verapamil and D-600 (methoxyverapamil) are known to reduce the amplitude of Ca^{2+} spikes induced by iontophoretic pulses of NMDA in hippocampal slice preparation. Verapamil also partially protects the kindled rats from subsequent kindling stimuli. In the present study verapamil (10 and 20 mg/kg) was protective only at the higher dose. The dihydropyridine CCI, nifidepine (2.5 and 5 mg/kg) was also ineffective and did not show any respite from the seizures. Amlodipine (5 and 10 mg/kg), another dihydropyridine CCI, with a long duration of action was found to be partially effective at 10 mg/kg dose in delaying the onset of seizures. In the EEG studies, the percent increase in amplitude at various time points with amlodipine (10 mg/kg) pretreatment was practically similar as that of controls.

Flunarizine (difluoro derivative of cinnarizine), a diphenylalkylamine, has a wide spectrum of pharmacological activity. Among these, actions which may account for its anticonvulsant properties are suppression of N- and T-type Ca^{2+} channel conductance, phenytoin-like effects on sodium channels, and inhibition of adenosine

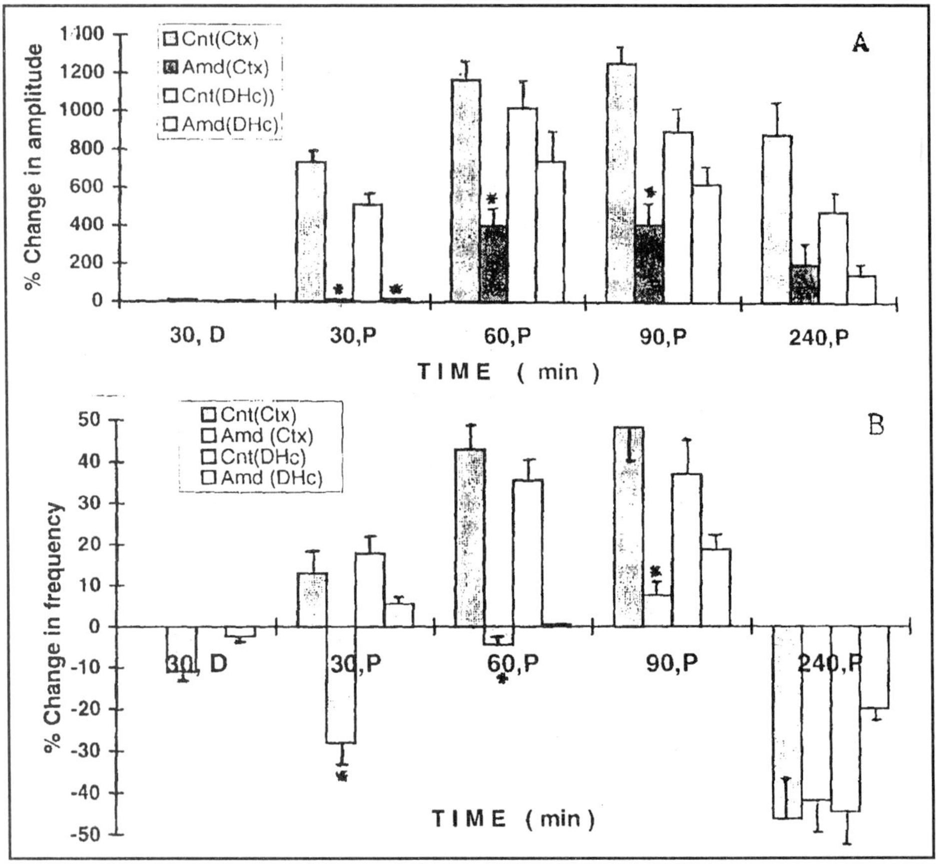

Fig.7. A. The percent change in amplitude observed after amlodipine (Amd: 10 mg/kg) pretreatment on cortical (Ctx) and dorsal hippocampal (DHc) EEG activity. **B.** Similarly, for percent change in frequency in Li-pilocarpine model. Each value represents mean±S.D. (n=4-6). $P<0.05$ [compared with respect to control values, one way ANOVA followed by Student's t-test.

reuptake. Flunarizine (10 and 20 mg/kg) dose dependently delayed the onset of F.C+R. The 20 mg/kg dose also brought down the mortality rate significantly.

The mechanism of action of CCIs in epilepsy is not well understood. The antiepileptic effects may be by either decreasing neuronal recruitment or abolishing the paroxysmal depolarization shift (PDS), an excitatory field potential recorded in groups of neurons during the process of seizure initiation. The PDS is believed to be the underlying generator of burst firing of neuronal groups that synchronize firing in discrete areas of the brain. CCIs, such as verapamil have been reported to reduce the amplitude of the PDS or possibly to decrease generation of such spikes in hippocampal slice preparation[14]. Ca^{2+} entry into neurons is involved in initiation of epileptiform activity by activating Ca^{2+} and calmodulin-dependent protein kinases. The subsequent cell damage is mediated largely through second messenger mechanisms.

Ca^{2+} ions also play a pivotal role in EAA-mediated events[15]. Combination therapy, opens new possibilities for some of the EAA receptor antagonists in the treatment of epilepsy[16]. In the present study, MK-801 (0.2 mg/kg) administered before the subeffective doses of CCIs in Li-pilocarpine model [diltiazem (5 mg/kg), verapamil (10 mg/kg), nifedipine (5 mg/kg), amlodipine (5 mg/kg), and flunarizine (10 mg/kg)] led to a potentiation of the antiseizure activity. The exact nature of the interaction between voltage-dependent calcium channels and EAA receptors remains to be determined. NMDA and non-NMDA receptors differ substantially in ion selectivity[17]. It is known that the NMDA receptor-mediated effects are calcium dependent due to the high permeability of the NMDA receptor to Ca^{2+} ions[18]. CCIs, therefore, may synergistically increase the protective action of competitive NMDA receptor antagonists against convulsions. It can be concluded that the anticonvulsant action of MK-801 can be enhanced by centrally acting CCIs. Such combinations may prove useful in rationalizing polypharmacological approaches in the treatment of epilepsy.

Dynamic regulation of Ca^{2+} signal transduction system may provide insight into the molecular mechanisms of altered neuronal excitability which are important not only in the development of better therapeutic strategies in pathologic processes such as epilepsy, but also in understanding the physiological development of neuronal plasticity.

REFERENCES

1. Desmedt LKC, Niemegeers CJF & Janssen PAJ, Anticonvulsant properties of cinnarizine and flunarizine in rats and mice. *Drug Res*, 25 (1976) 1408-1413.

2. Czuczwar SJ, Malek U & Kleinrok Z, Influence of calcium channel inhibitors upon the anticonvulsant efficacy of common antiepileptic agents against PTZ-induced convulsions in mice. *Neuropharmacology*, 29 (1990) 943-948.

3. Vezzani A. Wu Q, Stasi MA, Angelico P & Samanin R, Effect of various calcium channel blockers on three different models limbic seizures in rats. *Neuropharmcology*, 27 (1988) 451-458.

4. Porter RJ & Rogawski MA, New antiepilcptic drugs: from serendipity to rational discovery. *Epilepsia.* 33 (Suppl. 1) (1992) S I -S6.

5. Faingold CL, Overview of ion channels, antiepileptic drugs, and seizures in: *Drugs for control of epilepsy: Actions on neuronal networks involved in seizure disclosure.* Edited by Fangold CL, Fromm GH. (CRC Press, Boca Raton) 1992, 57-68.

6. Wurpel JN & Iyer SN, Calcium channel blockers verapamil and nimodipine inhibit kindling in adult and immature rats. *Epilepsia,* 35 (1994) 443-448.

7. Doble A & Martin IL, Multiple benzodiazepine receptors: no reason for anxiety. *Trends Pharmacol Sci,* 13 (1992) 76-81.

8. Meldrum BS, Excitatory amino acids in epilepsy and potential novel therapies. *Epilepsy Res,* 12 (1992) 189-196.

9. Griffiths T, Evans C & Meldrum BS, Status epilepticus: The reversibility of calcium loading and acute neuronal pathological changes in the rat hippocampus. *Neuroscience,* 12 (1984) 557-567.

10. Honchar MP, Olney JW & Sherman WR, Systemic cholinergic agents induce seizures and brain damage in lithium treated rats. *Science,* 220 (1983) 323-325.

11. Hirsch E, Snead OC, Vergnes M & Gille F, Corpus callosotomy in the lithium-pilocarpine model of seizures and status epilepticus. *Epilepsy Res,* 11 (1992), 183-191.

12. Paxinos G & Watson C, *The rat brain in stereotaxic coordinates.* (Academic Press. Sydney) 1982.

13. Tsien RW, Lipscombe D, Madison DV, Bley KR & Fox AP, Multiple types of neuronal calcium channels and their selective modulation. *Trends Neurosci,* 11 (1988) 431-438.

14. Dingledine RJ, NMDA activates voltage dependent calcium conductance in rat hippocampal pyramidal cells. *J Physiol.* 343 (1983) 385-405.

15. Gasior M, Kleinrok Z & Czuczwar S.I. Influence of BAY K-86444, a calcium channel agonist, on the anticonvulsant activity of conventional antiepileptics against electroconvulsions in mice. *Neurophamcology,* 34 (1995) 433-438.

16. Rogawski MA, in: *CNS neurotransmitters and neuromodulators.* Edited by Stone TW. (CRC Press, Boca Raton), 1995, 219.

17. Kullmann DM, Perkel DJ, Manabe T & Nicoll RA, Calcium entry via postsynaptic voltage-sensitive calcium channels can transiently potentiate

excitatory synaptic transmission in the hippocampus. *Neuron,* 9 (1992) 1175-1183.

18. Wroblewski JT &. Danysz W, Modulation of glutamate receptors: Molecular mechanisms and functional implications. *Ann Rev Pharmacol Toxicol,* 29 (1989) 441-474.

Paper Published In:
I.J.E.B. (Vol. 38, February 2000, pp 105-112)

6

Studies on anticonvulsant actions of L-deprenyl

MANU GUPTA & S. K. KULKARNI
Pharmacology Division, University Institute of Pharmaceutical Sciences, Panjab University, Chandigarh, 160 014, India

L-Deprenyl (Selegeline) introduced for use in Parkinson's disease, is implicated to show beneficial effects in epilepsy, Alzheimer's disease, cognition, depression and other age related neurological diseases. In this study, we investigated the CNS effects of L-deprenyl with special reference to epilepsy, anxiety and cognition and memory in mice. L-deprenyl (10, 20 and 40 mg/kg) showed a significant anticonvulsant activity against pentylenetetrazole (PTZ)- induced convulsions. Combination of L-deprenyl (10 mg/kg) with the sub-protective dose of diazepam (1 mg/kg) showed potentiation of the anticonvulsant effect. In the maximal-electroshock (MES)- induced convulsions, L-deprenyl (10 mg/kg) significantly delayed the onset and decreased the duration of extensor phase. Its combination with the lower dose of phenytoin (10 mg/kg) showed potentiation in response compared to the *per se* effect of both the drugs. However, L-deprenyl did not show any protective effect in lithium-pilocarpine induced status epilepticus. Acute treatment with L-deprenyl had no effect on learning and memory. In chronic treatment, L-deprenyl *per se* showed no effect on learning and memory but did improve the condition in mice with scopolamine induced memory deficit. L-Deprenyl *per se* was anxiogenic though in combination with diazepam (1 mg/kg) it potentiated the antianxiety effect of the latter. The above observations suggest that in epilepsy, L-deprenyl might be acting partially by influencing the $GABA_A$/benzodiazepine mechanism in the brain (similar to diazepam and phenytoin), and in cognition enhancing effect, the cholinergic system might be playing a role. Thus, L-deprenyl could prove to be an adjuvant in the antiepileptic therapy and beneficial in dementia associated with epilepsy.

L-Deprenyl (Selegiline), an irreversible inhibitor of MAO type B is being used in the therapy of Parkinson's disease (PD) since 1986 (ref. 1, 2). Besides inhibition of MAO type B, it also inhibits reuptake of dopamine and noradrenaline, increases the turnover of dopamine[3], enhances striatal enzymes, i.e., superoxide dismutase, catalase activity and is also involved in the detoxification of free radicals[1]. Stimulation of neurotropic factor synthesis and antagonistic modulation of polyamine binding site of N-methyl-D-aspartate (NMDA) -subtype of glutamate receptor by L-deprenyl has also been suggested [4].

Loscher and Honack were the first to report the anticonvulsant effect of L-deprenyl in kindled rats[5]. It also showed learning and memory improving effects in various cognitive test models in animals as well as in humans[6,7]. The aim of the present research was to study the protective effect of L-deprenyl in various animal models of epilepsy and memory deficit.

Materials and Methods

Animals– Laca mice of either sex weighing 20-25 g, bred in the Central Animal House facility of Panjab University were used in the present study. The animals were housed under standard laboratory conditions and were provided with food and water *ad libitum.*

Effect of L-deprenyl in chemical seizures– Acute administration of pentylenetetrazole (PTZ), 80 mg/kg, i.p. produced convulsions and death in control group of mice. Animals were observed for the onset of Straub's tail, jerks, clonic, tonic phase of convulsions and death/ recovery. Diazepam (1, 4 mg/kg, i.p.) was administered in two different groups, 30 min prior to PTZ challenge. In other groups of animals, L-deprenyl (10, 20, 40 mg/kg, i.p.) was given in different doses 30 min prior to PTZ. In combination studies, L-deprenyl (10 mg/kg) and the sub-effective dose of diazepam (1 mg/kg) were given to a group of mice, 30 min before PTZ challenge. All experimental groups consisted of 5-9 animals per treatment group. All experiments were carried out between 0900 and 1300 hrs.

Effect of L-deprenyl in electrical seizures– Application of electric-shock (50 mA for 0.2 sec) through corneal electrodes produced convulsions and death in the control group of mice. Phenytoin (10, 20 mg/kg, i.p.)

was administered in two different groups, 30 min prior to the electric-shock and the animals were observed for the onset and duration of tonic flexion, tonic extensor, clonus, stupor and death/recovery. In other group of animals, L-deprenyl (10, 20 mg/kg, i.p.) was given in different doses 30 min prior to the electric-shock and the animals were observed as for phenytoin groups. In combination studies, L-deprenyl (10 mg/kg) and the lower dose of phenytoin (10 mg/kg) were given to a group of mice, 30 min before the electric shock. All experimental groups consisted of 5-9 animals per treatment group. All administrations were done between 0900 and 1300 hrs, daily.

Effect of L-deprenyl in status epilepticus– Status epilepticus (SE) was induced in rats by Li (3 meq/kg, i.p.) followed 21 hr later by pilocarpine (30 mg/kg, s.c.), following which the animals were observed continuously for the occurrence of behavioral seizures. The animals were kept individually in plexiglas chambers (30 x 90 x 90 cm with partitions). The neuroprotective profile of L-deprenyl (10 mg/kg, i.p.) was studied by administering it 30 min prior to the pilocarpine challenge, subsequently the animals were observed for a period of 90 min to note the onset of forelimb clonus with rearing (FC+R). The mortality (if any) was observed for a period of 48 hrs. Both the experimental groups consisted of 7-9 animals.

Effect of acute treatment with L-deprenyl on learning and memory– To study the learning and retention of a learned task (short-term memory), a step-down (passive avoidance) task behavior paradigm was used.[8] The equipment consisted of an electric grid (24 x 30 cm), with a shock-free zone (SFZ) (2 x 3 x 1 cm) in the center and the electric grid having a perflex enclosure. Mice were put individually on the SFZ (a wooden block) and allowed to explore for about 1 min. Then the animal was placed on SFZ and the time it took to step onto the grid was noted. As soon as it stepped on the grid, an electric stimulus (20 V) was given for a fixed period of 80 sec. After 1 hour and 24 hrs of the first trial i.e. learning, each animal was again put individually on the SFZ and the latency in reaching the grid was recorded, in both, the control and the drug treated groups. Drug treated groups consisted that of physostigmine (a cholinergic nootropic), L-deprenyl, scopolamine (an anticholinergic amnesic drug), scopolamine plus physostigmine and scopolamine plus L-deprenyl. All experimental groups consisted of 5 animals per treatment group.

Physostigmine and L-deprenyl were administered just after training while scopolamine was administered 30 min after the training, so that the effect of physostigmine and L-deprenyl could be observed 1 hr after training, while that of scopolamine after 30 min of its injection.

Effect of chronic treatment with L-deprenyl on learning and memory– The equipment used was same as for acute effect on learning and memory. The animals were trained as for acute study. The experiments were done on three groups and one served as a control. Treatment groups consisted of L-deprenyl (10 mg/kg), scopolamine (0.3 mg/kg) and scopolamine plus L-deprenyl. L-deprenyl was given to group I just after training, scopolamine to group II 30 min after training while group III received L-deprenyl just after training followed 30 min by scopolamine. Same drugs were administered to respective animal groups once a day for 8 days at a gap of 24 hrs. Latency was noted on day one, 1 hr after the training and on days 2 and 8, 1 hr after L-deprenyl injection or 30 min after scopolamine injection.

Effect of L-deprenyl on anxiety– Anxiety was measured on elevated plus-maze, a model described and validated by Lister [9] and Sharma and Kulkarni [10] for mice.

L-deprenyl (10, 20 mg/kg, i.p.) and diazepam (1, 2 mg/kg, i.p.) were administered to different groups of animals, and 30 min later, the animals were tested on elevated plus-maze for acute effect. In combination studies, L-deprenyl (10 mg/kg, i.p.) and diazepam (1 mg/kg, i.p.) were administered to a group of animals and 30 min later, the animals were tested on elevated plus-maze for acute effect. Control animals were treated with normal saline. All experiments were done between 0900 and 1300 hrs, daily.

Drugs– The drugs used for pharmacological interventions were diazepam injection (Ranbaxy Laboratories Ltd., New Delhi), PTZ (Sigma Chemicals, St. Louis, USA), L-deprenyl (Chinoin, Budapest), phenytoin sodium injection (Cadila healthcare Pvt. Ltd., Ahmedabad, India), Lithium chloride (Merck, Germany), pilocarpine nitrate (Boehringer Ingelheim, Germany), scopolamine (Merck & Co. Inc., Rahway, USA), physostigmine hemisulfate (Sigma Chemical Co., USA). All the drugs were directly dissolved in freshly distilled water except for phenytoin injection which was first wetted in a drop or so of tween-80 and then suspended in distilled water. All the drugs were given intraperitoneally (i.p.) except for pilocarpine hemisulfate which was given subcutaneously (s.c.), in a constant volume of 1 ml/100 g of body weight for mice and 0.5 ml/ 100g of body weight for rats.

Statistical analysis– The non-parametric Mann-Whitney test was used to evaluate the statistical significance of the difference between the values of each group and that of the corresponding control group in chemical and electrical seizure test and in test for status epilepticus and $P < 0.05$ was considered statistically significant. For memory and anxiety tests, the data was presented as mean ± SE and analyzed using one way analysis of variance (ANOVA) followed by Dunnet's test and $P < 0.05$ was considered statistically significant.

Results

Evaluation of anticonvulsant activity in chemical seizures– L-Deprenyl (10, 20 and 40 mg/kg) showed a significant anticonvulsant activity against PTZ-induced convulsions as it delayed the onset of Straub's tail and jerks. Diazepam (4 mg/kg) offered complete protection against convulsions while a lower dose of diazepam (1 mg/kg) significantly delayed the onset of Straub's tail, jerks, clonic convulsions and complete abolition of the tonic extensor phase. The combination of subprotective doses of L-deprenyl (10 mg/kg) and diazepam (1 mg/kg) showed a significant potentiation of the anticonvulsant effect as the combination delayed the onset of jerks, clonic and tonic convulsions.

Evaluation of anticonvulsant activity in electrical seizures– L-Deprenyl (10 and 20 mg/kg) delayed the onset of extensor phase (the effect being nonsignificant) while L-deprenyl (10 mg/kg) significantly decreased the duration of extensor phase when compared to the control group. Phenytoin (20 mg/kg and not 10 mg/kg) showed a significant protection against the onset of extensor phase and its duration when compared to control animals. Combined administration of L-deprenyl (10 mg/kg) and phenytoin (10 mg/kg) showed a significant delay in the onset of extensor phase as well as decrease in its duration as compared to the *per se* effect of both the drugs (Fig. 1).

Evaluation of anticonvulsant activity in status epilepticus– Consecutive treatment with L-deprenyl did not affect the time of onset of forelimb clonus and rearing (FC + R) and its duration due to the administration of lithium and pilocarpine, statistically. Also, it did not affect the mortality rate by lithium and pilocarpine.

Acute effect of L-deprenyl on learning and memory– Scopolamine, *per se,* significantly decreased the latency while physostigmine significantly increased the latency to reach the grid compared to the control animals. L-Deprenyl did not significantly affect the latency. In scopolamine treated animals, L-deprenyl did not significantly affect the latency 1 hr after its administration as compared to scopolamine treated animals. However, physostigmine significantly increased the latency after 1 hour of training in scopolamine treated mice (Fig 2). After 24 hr of training, none of the five drug treated animal groups showed any significant difference in latency (Fig. 3).

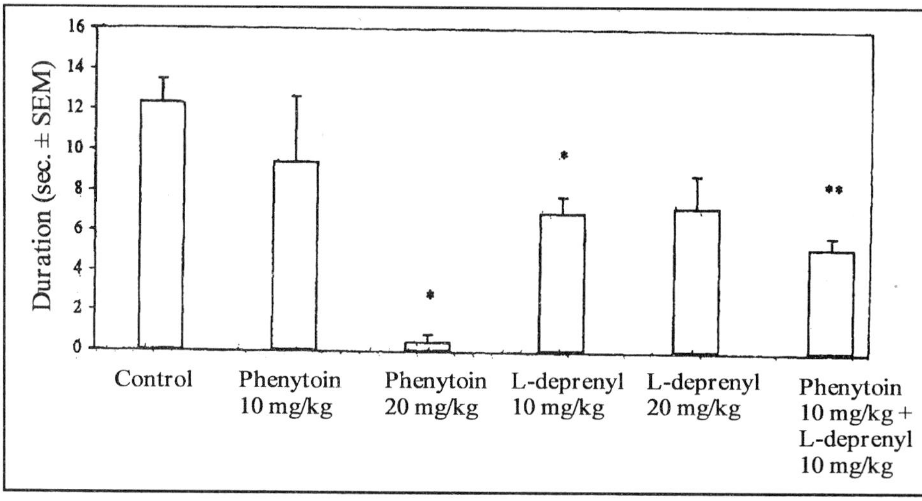

Fig 1. Effect of various drugs on the duration of tonic extensor phase in MES-induced convulsions in mice. Values are mean ± SE. * P < 0.05 compared to control, ** P < 0.05 compared to L-deprenyl (10 mg/kg) and phenytoin (10 mg/kg).

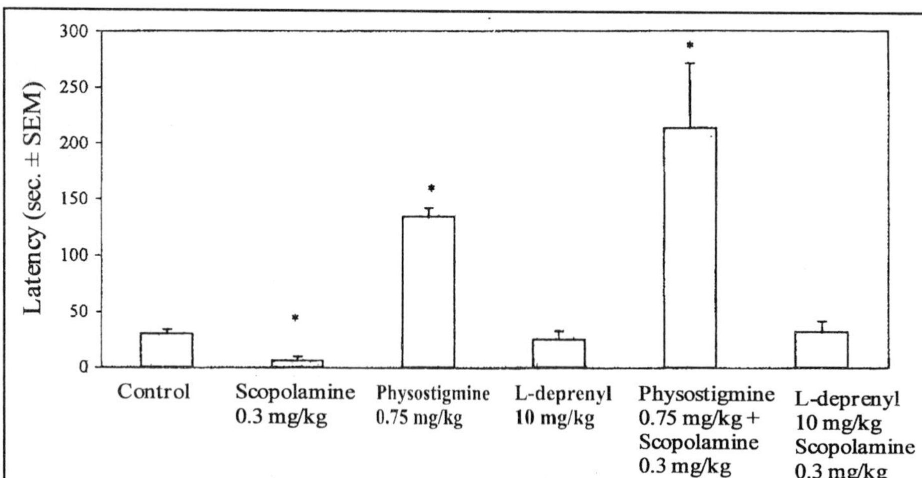

Fig 2. Effect of acute treatment with various drugs on learning (tested 1 hr after training) in mice. Values are mean ± SE. * P < 0.05 compared to control value.

Effect of chronic treatment of L-deprenyl on learning and memory- Scopolamine (0.3 mg/kg) produced a significant memory deficit in mice on days 1, 2 and 8 as compared to control animals. Compared to control animals, L-deprenyl (10 mg/kg) *per se* did not show a significant effect on latency on day 1, 2 and 8. When given concurrently with scopolamine, L-deprenyl did not show any significant increase in latency compared to scopolamine treated animals on day 1 and 2. However, on day 8, there was a significant increase in latency of mice to step onto the grid (Fig 4).

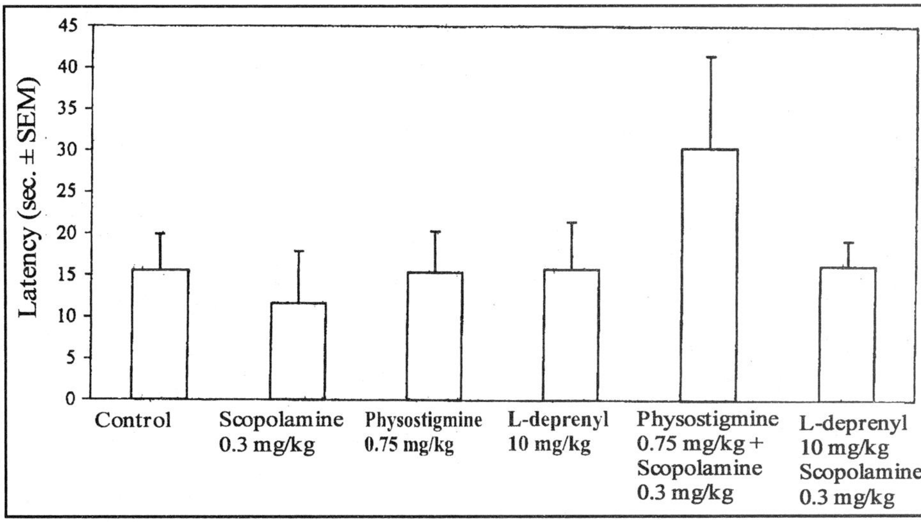

Fig. 3. Effect of acute treatment with various drugs on memory paradigm (tested 24 hr after training) in mice. Values are mean ± SE. No significant difference was observed between different groups

Effect of L-deprenyl treatment on anxiety response- In the control group, the percentage preference of mice for the open arm was 40%. In L-deprenyl (10, 20 mg/kg) treated group, it was 0%. In diazepam (2 mg/kg) group, it was 60% while in diazepam (1 mg/kg) group, it was 0%. Combination of L-deprenyl (10 mg/kg) and diazepam (1 mg/kg) increased the percentage preference for the open arm to 40%.

Diazepam (2 mg/kg) significantly increased the mean total number of entries and the mean total time spent by mice in the open arm of the maze while L-deprenyl (10, 20 mg/kg) and diazepam (1 mg/kg) did not affect both the parameters, significantly. Combination of L-deprenyl (10 mg/kg) and diazepam (1 mg/kg) did not significantly affect the number of entries in the open arm as compared to control or the *per se* effect of either L-deprenyl (10 mg/kg) or diazepam (1 mg/kg) but significantly increased the mean total time spent in the open arm compared to the *per se* effects of both the drugs.

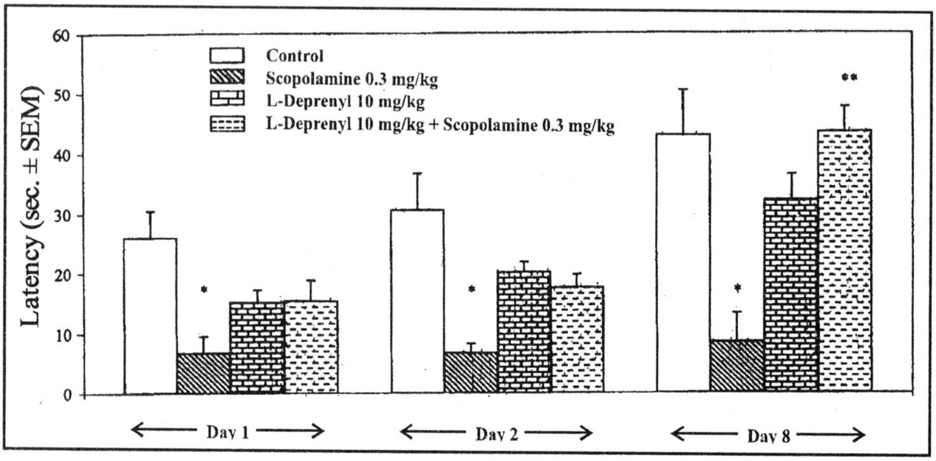

Fig. 4. Effect of L-deprenyl on scopolamine-induced memory deficit in mice when tested on days 1, 2 and 8, respectively. Values are mean ± SE. * $P < 0.05$ compared to control. ** $P < 0.05$ compared to scopolamine (0.3 mg/kg) *per se.*

Discussion

In the present study, L-deprenyl exhibited anticonvulsant effect at all the doses studied as it blocked the appearance or delayed the onset of Straub's tail and jerks. However, the onset of clonic convulsions or tonic extensor phase was not significantly delayed due to wide variation in responses of animals within the groups. When L-Deprenyl was administered with a sub-effective dose of diazepam, it potentiated the anticonvulsant effect. The previous studies have reported controversial results. While Loscher and Lehmann[11] found L-deprenyl (1, 2.5 and 5 mg/kg) to significantly increase the myoclonic and clonic convulsive thresholds due to PTZ 30 min after its administration, Hoffman *et al.*[12] found repeated treatment and not the single dose treatment with L-deprenyl to affect the PTZ-induced convulsions. Similarly, in MES-convulsions, L-deprenyl (10 mg/kg and not 20 mg/kg) pretreatment showed a significant anticonvulsant profile. Co-administration of lower dose of L-deprenyl with phenytoin (10 mg/kg) showed advantage over the *per se* effect of both the drugs. Thus, L-deprenyl *per se* or its combination with phenytoin exhibited a potent anticonvulsant activity.

Although, till now, there are no reports of any pathophysiological significance of MAO-B in epilepsy, the finding of anticonvulsant activity of L-deprenyl (MAO-B inhibitor) suggests that the role of MAO-B in epilepsy should be investigated in more detail. Recently, Loscher *et al*[13] have proposed that L-deprenyl also inhibits MAO-A at a higher dose (>10 mg/kg) and it is this inhibition of MAO-A which is responsible for the anticonvulsant effect and not the inhibition of MAO-B mechanism. Hoffman *et al* proposed the mechanism for this effect of L-deprenyl not to be associated with dopaminergic or cholinergic mechanism.

Effect of L-deprenyl on lithium-pilocarpine induced convulsions was studied to determine its protective effect in SE and its mechanism of action. Since L-deprenyl did not affect the onset of FC + R or its duration, it suggests that when given as a single dose, it does not protect the animals against SE. This is supported by a report from Hoffman *et al.*[12] who showed that the mechanism for the anticonvulsant effect of L-deprenyl is not related to the changes in acetylcholine levels since prolonged treatment with L-deprenyl did not attenuate the brain sensitivity to pilocarpine-induced seizures. However, in another experiment, chronic treatment with L-deprenyl could improve the scopolamine-induced deficit in learning and memory i.e. by acting through cholinergic mechanism. So, the effect of chronic treatment with L-deprenyl on SE should be determined as the chronic treatment may build up the concentration of acetylcholine in the CNS that might show protective effect.

Inhibition of cholinergic neurotransmission plays a predominant role in dementia. Scopolamine, a cholinergic muscarinic receptor antagonist is known to produce short term amnesia in humans and animals. In the present study, acute administration of deprenyl *per se* did not affect acquisition or memory nor did it modify scopolamine-induced memory deficit. In the chronic 8-day treatment schedule, scopolamine produced a significant decrease in acquisition and retention on day 1, 2 and 8. L-deprenyl did not affect learning and memory on day 1 and 2 but significantly improved memory on day 8 in scopolamine treated animals. This is in agreement with the previous reports[14,15.] Thus, chronic treatment and not the acute treatment with L-deprenyl improved the memory in scopolamine-induced memory deficit. The data suggest that L-deprenyl may have beneficial effect in epilepsy as an adjuvant therapy with major anticonvulsants and it possessed cognitive enhancement abilities. Though the exact mechanism is far from clear, L-deprenyl might be modulating cholinergic activity in the brain.

L-deprenyl, tested at both the doses showed an anxiogenic effect as it decreased the percent preference of animals for the open arm from 40% (in controls) to 0%. However, the combination of L-deprenyl and diazepam (both at lower doses) was anxiolytic as compared to the *per se* effects of both the drugs. It may be concluded that L-deprenyl (10 mg/kg and 20 mg/kg) *per se,* increased the anxiety in animals. This effect could be because of the metabolites of L-deprenyl i.e. amphetamine and methamphetamine, which may cause anxiety, insomnia, and other adverse symptoms[16]. When in combination with diazepam (1 mg/kg), it enhanced its antianxiety effect. A direct mechanism could not be proposed from these studies, however, it seems that deprenyl facilitated the antianxiety effect of diazepam through its central action.

REFERENCES

1. Knoll, J. The pharmacological profile of (-)-deprenyl (selegiline) and its relevence for humans. A personal view. *Pharmacol Toxicol,* 70 (1992) 317.
2. Wessel, K & Szelenyl, I. Selegiline- an overview of its role in the treatment of Parkinson's disease. *Clin Invest,* 70 (1992) 459.
3. Heinonen, E H & Lammintausta, R. A review of pharmacology of selegiline. *Acta Neurol Scand,* 84 (1991) 44.
4. Gerlach, M, Youdim, M B H & Riederer, P. Is selegiline neuroprotective in Parkinson's disease? *J Neural Trans,* 41:Suppl (1994) 177.
5. Loscher, W & Honack, D, Anticonvulsant effect of L-deprenyl (selegiline) in the kindling model of epilepsy. *J Pharmacol Exp Ther,* 274 (1995) 307.
6. Brandeis, R, Sapir, M, Kapon, Y, Borelli, G, Cadel, S & Valsecchi, B. Improvement of cognitive function by MAO-B inhibitor L-deprenyl in aged rats. *Pharmacol Biochem Behav,* 39 (1991) 297.
7. Head, E, Hartley, J, Kameka, A M, Mehta, R, Ivy, G O, Ruehl, W W & Milgram, N W. The effect of L-deprenyl on spatial long term memory in young and aged dogs. *Prog Neuropsychopharmacol Biol Psychiatry,* 20 (1996) 515.
8. Sharma, A C & Kulkarni, S K. Evidence for GABA-BZ receptor modulation in short-term memory passive avoidance task paradigm in mice. *Meth Find Exp Clin Pharmacol,* 12 (1990) 175.
9. Lister, R G. The amnesic action of benzodiazepines in man. *Neurosci Biobehav Rev,* 9 (1985) 87.

10. Sharma, A C & Kulkarni, S K. MK-801 produces anti-anxiety effect in elevated plus-maze in mice. *Drug Dev Res,* 22 (1991) 251.

11. Loscher, W & Lehmann, H. L-deprenyl (selegiline) exerts anticonvulsant effects against different seizure types in mice. *J Pharmacol Exp Ther,* 277 (1996) 1410.

12. Hoffman, A, Afargan, M, Backon, J & Pearlstein, I. The anticonvulsant effect of deprenyl on pentylenetetrazole-induced seizure in lewis rats. *Int J Neurosci,* 90 (1997) 223.

13. Loscher, W, Lehmann, H, Teschendorf, H J, Trant, M & Gross, G. Inhibition of monoamine oxidase type A, but not type B, is an effective means of inducing anticonvulsant activity in the kindling model of epilepsy. *J Pharmacol Exp Ther,* 288 (1999) 984.

14. Finali, G, Piccirilli, M, Oliani, C & Piccinin, G L. Alzheimer's-type dementia and verbal memory performance: influence of selegiline therapy. *Ital J Neurol Sci,* 13 (1992) 141.

15. Lawlor, B A, Aisen, P S, Green, C, Fine, E & Scheidler, J. Selegiline in the treatment of behavioural disturbance in Alzheimer's disease. *Int J Geriatr Psychiatry,* 12 (1997) 319.

16. Standaert, D G & Young, B A. Treatment of Central Nervous System Degenerative Disorders : *in: Goodman & Gilman's: The Pharmacological Basis of Therapeutics.* (McGraw Hill, New York.) 1996, 503.

Paper Published In:
I.J.E.B. (Vol. 38, April 2000, pp. 332-337)

7

Pentylenetetrazol-induced kindling in animals: Protective effect of BR-16A

S.K. KULKARNI & B. GEORGE
Pharmacology Division, University Institute of Pharmaceutical Sciences,
Panjab University, Chandigarh 160 014, India

Repeated administration of pentylenetetrazol (PTZ, 30 mg/kg, thrice a week) to mice for 9 weeks and subsequent challenge of the animals with the same dose of PTZ on the last chronic dose produced chemical kindling. The mice showed myoclonic jerks, clonus, Straub's tail, falling back response and full blown convulsions. The anticonvulsant profile of chronic administration of BR-16A (100 and 500 mg/kg) was studied in this model of epilepsy. BR- 16A offered protection against PTZ-induced chemical kindling. The percent animals showing myoclonic jerks and clonus was reduced to 40 and 34 with 100 mg/kg and 54 and 27 with 500 mg/kg of BR-16A, respectively. The protective effect was compared with diazepam (1 mg/kg, ip). The results demonstrated $GABA_A$ receptor mediated PTZ-induced kindling and protective effect of BR-16A therein.

Kindling is a model of epilepsy and epileptogenesis. Kindled seizures in animals after daily electrical stimulation of the amygdaloid complex through low-intensity electric current have been described[1]. Repeated application of subconvulsive doses of CNS stimulants like pentylenetetrazol (PTZ)[2], cocaine[3], picrotoxin[4], strychnine[5] and bicuculline[6] once every 24 or 48 hr over a period of time is also known to induce a permanent change in the epileptogenic sensitivity of forebrain structures, such that initially subconvulsive stimuli become capable of evoking fully developed seizures. PTZ-induced kindling is related to the down regulation of $GABA_A$-ergic transmission in the CNS. PTZ is reported to inhibit $GABA_A$-induced chloride conductance in cultured mouse spinal-cord neurons[7], and also ^{35}[S]TBPS binding in rat brain homogenates in a concentration-dependent manner[8].

BR-16A, a herbal psychotropic preparation contains various ingredients reputed in the ancient system of Ayurvedic medicine to be useful in the management of nervous disorders. These include: brahmi *(Hydrocotyl asiatica)*, shatavari *(Asparagus racemosus)*, buchh *(Acorus calamus)*, jatamansi *(Nardostachys jatamansi)*, ashwagandha *(Withania somnifera)*, shankpushpi *(Evolvulus alsinoides)*, kuth *(Sausurea lappa)* and triphala *(Terminalia chebula)*[9]. Some of the CNS activities of BR-16A have been related to its modulatory action on $GABA_A$-ergic transmission[10]. BR-16A has been recently tried as an adjuvant to the commonly used antiepileptic drugs in clinical trials and was found to significantly reduce seizure frequency (personal communication, from Himalaya Drug Co). In the present study therefore, an attempt has been made to study the protective effect of BR-16A in a laboratory model of epilepsy, i.e., PTZ-induced kindling in mice.

Materials and Methods

Animals– Laka mice of either sex, weighing between 20 and 25 g, (bred in the Central Animal House facility of the Panjab University), were used. Animals were housed under standard laboratory conditions and were supplied with food and water *ad libitum*. The animals were maintained at 12 hr day/night cycle and all experiments were carried out between 0900 and 1700 hrs.

Chemical kindling in mice– Pentylenetetrazol (PTZ) was given in a subconvulsive dose of 30 mg/kg, ip, thrice a week for 9 weeks in control mice. After each injection of PTZ, occurrence of CNS excitation was noted over 10-15 min by observing the mice in a plexiglass chamber (30 x 24 x 22 cm) with partitions in between. The intensity of behavioural seizures was evaluated using a six point scoring system: 0 =no effect; 1=jerks; 2 = Straub's tail; 3 =clonus. The degree of behavioural response increased progressively over the weeks until the animals exhibited full motor seizures. Cumulative kindling score (calculated by taking the average of all the individual behavioural scores and then dividing them with the number of subjects) was plotted against duration of treatment.

These chronically-treated mice were then challenged with the same subconvulsive dose of PTZ (30 mg/kg, ip) on the 3rd and 10th day of the last chronic dose. These mice showed different phases of CNS excitation and convulsions, which were recorded. The onset, and the percentage of animals showing jerks and clonus were also recorded.

In order to study the involvement of GABA/benzodiazepine receptors in PTZ-induced kindling, on the 3rd day after the last chronic dose a group of these animals were challenged with FG-7142 (20 mg/kg, ip), an inverse agonist of BZ-receptor, given 30 min prior to PTZ (30 mg/kg, ip). Cumulative kindling score was compared with the control group. Separate groups of mice were pretreated with BR-16A (100 and 500 mg/kg, po), given 30 min prior to chronic treatment with PTZ for 9 weeks. Behavioural seizure were scored as described earlier. These chronically pretreated animals were again challenged with PTZ (30 mg/kg) on the 3rd and 10th day of the last PTZ challenge dose.

Drugs– Pentylenetrazol (PTZ) - Sigma Chemicals, St. Louis, USA; diazepam - Ranbaxy, New Delhi; and FG-7142 - Schering, Germany were used. BR-16A (Mentat)[R] was a gift from Himalaya Drug Company, Bangalore.

Statistical analysis– The kindling scores expressed as the arithmetic mean ±SD were analysed by Student's *t* test (independent). One way analysis of variance (ANOVA) was performed on the cumulative kindling score at (i) different weeks of treatment (3rd, 6th, and 9th week), and (ii) the last day of 9th week, and the 3rd and 10th days after the last challenge dose. Posthoc comparisons were made using Duncan's new multiple range test. Probability levels < 5% were considered significant.

Results

PTZ-induced kindling in mice– PTZ (30 mg/kg ip thrice a week) when given for 9 weeks produced different phases of CNS excitation and convulsions. These episodes included Straub's tail, jerks, clonus, and circling. When these chronically treated animals were further challenged with the same subconvulsive dose of PTZ on the 3rd and 10th day of the last chronic dose (9 weeks), they exhibited frank convulsions (jerks, clonus, extensor and falling back) (Figs 1-3). The percent animals showing jerks and clonus were 100 and 64.3, respectively on both 3rd and 10th day of challenge (Tables 1 and 2). These kindled eflects were blocked by diazepam (1 mg/kg, ip) when given prior to PTZ challenge (Figs 1-3).

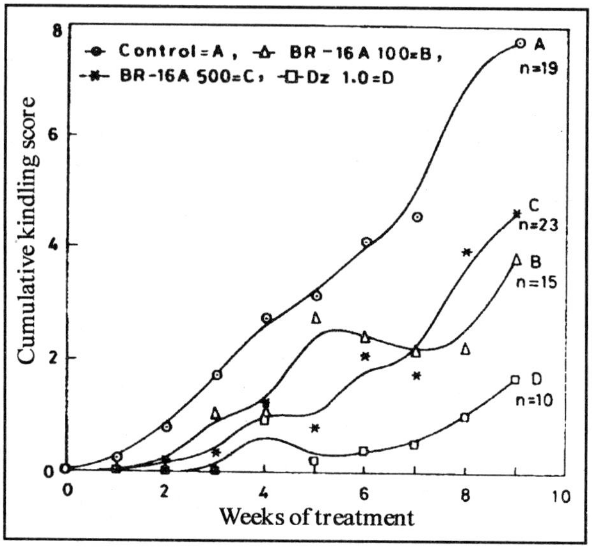

Fig. 1. Modification of PTZ-induced kindling in mice (as observed during 9 weeks of treatment) by BR-16A and diazepam. [During 3rd week: F(3,63) = 4.27. (P < 0.05). At 5% level, (A and C), (A and D) are statistically significant. During 6th week: F (3, 63) = 6.36, (P < 0.05). At 5% level, (A and C), (A and D) are statistically significant. During 9th week: F(3,63) = 3.12, (P < 0.05)]

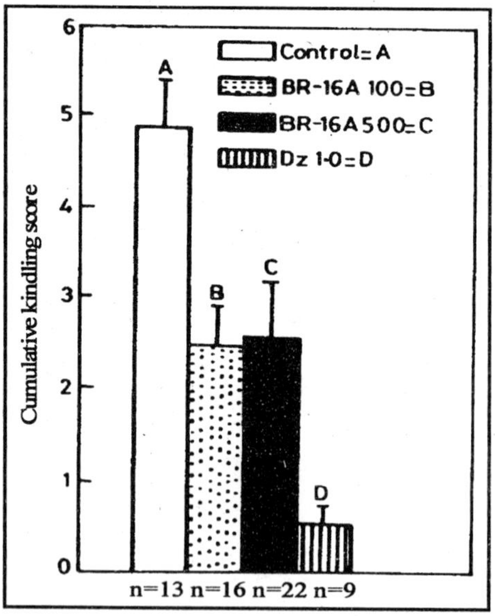

Fig. 2. Protective effect of BR-16A and diazepam on PTZ-induced kindling (cumulative kindling score) on the 3rd day after the last chronic dose. [F(4,41) = 17.76, (P < 0.05). At 5% level, (A and C), (A and D), (C and D) are statistically significant]

Pretreatment of BR-16A on PTZ induced kindling in mice– BR-16A (100 and 500 mg/kg, po) was given 30 min prior to each (chronic) treatment with PTZ for 9 weeks. These animals showed a milder degree of CNS excitation all throughout 9 weeks as compared to control group which received only PTZ (Fig. 1). Further, these BR-16A pretreated animals, when challenged with PTZ (30 mg/kg) on the 3rd and 10th day of the last challenge dose of PTZ, showed a significant attenuation of seizures to PTZ (Fig. 3). The percentage of animals showing jerks and clonus was decreased to 40 and 33 for the 100 mg/kg dose, and 54 and 27 for the 500 mg/kg dose, respectively, on the 3rd day of challenge (Table 1). Similarly, on the 10th day, it was reduced to 53 and 7 for 100 mg/kg and 57 and 21 for 500 mg/kg dose of BR-16A, respectively (Table 2).

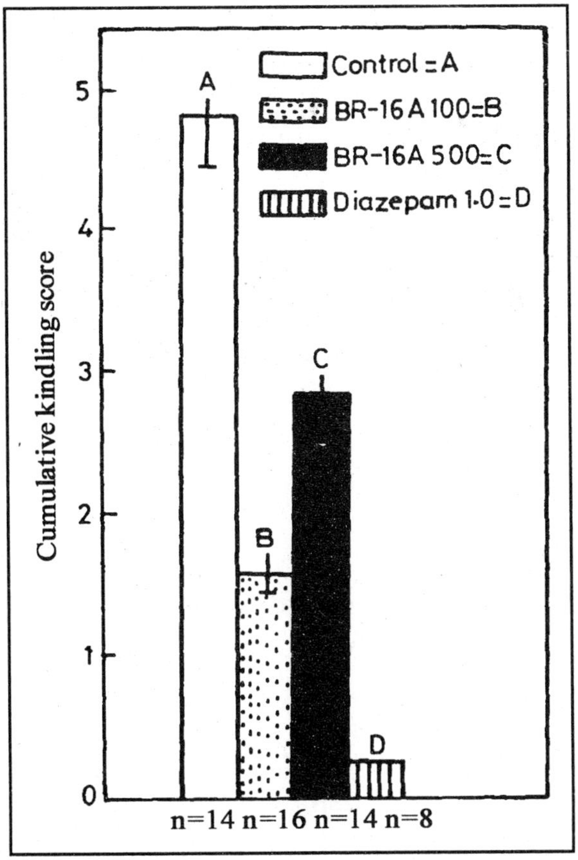

Fig. 3. Protective effect of BR-16A and diazepam on PTZ-induced kindling (cumulative kindling score) on the 10th day after the last chronic dose. [F(3,38)=14.16, (P<0.05). At 5% level, (A and D) is statistically significant]

Discussion

The kindling phenomenon described by Goddard[1] is now generally accepted as an experimental model of epilepsy and epileptogenesis. In kindling, repeated administration of an initially subconvulsive stimulus causes a progressive intensification of seizure activity leading to a distinct generalized seizure[11]. Kindled seizures have been induced in rats, cats, monkeys, dogs, rabbits and frogs[1,12-16].

The CNS stimulant and convulsant actions of PTZ are reported to be mediated through specific interaction with $GABA_A$-gated chloride ionosphore. PTZ inhibited the binding of [^{35}S]-TBPS in rat brain homogenates in a concentration dependent manner[17,18]. It also inhibited GABA-induced chloride conductance in functional assays in cultured spinal cord neurons[7].

Table 1- Protective effect of BR-16A on PTZ-induced kindling in mice, on 3rd day of last PTZ challenge dose [Values expressed in sec are mean ±SD. Figures in parentheses are no. of mice, out of total used in that particular treatment, showing jerks/clonus]

Treatment (mg/kg)	N	Onset		Severity of clonus
		Jerks	Clonus	
Control PTZ	14	173.1 ± 100.91	331.2 ± 95.4	+ +
30 ip		(14)	(9)	
FG-7142	3	130 ± 17.32	485.5 ± 495.68	+ +
20 ip		(3)	(2)	
BR-16A	15	210.4 ± 80.53	422.0 ± 238.36	+
100 po		(6)	(5)	
BR-16A	22	222.9±35.95	259.2 ± 59.47	+
500 po		(12)	(6)	
Diazepam	9	435	-	-
1 ip		(I)		

Time of onset was taken as the time when the animal first starts showing jerks/ clonus.

The role of GABA receptors in kindling is further substantiated by the observation that FG-7142, a beta-carboline potentiated the convulsive response of subconvulsive dose of PTZ. Repeated administration of this negative ligand of benzodiazepine receptor is known to produce generalized seizures in rats and mice[19]. Concurrent administration of diazepam inhibited PTZ-induced kindling. Moreover, Ro15-1788, a benzodiazepine receptor antagonist when given concurrently with FG-7142 prevented kindling[20]. suggesting that the

Table 2. Protective effect of BR-16A on PTZ-induced kindling in mice, on 10th day of last PTZ challenge dose

[Values expressed in sec are mean ± SD. Figures in parentheses are no. of mice, out total used in that particular treatment, showing jerks/clonus]

Treatment (mg/kg)	N	Onset		Severity of clonus
		Jerks	Clonus	
Control PTZ	14	194.1 ± 96.68	324.8 ± 177.84	+ +
30 ip		(14)	(9)	
BR-16A	15	295.6 ± 122.18	275	+
100 po		(8)	(1)	
BR-16A	14	235.3 ± 47.71	266.7 ± 20.19	+
500 po		(8)	(3)	
Diazepam	8	–	–	–
1 ip				

Details are same as in Table 1.

beta-carboline-induced kindling is mediated by the benzodiazepine-receptors[21]. The inverse agonist FG-7142 (20 mg/kg, ip) potentiated the convulsive response of subconvulsive dose of PTZ as these animals showed quick onset of jerks.

BR-16A, a herbal psychotropic preparation contains besides many other indigenous ingredients, Brahmi *(Hydrocotyl asiatica)* and Aswagandha *(W. somnifera)*. In Ayurvedic medicine, Brahmi has been extensively used in insanity and epilepsy[22]. The extract of Brahmi has also been found to enhance pentobarbitone-induced sleep time and protect animals from maximal electroshock seizures[23]. The methanolic extract of the roots of *W. somnifera* has been shown to potentiate pentobarbitone-induced narcosis and increase PTZ-induced seizure latency following chronic administration[24]. Pretreatment with BR-16A offered a significant protection both during the development of kindling and also once kindling was established in these animals. The protection against kindling-induced epilepsy draws further support from the observation that BR-16A reversed ethanol withdrawal-induced anxiety and the proconvulsive action of PTZ in rats and mice[25], a behavioural phenomenon known to involve GABA/BZ receptors[26]. In this study nonconvulsive doses of PTZ were able to produce full blown convulsions and increased mortality in ethanol withdrawn animals, a phenomenon known to involve $GABA_A$-ergic mechanism and susceptible to blockade by both acute and chronic treatment of BR-16A.

The present study demonstrated that PTZ-induced chemical kindling is a reliable and reproducible model of chronic epilepsy, the phenomenon being demonstrable for several weeks. Further, a decreased $GABA_A$-ergic tone caused by PTZ is responsible for the epileptogenesis. Chronic treatment with BR-16A offered a significant protection against PTZ-induced kindling. The preparation, may find an useful application as an adjunct in the management of epilepsy.

Acknowledgement

The study was supported by the financial grants of Himalaya Drug Co., Bangalore.

REFERENCES

1. Goddard G V, *Nature,* 214 (1967) 1020.
2. Corda M G, Orlandi M, Lecca D & Giorgi O, *J Pharmacol Exp Ther,* 262 (1992) 792.
3. Post R M & Rose H. *Nature,* 261 (1976) 731.
4. Roberts E, Kuriyama K & Halter B, *Advances in biochemical psychopharmacol,* (Raven Press, New York) 1970, 131.
5. Silvestrini B & Longo V G, *Arch Intern Pharmacodynamie,* 119 (1959) 359.
6. Drugan R C, McIntyre T D, Alpern H P & Maier S F, *Brain Res,* 34 (1985) 9.
7. De Deyn P P & Macdonald R L, *Epilepsia,* 30 (1989) 17.
8. Kulkarni S K, Sharma A, Verma A & Ticku M K, *Indian Drugs,* 30 (1993) 305.
9. Iyengar M A, in *Study of crude drugs,* edited by M A Iyengar (Manipal Power Press, India) 1991.
10. Kulkarni S K & Verma A, *Indian J Physiol Pharmacol,* 36 (1992) 29.
11. McNamara J O, Byrne M C, Dasheiff R M & Fitz J G, *Prog Neurophysiol,* 15 (1980) 139.
12. Goddard G V, McIntyre D & Leech C, *Exp Neurol,* 25 (1969) 295.
13. Wada J A & Sato M, *Neurology,* 24 (1974) 565.
14. Morrell F & Tsuru N, *Electroencephalogr Clin Neurophysiol,* 40 (1976) 1.
15. Stach R, Lazarova M & Kacz D, *Acta Neurobiol Exp,* 38 (1978) 227.
16. Wauquier A, Ashton D & Melis W, *Exp Neurol,* 64 (1979) 579.
17. Corda M S, Giorgi O, Longoni M & Biggio G, *J Neurochem,* 55 (1990) 1216.

18. Ramanjaneyulu R & Ticku M K, *Eur J Pharmacol,* 98 (1984) 337.

19. Stephens D N, Turski L A, Turner J D & Schneider H H, *Br J Pharmacol,* 101 (1990) Suppl, 837p.

20. Little H J, Nutt D J & Taylor S C, *Br J Pharmacol,* 83 (1984) 951.

21. Morin A M. *Brain Res,* 321 (1984) 151.

22. Chopra R N, Nayar S L & Chopra I C, *Glossary of Indian medicinal plants,* (CSIR, New Delhi) 1956, 217.

23. Sakina M R & Dandiya P C. *Fitoterapia,* 61 (1990) 291.

24. Prabhu M Y, Rao A & Karanth K S, *Fitoterapia,* 61 (1991) 237-240.

25. Kulkarni S K & Verma A. *Indian J Exp Biol,* 31 (1993) 435.

26. Ticku M K, Mehta A K, Mhatre M & Kulkarni S K, in *GABA-benzodizepine receptors: Chloride channels,* edited by R A Deitrich and A A Pawlowski (NIAAA Research Monograph-20, Bethseda, USA) 1990, 401.

Paper Published In:
I.J.E.B. (Vol. 33, June 1995, pp. 424-427)

8

Altered response to GABAergic agents following electro and chemo convulsions in mice

K.O. ALEY & S.K. KULKARNI
Pharmacology Division, Department of Pharmaceutical Sciences,
Panjab University, Chandigarh, 160 014, India

Effects of GABAergic agents and that of electroconvulsive shock (ECS) treatment were studied on bicuculline and picrotoxin (PTX)-induced convulsions in mice. Neither acute nor chronic ECS had any significant effect on bicuculline-induced convulsions, whereas the latency for PTX-induced convulsions was delayed by both acute and chronic ECS. Baclofen treatment delayed significantly the latency for PTX-induced convulsions in animals which were subjected to both acute and chronic ECS, whereas in bicuculline-induced convulsions, it shortened the latency of convulsions 24 hr after acute ECS. Progabide delayed the bicuculline-induced convulsions except in the case of 24 hr after acute ECS and PTX-induced convulsions except in the case of animals treated chronically with ECS. Fengabine showed no significant effect on bicuculline-induced convulsions. However, on PTX-induced convulsions, the latency was delayed in animals not subjected to ECS and in those subjected to chronic ECS. The possible explanations for the alterations in the effect of GABAergic agents following electro and chemo convulsions are (i) differences in the nature of antagonism by bicuculline and PTX, (ii) alterations in receptor sensitivity or number, and (iii) alterations in the levels of endogenous neurotransmitters, the latter two resulting as a result of acute or chronic ECS.

ECS (Electroconvulsive shock) treatment has been extensively employed for many years to treat psychiatric illness. But the mechanism of its action is still unknown. Reports on the effects of ECS on biogenic amines in the brain are contradictory both after single and multiple shocks in rats[1]. Repeated but not single ECS is shown to cause (1) an enhancement in catecholaminergic postsynaptic activity[2], (ii) an inhibition of potassium evoked release of 5-hydroxytryptamine (5-HT) and norepinephrine (NE) from cortical slices[3], (iii) an increase in postsynaptic 5-HT_2 receptor number[4], (iv) an increase in gamma aminobutyric acid (GABA) content in several brain regions[3], and (v) an alteration in $GABA_B$ receptor function in mouse frontal cortex[5,6].

A sudden decrease in abnormally elevated levels of GABA is shown to generate epileptogenic processes[7]. Further, change in $GABA_B$ receptor function is shown to alter 5-HT mediated behaviour in rats[8]. Clonidine, an $alpha_2$ agonist and fengabine a GABA agonist are shown to have anticonvulsant activity[9,10]. Yohimbine, an $alpha_2$ antagonist is demonstrated to block the anticonvulsant action of intranigral muscimol[11]. In the present study, alterations in the effect of GABAergic agents after acute and/or chronic ECS have been investigated. Also the effect of acute and/or chronic ECS on the convulsant and anticonvulsant effects of GABAergic agents has been studied with a view to assess the alteration in receptor sensitivity due to ECS treatment.

Materials and Methods

Animals: Male Wistar albino mice (25-30 g) obtained from Panjab University Central Animal House Facility, Chandigarh were maintained at diurnal conditions with free access to food and water. All experiments were carried out between 10.00 and 14.00 hrs.

Experimental design: Animals were divided into 8 main groups of minimum of 18-24 animals each. Groups 1 and 2 served as control groups and had four (a,b,c, and d) subgroups. Animals in subgroup(a) received a single ECS and 30 min after this they were challenged with convulsive doses of bicuculline or PTX. Animals in subgroup (b) were given a single ECS, 24 hr after which they were challenged with convulsive doses of bicuculline or PTX. Animals in subgroup (c) were exposed to chronic ECS, once daily for 7 days and 30 min after the last (7th) ECS they were challenged with bicuculline or PTX. Animals in subgroup (d) were challenged with bicuculline or PTX without prior ECS treatment (but sham treated). Animals in the main groups 3-8 served as the test groups. Each of them had three subgroups (a,b, and c). Animals in each of these subgroups were treated with ECS in a similar manner as in the case of the control groups, but 30 min prior to the administration of bicuculline or PTX, they were treated with the respective test drugs. In all these, the parameter observed was the latency of convulsions.

ECS: Animals were given ECS treatment by passing a constant current of 48 mA (Techno Convulsometer) for 0.2 sec via saline wetted corneal electrodes. In chronic ECS study, animals were exposed to ECS once a day for seven consecutive days at an interval of 24 hr.

Drugs: Bicuculline methiodide (Sigma, St Louis, MO, USA), picrotoxin (BDH, Poole, Dorset, England), baclofen (Ciba-Geigy, Basel, Switzerland), fengabine and progabide (L.E.R.S.. Paris) were used. Fengabine and progabide were suspended with the help of tween 80 and diluted with deionised water. All the other drugs were dissolved in deionised water. All the drugs were administered (ip) at a constant volume of 1ml/100g body weight of the animals. The doses of the drugs were chosen based on the previous work done in our laboratory.

Data were analysed employing Student's t test with $P < 0.05$ as the level of significance.

Results

Effect of ECS/GABAergic agents on bicuculline-induced convulsions in mice: Bicuculline (4 mg/kg) produced tonic clonic convulsions leading to 100% mortality. The latency of convulsion was 3.0±0.2 min. Acute or chronic ECS did not produce any significant effect on the latency of bicuculline-induced convulsions. Baclofen (5 mg/kg) reduced the latency 24 hr after acute ECS. Progabide (100 mg/kg) significantly delayed the latency of convulsions regardless of whether the animals were subjected to prior ECS treatment or not except in the case of 24 hr after acute ECS. Fengabine (80 mg/kg), had no significant effect on bicuculline-induced convulsions whether the animals were subjected to prior ECS treatment or not (Table 1).

Effect of ECS/GABAergic agents on PTX-induced convulsions in mice: PTX (6 mg/kg) produced tonic clonic convulsions in 100% of the animals with 56% mortality. This mean latency for convulsion was 9.4±0.8 min. The period was increased significantly after chronic treatment with ECS. Baclofen significantly delayed the latency of convulsions in animals subjected to both acute and chronic ECS. Progabide delayed the latency of convulsions in all cases except in the case of animals chronically treated with ECS. Fengabine delayed the latency of convulsions in animals subjected to chronic ECS and those not treated with ECS (Table 2).

Discussion

Acute ECS is shown to result in potassium-evoked release of endogenous NE, 5-HT and an inhibition of endogenous GABA release[3]. But chronic ECS is shown to increase catecholamine postsynaptic activity[2], inhibit 5-HT and NE release[3], increase 5-HT_2 postsynaptic receptor density[4], increase GABA content in different brain regions of rats[3], and alter GABA content in the frontal cortex of mouse[5,6]. Further, selective damage to the polymorphic neurons on the innermost aspect of the dentate granule cell layer has been described as a consequence of sustained limbic seizures induced by kainic acid[12]. A similar pattern of damage is reported to be induced by sustained electrical stimulation of the perforant path in the rat[13].

In the present study, the convulsant effect of bicuculline and PTX was differently affected following ECS and GABAergic treatment. Baclofen, a bicuculline-insensitive $GABA_B$ agonist[14-15] shortened the latency of bicuculline-induced convulsions, 24 hr after acute ECS, whereas it delayed the latency of PTX-induced convulsions in ECS treated animals. Progabide, an agonist at both $GABA_A$ and $GABA_B$ receptors[16] delayed the latency of both bicuculline and PTX-induced convulsions except in the case of 24 hr after acute and 30 min after chronic ECS respectively. Fengabine, an agonist at $GABA_A$ receptors[17] showed no effect on the latency of bicuculline-induced convulsions, whereas it delayed the latency of PTX-induced convulsions in animals not treated with ECS and in those chronically treated with ECS. Baclofen has both pre- and postsynaptic involvement[18], and in contrast to the $GABA_A$ receptors, $GABA_B$ receptors do not contain an integral ion channel. However, a linking of phospholipase A_2-coupled $GABA_B$ receptors to protein kinase C and to potassium channels is considered possible[19]. The possible negative control of $GABA_B$ receptor potassium channels by ECS may alter the action of other transmitter systems like NE and 5-HT. But this speculation needs further elucidation. The stereospecificity for $GABA_B$ receptors[20] is indicative of subtypes for $GABA_B$ receptors and the heterogeneity of the receptors may have also influenced the results. However, specific and potent antagonist of $GABA_B$ is still not available to assess the specificity of the action. $GABA_A$ receptors are already demonstrated to be heterogenous in nature[21].

In conclusion, it may be suggested that the altered response to GABAergic agents following electro and chemo convulsions may be due to the difference in the nature of antagonism of bicuculline and PTX, variation in the specificity of different agonists employed in the study, alteration in the receptor sensitivity or density, or alterations in the levels of endogenous neurotransmitters, the latter two resulting as a consequence of acute or chronic ECS.

Table 1. Effect of ECS and GABAergic agents on bicuculline-induced convulsions in mice [Values (min) are mean ± SE. Figures in parentheses are no. of mice used]

Treatment	Dose mg/kg, ip	Without ECS	Latency		
			30 min post acute ECS	24 hr post acute ECS	30 min post chronic ECS
Bicuculline (14)	4	3.0±0.2	2.9±0.1	3.8±0.2	3.0±0.4
Baclofen	5	3.4±0.1	2.6±0.1	2.1±0.1*	2.9±0.3
+ bicuculline (6)	4				
Progabide	100	5.4±0.3††	7.6±0.2††	4.1 ±0.1	6.9±1.3†
+ bicuculline (6)	4				
Fengabine	80	3.5±0.3	3.6±0.3	2.9±0.3	2.4±0.5
+ bicuculline (6)	4				

P values: * <0.05 and † <0.01 and †† <0.001

Table 2. Effect of ECS and GABAergic agents on PTX-induced convulsions in mice [Values are mean± SE. Figures in parentheses are no. of mice used]

Treatment	Dose mg/kg, ip	Without ECS	Latency		
			30 min post acute ECS	24 hr post acute ECS	30 min post chronic ECS
PTX (16)	6	9.4±0.8	13.7±1.2	7.9±0.4	17.7±1.8†
Baclofen	5	11.5±0.6	17.9±1.1†	15.7±5.4*	18.0±2.1†
+PTX (6)	6				
Progabide	100	16.3±0.3†	17.4±0.2†	14.5±2.3*	10.4±0.3
+PTX (6)	6				
Fengabine	80	16.4±0.2†	13.2±1.3	14.0±1.4	19.4±0.5†
+ PTX (6)	6				

P values: * <0.05 and † <0.01

REFERENCES

1. Essman W B, *Neurochemistry of cerebral electroshock flushing* (Spectrum Publications, New York) 1973.
2. Modigh K J, *Neural Trans,* 36 (1975) 19.
3. Green A R, Minchin M C W & Vincent N D. *Br J Pharmacol,* 92 (1987) 13.
4. Kellar K M, Cascio C S, Butler J A & Kurtzke R W, *Eur J Pharmacol,* 69 (1981) 515.
5. Lloyd K G, Thuret F & File A, *J Pharmac Exp Ther,* 235 (1985) 191.
6. Gray J A & Green A R, *Br J Pharmacol,* 92 (1987) 357.
7. Brailowsky S, Kunimoto M, Menini C, Silva-Barrat C, Riche D & Naquet R, *Brain Res,* 442 (1988) 175.
8. Gray J A, Metz A, Goodwin G M & Green A R, *Neuropharmacology,* 25 (1986) 711.
9. Kulkarni S K, *Arch Int Pharmacodyn,* 252 (1981) 124.
10. Aley K O & Kulkarni S K, *Method Find Exp Clin Pharmacol* 10 (1988) 563.
11. Kenneth P, Linda S B, Bonhaus D W & McNamara J O, *J Pharmac Exp Ther,* 241 (1987) 751.
12. Sloviter R S & Damiano B P, *Neuropharmacology,* 20(1981) 1003.
13. Sloviter R S, *Brain Res Bull,* 10 (1983) 675.
14. Hill D R & Bowery N G, *Nature,* 290 (1981) 149.
15. Bowery N G, Hudson A L, Hill D R & Price G W, *Proc of the 9th Int Congr of Pharmacology* (Macmillan. London) 1985, 159.
15. Lloyd KG, Morselli PL, Depoortere H, Fourmer V, Zivkovic B, Scatton B, Brookkamp C, Worms P & Bartholini G, *Pharmacol Biochem Behav,* 18 (1983) 957.
17. Lloyd K G, Zivkovic B, Sanger D, Depoortere H & Bartholini G, *J Pharmac Exp Ther,* 241 (1987) 245.
18. Newberry N R & Nicoll R A, *Physiology,* 360 (1985) 161.
19. Duman RS, Karbon E V, Harrington C & Enna S J, *J Neurochemistry,* 47 (1986) 800.
20. Aley K O & Kulkarni S K, *Arch Int Pharmacodyn,* (in press).
21. Levitan E S, Schofield P R, Burt D R, Rhee L M, Wisden W, Kohler M, Fujita N, Rodriguez H F, Stephenson A, Darlison M G, Barnard E A & Seehurg P H, *Nature,* 335 (1988) 76.

—•—

Paper Published In:

I.J.E.B. (Vol. 29, March 1991, pp. 241-243)

9

Effect of chronic treatment of Ro 15-1788 and its withdrawal on cortical and hippocampal EEG activity in rats

K.O. ALEY & S.K. KULKARNI
Pharmacology Division, Department of Pharmaceutical Sciences,
Panjab University, Chandigarh 160 014, India
R. MATHUR & U. NAYAR
Department of Physiology, All India Institute of Medical Sciences,
New Delhi 110 029, India

Effect of chronic treatment with Ro 15-1788, a benzodiazepine (BZ) receptor antagonist, and its withdrawal, on the cortical and hippocampal electroencephalogram (EEG) was investigated in rats. Chronic treatment with Ro 15-1788 and its withdrawal (24 and 48 hr) were found to reduce the EEG amplitude in both cortical and hippocampal regions. This reduction in cortical and hippocampal EEG amplitude produced by chronic treatment with Ro 15-1788 and its withdrawal was reversed by gamma aminobutyric acid (GABA), pentobarbitone and picrotoxin, agents known to modulate the GABA/BZ synaptic events by acting at different sites on the complex. Baclofen a $GABA_B$ agonist and FG 7142, a BZ inverse agonist were found to further reduce the EEG amplitude in the cortical and hippocampal regions of these rats, chronically treated with Ro 15-1788. Diazepam, a BZ agonist was found to have no significant effect on the alteration produced in the cortical and hippocampal EEG amplitude by chronic treatment with Ro 15-1788 or its withdrawal. It is suggested that the conformational changes produced on the GABA/BZ receptor complex by BZ receptor occupation, has a facilitatory effect on the actions of those drugs which act on the GABA/BZ receptor complex and the direction of this enhancement depended on the nature of the drug.

Introduction

Ro 15-1788 (Flumazenil), an imidazodiazepine is demonstrated to antagonise a wide spectrum of behavioural effects of BZs. It is also known to antagonize the intrinsic effects of beta-carbolines that are inverse agonists at the BZ binding sites[1]. Recently, some behavioural, neurological, electrophysiological and biochemical studies have shown that Ro 15-1788 also possesses intrinsic activity[2,3]. The agonist-like and/or antagonist-like actions of Ro 15-1788 are reported to be related to the dose of the drug, but the results are not found to be consistent[4,5]. Such inconsistent results also lead to the speculation that the compound may be influencing the binding sites of the GABA/BZ receptor complex or other neurotransmitter mechanisms. Moreover, unlike the BZ agonists, a very few reports are available regarding the chronic use of Ro 15-1788. Some recent studies have demonstrated the upregulation of BZ sites in rat cerebral cortex[6], and upregulation of inverse agonist sites in rat cerebral cortex and hippocampus following chronic treatment with Ro 15-1788 and its withdrawal[7]. If the inverse agonistic sites are upregulated during the withdrawal period of Ro 15-1788, one may expect both behavioural and EEG excitation in these brain areas. In the present study, therefore, effect of chronic treatment and its withdrawal due to Ro 15-1788 was studied on cortical and hippocampal EEG discharges in conscious rat brain. The possible modification of the activities by agents acting at BZ (agonist-diazepam), picrotoxin site (convulsant-picrotoxin), barbiturate site (pentobarbitone), inverse agonist site (FG 7142) and GABA were investigated.

Materials and Methods

Animals: Wistar albino rats (200-250 g) obtained from AIIMS, New Delhi were employed for the study. They were maintained at constant room temperature (26°± 1°C) and light on period from 5.00-19.00 hrs with free access to food and water.

Experimental design: Rats were anaesthetised with ketamine (60 mg/kg, ip) for chronic implantation of electrodes. Three screws with connecting leads were implanted stereotaxically on the hippocampus, cortex and the far anterior part of the frontal cortex with the following co-ordinates[8]. Hippocampus: 3.8 mm behind bregma, 2 mm lateral to the mid sagital suture and 3 mm deep on the right side. Cortex: 2.8 mm behind bregma, 2 mm lateral to the mid sagital suture, on the surface of the skull on the left side. The third (grounding electrode) was implanted on the surface, on the far anterior part of the frontal cortex. These electrodes were fixed with dental cement (Stellon denture material) and the connecting leads were drawn under the skin and fixed dorsally. The animals were housed individually in separate cages.

Drug treatment and EEG recording: On recovery from the surgery (3 days), the animals were treated with the vehicle or Ro 15-1788 (4 mg/kg, ip) daily for a period of 14 days. The Ro 15-1788 treated animals were divided into 7 groups and C of these groups served as the test groups for the various drugs (GABA, baclofen, diazepam, FG 7142, pentobarbitone and picrotoxin) employed in the study. After 14th injection (vehicle or Ro 15-1788) EEG of all the animals were recorded from the cortical and hippocampal regions. For EEG recording, the electrodes were connected by means of a cable to a Grass Model 7D polygraph (Grass Instrument Co., Quincy, Mass, USA); permitting free movement of the rat within the home cage. The direct and integrated EEG signals were recorded on a chart paper (paper speed 25 mm/sec) with the help of a pen oscillograph. Each integrator reset occurred when the area under EEG trace reached a pre-set fixed value. The changes in EEG pattern were recorded continuously from the hippocampal and cortical areas in the control and test groups. The six test -groups were treated with the respective drug thirty min after the last (14th) dose of Ro 15-1788 and the EEG recording was continued for a period of one hour. Similar recording schedule of EEG recording was followed for 24 and 48 hr withdrawal period of either vehicle or Ro 15-1788 treated groups. The six test groups received the respective drug treatment also at 24 and 48 hr of the withdrawal of Ro 15-1788. The EEG recording was done before and after these drug treatment, for 30 min and 60 min respectively. The recording periods were divided into bins of 5 min.

Drugs: Ro 15-1788 (F. Hoffman-LA, Basle, Switzerland), baclofen (Ciba-Geigy, Basle, Switzerland), diazepam (Ranbaxy, New Delhi, India), pentobarbitone sodium (Loba Chemicals, Bombay), FG 7142 (Scherling, Berlin), picrotoxin (BDH, Poole, Dorest, England), GABA (Sigma, St. Louis, USA) and ketamine HCl (Parke Davis, Bombay) were employed for the study. Ro 15-1788 and FG 7142 were dissolved in dimethyl sulfoxide and administered intraperitoneally (ip) at a constant volume of 1 ml/kg. Diazepam was dissolved with the help of propylene glycol. All the other drugs were dissolved either in distilled water or normal saline and administered ip. Chronic study consisted of a daily injection of Ro 15-1788 (4 mg / kg) for fourteen days.

Each test group consisted of a minimum of four animals.

Results

Effect of chronic treatment with Ro 15-1788 and its withdrawal on cortical and hippocampal EEG of rats: Control animals which received chronic vehicle treatment manifested desynchronized EEG activity in both cortex and hippocampus (Fig. 1).

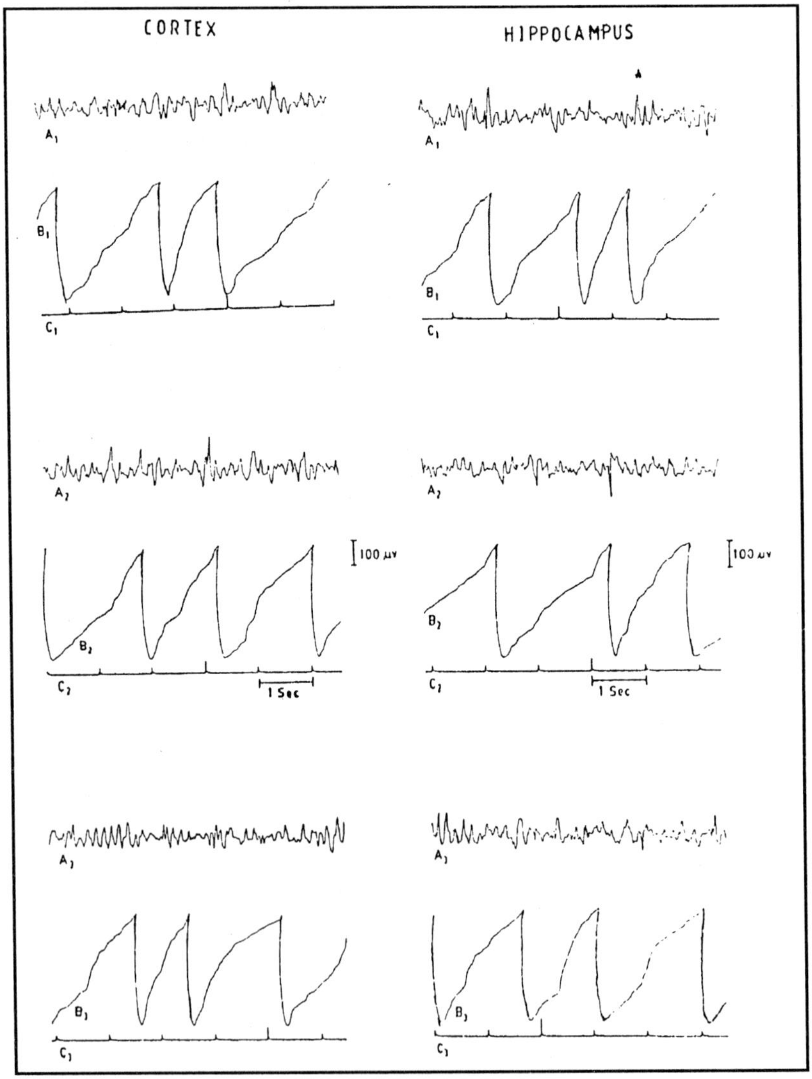

Fig. 1. Control cortical and hippocampal EEG. A: original. B: integrated voltage. C: time calibration. 1, 2, 3 represent effects at 30 min, 24 hr and 48 hr after 14th day treatment with vehicle.

Animals chronically treated with Ro 15-1788 also manifested desynchronized EEG activity in both cortex and hippocampus, at all stages, i.e., 30 min, 24 or 48 hr after the last (14th) dose of Ro 15-1788 treatment. However, the EEG amplitude was found to be decreased as compared to control value (Fig. 2) at all times of testing.

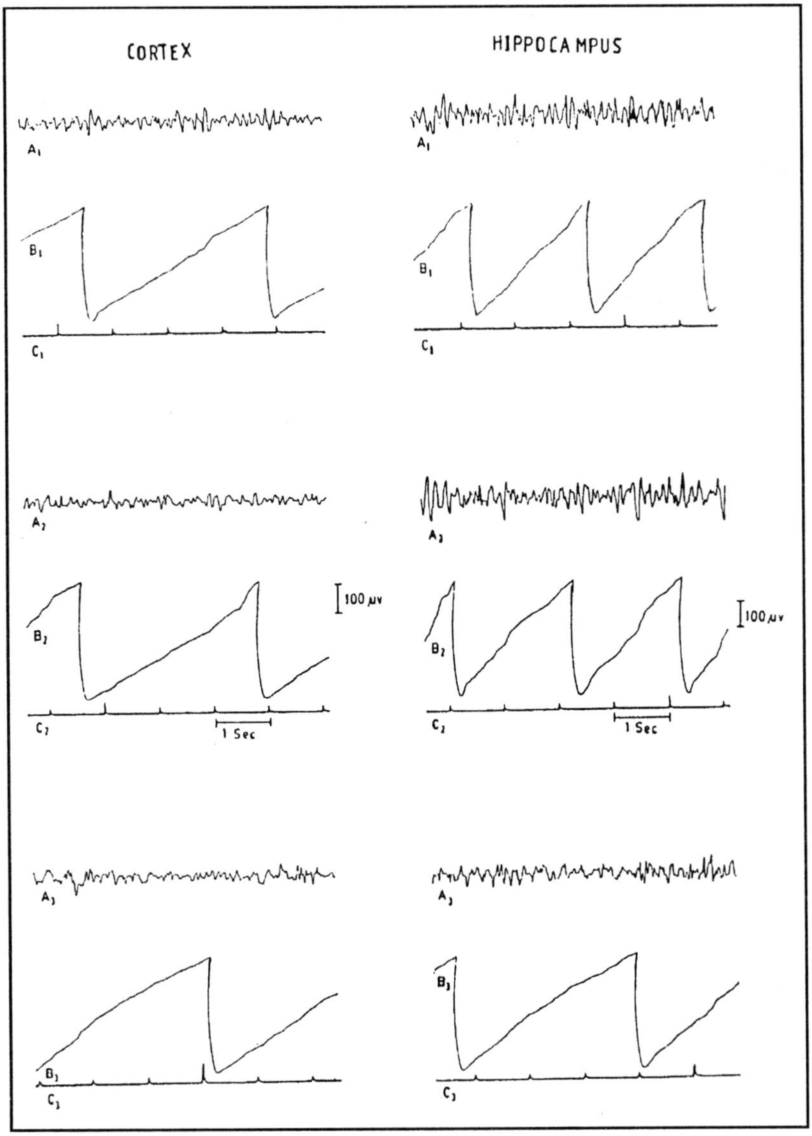

Fig. 2. Cortical and hippocampal EEG of rats chronically treated with Ro 15-1788. A: original EEG, B: integrated voltage. C: time calibration. 1, 2, 3 represent effects at 30 min, 24 hr and 48 hr after 14th dose of Ro 15-1788.

Effect of GABA: Treatment with GABA (100 mg/kg, ip) significantly reversed the effect of chronic treatment with Ro 15-1788 on cortical EEG amplitude at all time periods of testing. But it showed no significant effect on the alteration produced by chronic Ro 15-1788 treatment and its withdrawal on hippocampal EEG activity (Fig. 3).

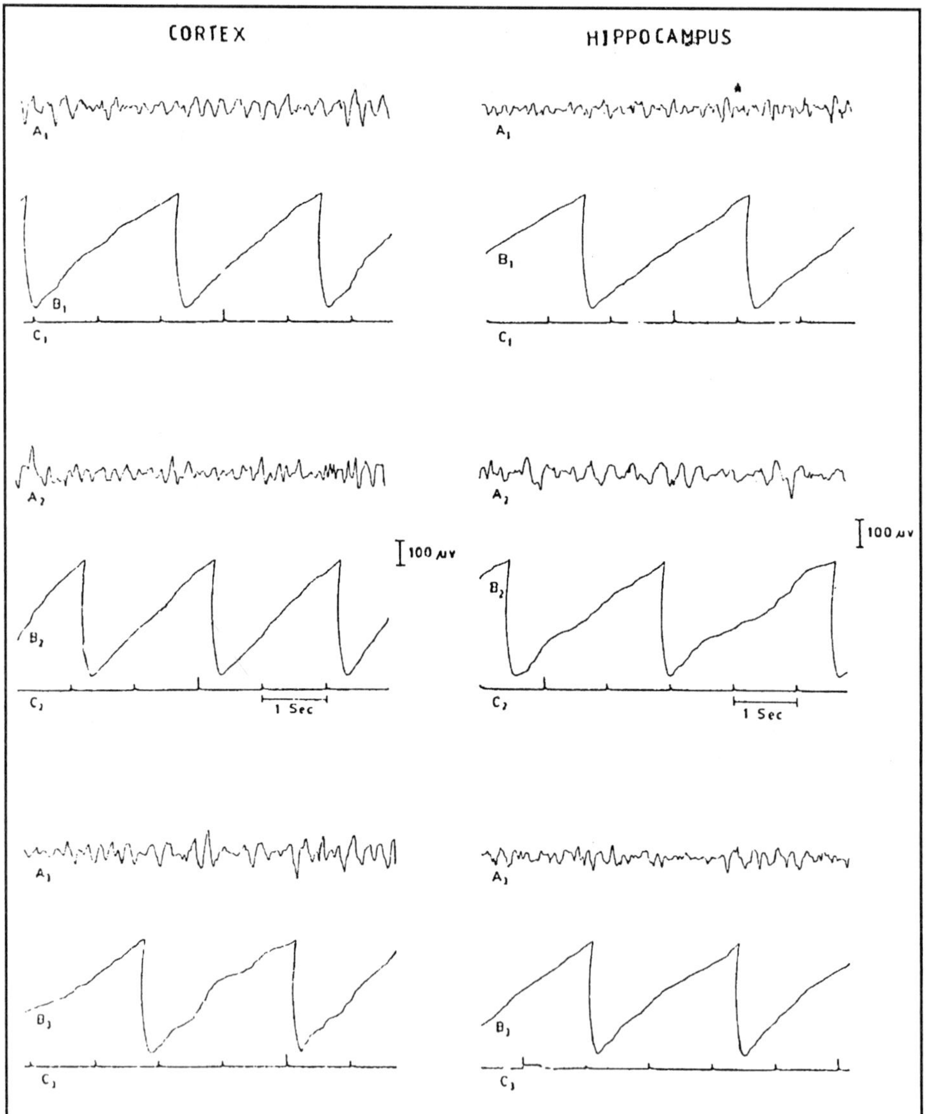

Fig. 3. Effect of GABA on cortical and hippocarmpal EEG of rats chronically treated with Ro 15-1788. A: original EEG, B: integrated voltage, C: time calibration. 1, 2, 3 represent effects at 30 min, 24 hr and 48 hr after 14th dose of Ro 15-1788.

Effect of baclofen: The reduction in EEG amplitude produced by chronic Ro 15-1788 treatment and its withdrawal was further increased (17 to 30%) by baclofen (5 mg/kg, ip) both in the cortical and hippocampal region (Fig. 4).

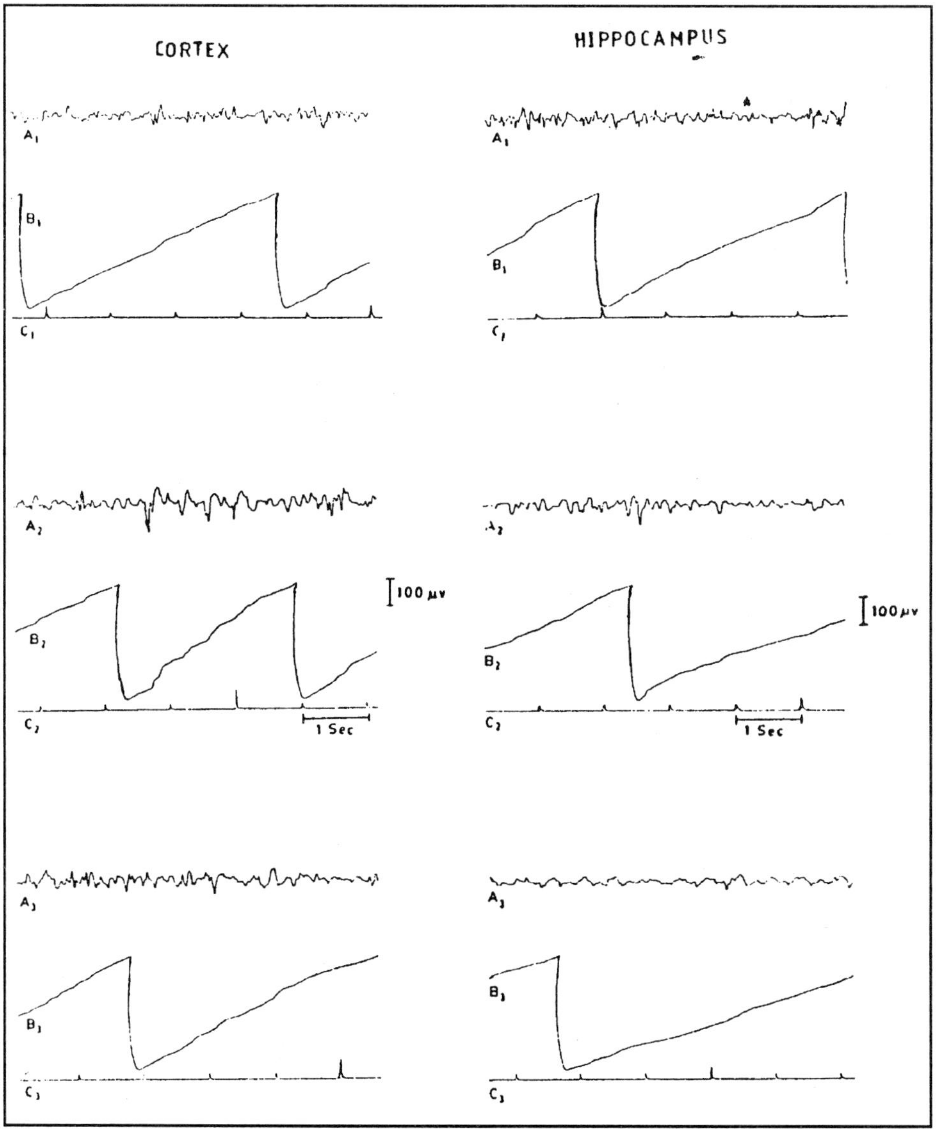

Fig. 4. Effect of baclofen on cortical and hippocampal EEG of rats chronically treated with Ro 15-1788. A: original EEG. B: integrated voltage, C: time calibration 1, 2, 3 represent effects at 30 min, 24 hr and 48 hr after 14th dose of Ro 15-I788.

Effect of diazepam: Diazepam (4 mg/kg, ip) did not produce any significant alteration on the effect of cortical and hippocampal EEG activity produced by chronic treatment with Ro 15-1788 or its withdrawal (Fig. 5).

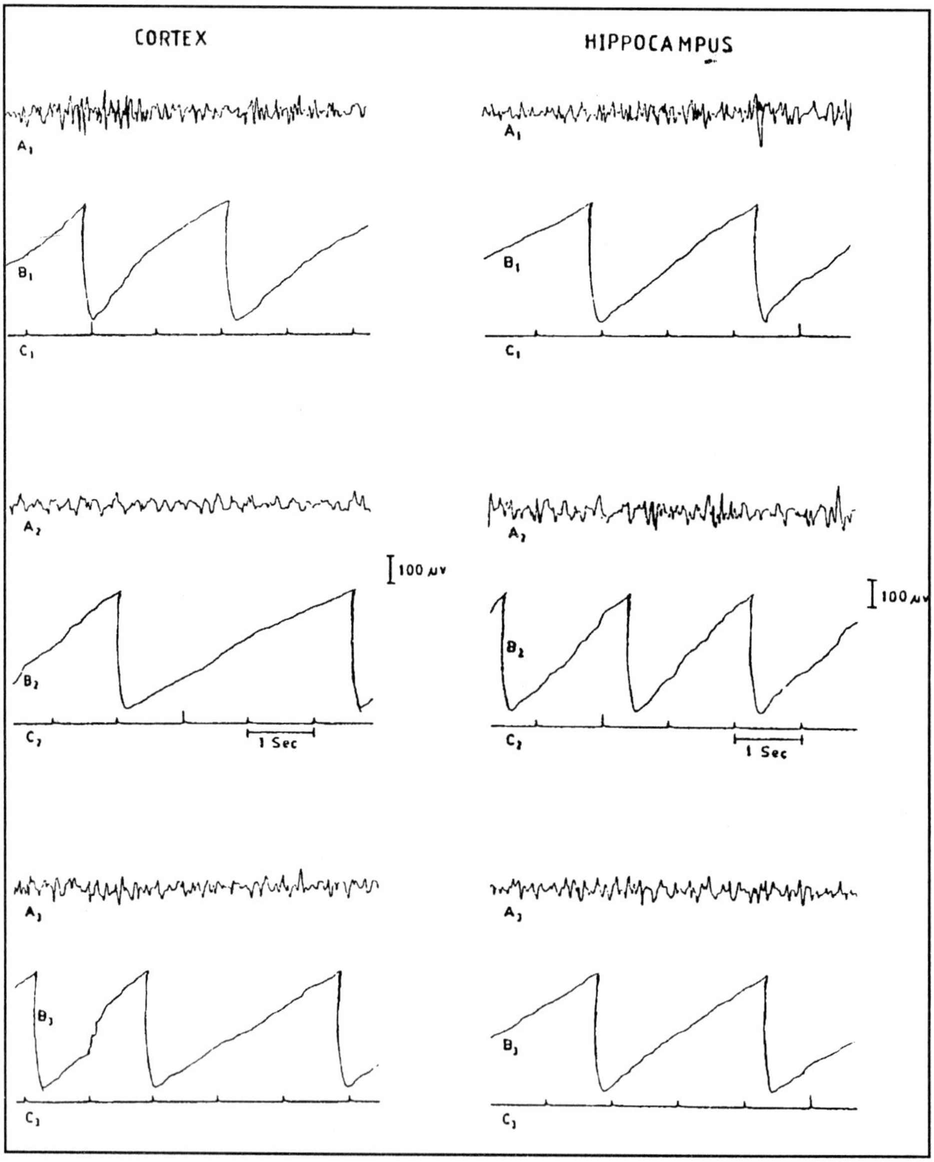

Fig. 5. Effect of diazepam on cortical and hippocampal EEG of rats chronically treated with Ro 15-1788. A: original EEG, B: integrated voltage, C: time calibration. 1, 2, 3 represent effects at 30 min 24 hr and 48 hr after 14th dose of Ro 15-1788.

Effect of FG 7142: The reduction in the cortical and hippocampal EEG amplitude produced by chronic treatment with Ro 15-1788 and its withdrawal was further increased (30-40%) by treatment with 10 mg/kg, ip FG 7142 (Fig. 6).

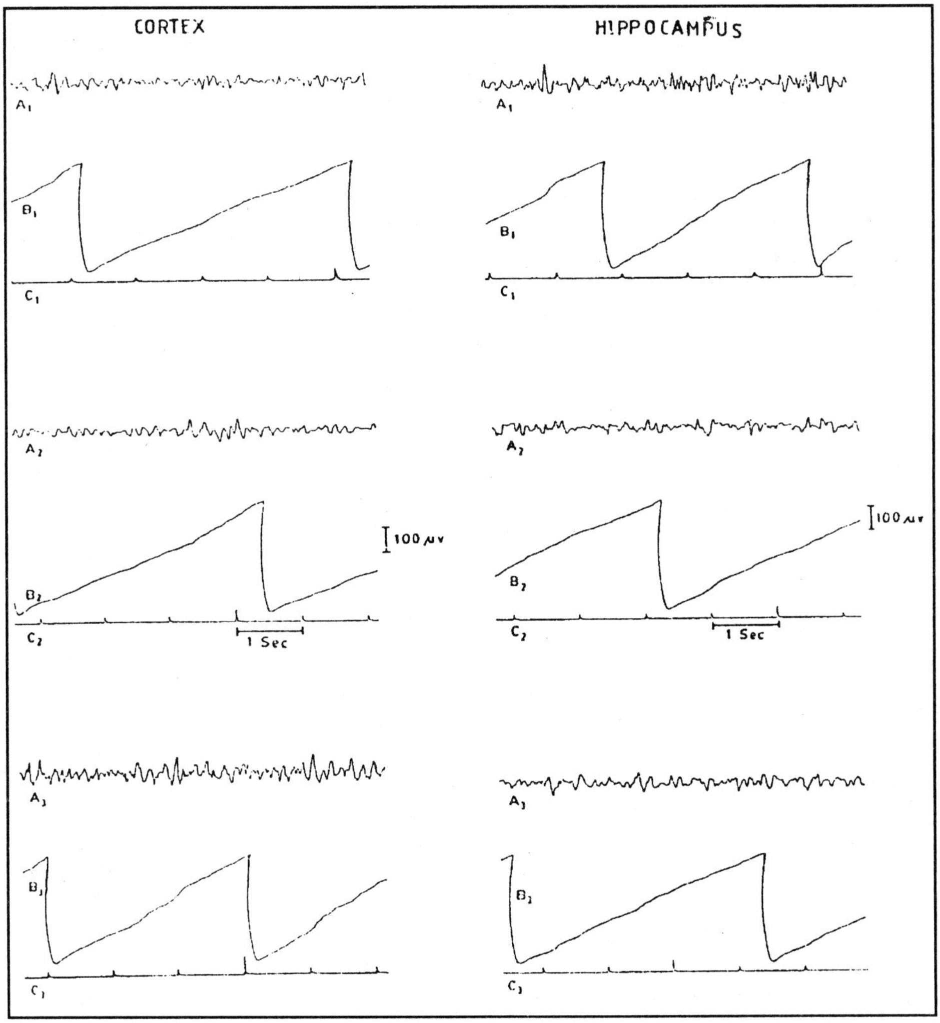

Fig. 6. Effect of FG 7142 on cortical and hippocampal EEG of rats chronically treated with Ro 15-1788. A original EEG, B: integrated voltage, C : time calibration. 1, 2, 3 represents effects at 30 min, 24 hr and 48 hr after 14th dose of Ro 15-1788.

Effect of pentobarbitone: Pentobarbitone (5 mg/kg, ip) totally reversed the effect of chronic treatment with Ro 15-1788 and its withdrawal on cortical and hippocampal EEG amplitude. Moreover, at 30 min past the last Ro 15-1788 treatment, pentobarbitone increased (30-60%) the EEG amplitude even from that of the control value (Fig.7). Also at times, the wave frequency, altered from that of the theta to the alpha rhythm, retaining the desynchronized nature of the wave. At a 10 mg/kg ip dose of pentobarbitone, the animals remained in a stupor stage which lasted for over 3 hr (Personal observation).

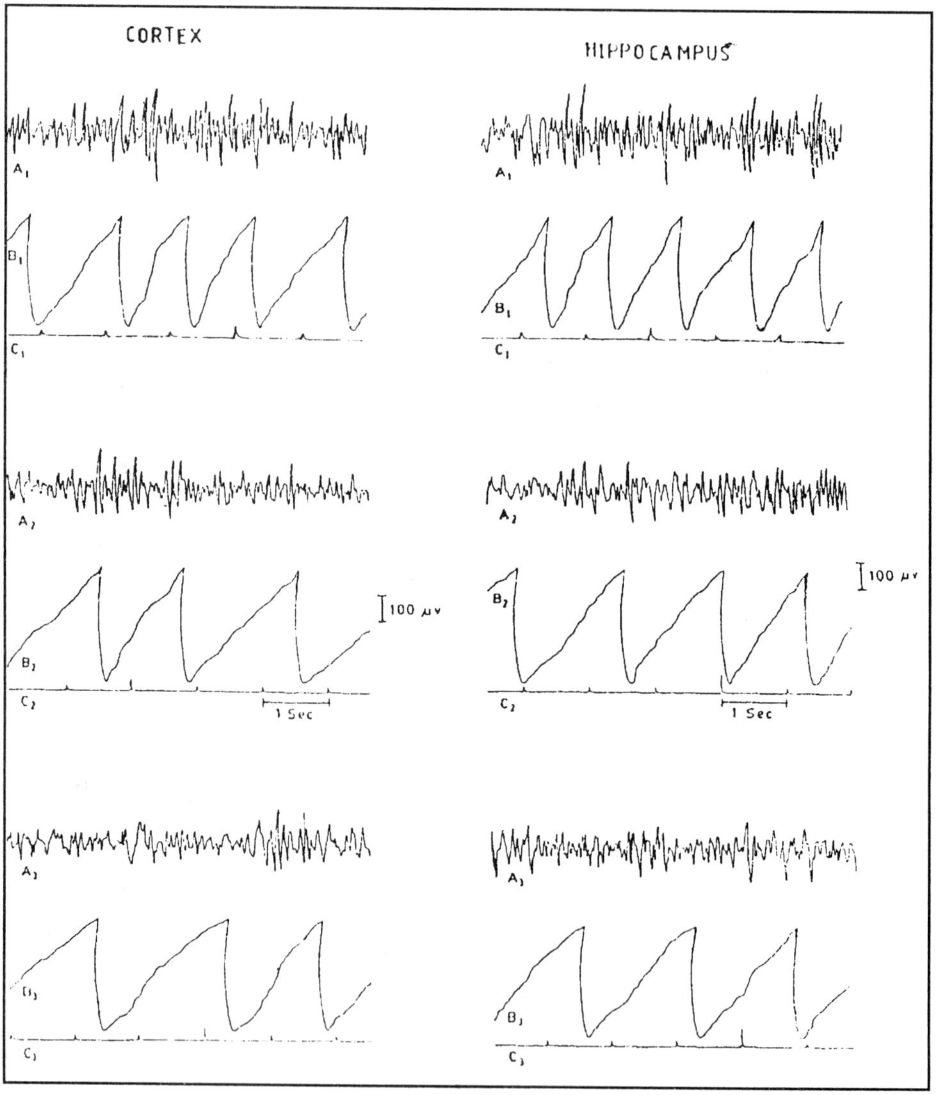

Fig. 7. Effect of pentobarbitone on cortical and hippocampal EEG of rats chronicallv treated with Ro 15-1788. A: original EEG, B: integrated voltage, C: time calibration 1, 2, 3 represent effects at 30 min, 24 hr and 48 hr after 14th dose of Ro 15-1788.

Effect of picrotoxin– Picrotoxin (2 mg/ kg, ip) not only reversed the effect of chronic treatment with Ro 15-1788 and its withdrawal on cortical and hippocampal EEG amplitude, but it also increased (30-60%) the EEG amplitude from that of the control value (Fig. 8). Further, at this low dose level, picrotoxin produced severe tonic clonic convulsions in animals chronically treated with Ro 15-1788. However, none of the animals succumbed to death.

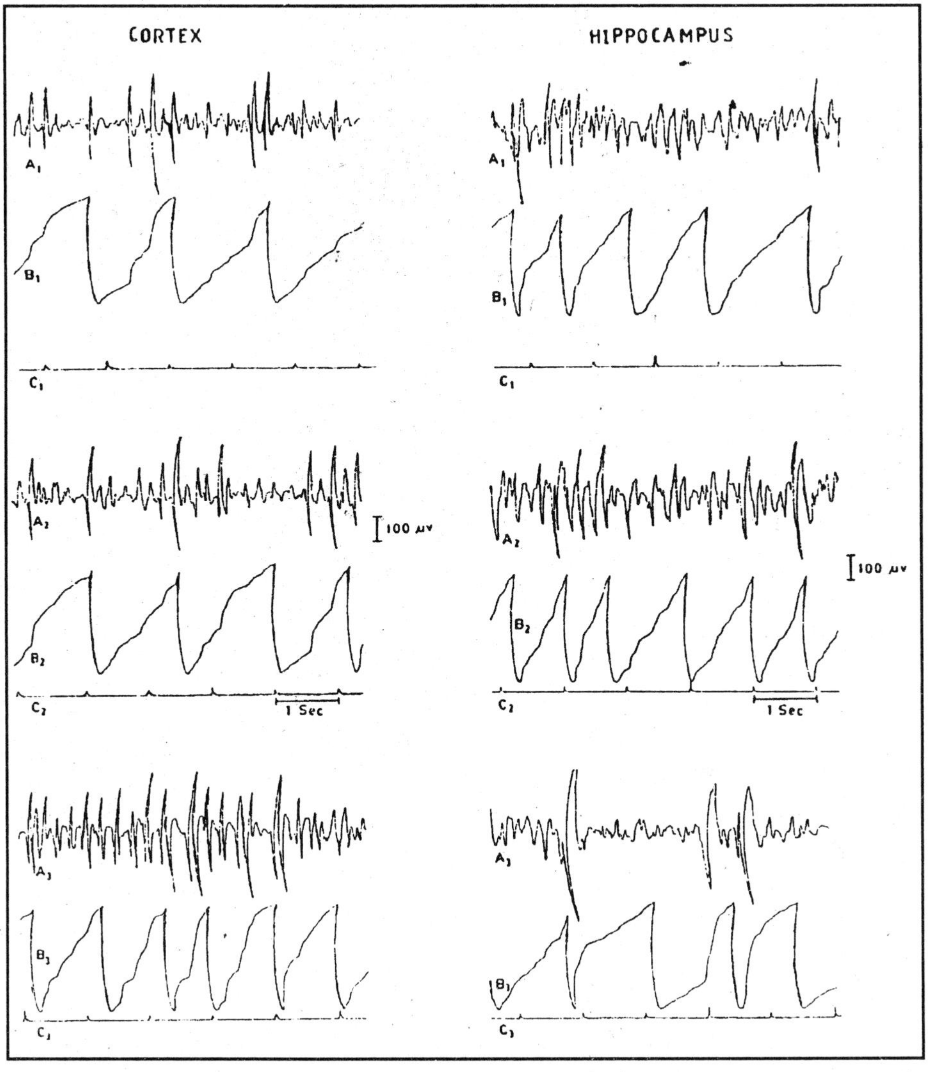

Fig. 8. Effect of picrotoxin on cortical and hippocampal EEG of rats chronically treated with Ro 15-1768. A: original EEG. B: integrated voltage. C: time calibration. 1, 2, 3 represent effects at 30min, 24 hr and 48 hr after 14th dose of Ro 15-1788.

Discussion

The GABA-receptor/ionophore supramolecular complex includes binding sites for GABA, benzodiazepines, barbiturates, picrotoxin, and the chloride channel. The benzodiazepine receptors are involved in regulating the coupling between the $GABA_A$-agonist recognition site and the opening of the chloride channels. Different ligands for benzodiazepine receptors can either enhance the effect of $GABA_A$-receptor activation (agonists, positive efficacy), reduce this effect (inverse agonists, negative efficacy)[10-12] or have little direct effect but block the actions of both agonists and inverse agonists (antagonists, no efficacy)[13,14]. Compounds possessing partial agonist and partial inverse agonist properties also have been described[15,16].

Chronic treatment with benzodiazepine ligand reduce the efficacy of coupling between benzodiazepine and $GABA_A$-receptors[17]. Flumazenil is a neutral antagonist at pharmacologically relevant doses. It antagonizes behavioural, biochemical, and electrophysiological actions of benzodiazepines[18-20] . However, many recent studies have shown that flumazenil possessed intrinsic activity in a variety of behavioural, neurological and electrophysiological parameters[2].

It has proconvulsant[21], anxiogenic[3], and at high doses partial agonist properties at benzodiazepine receptors[22].

In the present study, chronic treatment with Ro 15-1788 and its withdrawal reduced the cortical and hippocampal EEG amplitude as compared to the control group. Further, in rats chronically treated with Ro 15-1788, a low (non-convulsant) dose of picrotoxin produced severe tonic-clonic convulsions, and pentobarbitone (10 mg/kg, ip) caused prolonged (> 3 hr) stupor. In both these cases the effects of the drugs (picrotoxin and pentobarbitone) were potentiated, regardless of the particular nature of the drug. Since the effects of both the agonist and that of the antagonist are potentiated, it cannot be said that Ro 15-1788 is having an intrinsic activity. Conversely, it may be rendering the GABA/benzodiazepine supramolecular complex supersensitive and thus potentiating the effects of the drugs (agonist and antagonist) administered thereafter.

In animals, chronically treated with Ro 15-1788, diazepam (4 mg/kg) did not produce any significant effect. In this case, it is possible that the antagonistic nature of Ro 15-1788 is at play and hence no further effect, as both of them occupy the same receptors.

Recently, it has been reported that chronic treatment with Ro 15-1788 increases the binding of [^{3}H] Ro 15-1788 [^{3}H] flunitrazepam, [^{35}S] TBPS and [^{3} H] Ro 15-4513 in the cerebral cortex of rats. This increase in receptor density is reported to remain upregulated during the withdrawal period as well[23-25]. The specific binding of [^{3}H] Ro 15-1788 is reported to be increased in hippocampus also[7]. These findings and the EEG changes of cortical and hippocampal area observed in the present studies tend to suggest that chronic treatment with Ro 15-1788 and its withdrawal alter the receptor sensitivity of various binding sites on GABA/BZ receptor complex. These observations may have some implications in the development of drug discontinuation syndrome observed in man and animals due to BZ-like drugs. However, an extensive study with different doses of Ro 15-1788 and its interactions with different classes of drugs (agonists to inverse agonists) is required to unravel the nature of this compound.

In animals chronically treated with Ro 15-1788, GABA reversed the effect of chronic Ro 15-1788 treatment while, baclofen, a $GABA_B$-agonist and FG 7142, a benzodiazepine inverse agonist enhanced the effect. This may be due to the allosteric interactions at GABA/BZ receptor complex. Biochemical studies have demonstrated that various sites on the macromolecular GABA receptor complex, bear a relationship with each other in an allosteric manner[26,27].

In conclusion, it is suggested that the conformational changes produced on the GABA/BZ receptor complex by chronic Ro 15-1788 treatment has a facilitatory effect on the actions of other drugs which act on the oligomeric GABA/BZ receptor complex and the direction (positive or negative) of this enhancement will depend on the nature of the drug.

REFERENCES

1. Nutt D J, Cowen P J & Little H J, *Nature,* 295 (1982) 436.
2. File S E & Pellow S, *Psychopharmacology,* 88 (1986) I.
3. File S E, Lister R G & Nutt D J, *Neuropharmacology,* 17 (1982) 747.
4. Liljequist S & Engel J A, *Life Sci,* 34 (1984) 2525.
5. Jensen L H, Petersen E H, Braestrup C, Honore T, Kehr W, Stephens D N, Schneider H, Seidelmann D & Schmiechen R, *Psychopharmacology,* 83 (1984) 249.
6. Medina J H, Novas M L & DeRobertis E, *Eur J Pharmacol,* 90 (1983) 125.

7. Kulkarni S K & Ticku M K, *Brain Res,* 519 (1990) 6.
8. Paxinos G & Watson C, *The brain in stereotaxic coordinates,* (Academic Press, Sydney), 1982.
9. Olsen R W, *Annu Rev Pharmac Toxicol,* 22 (1982) 245.
10. Oakley N R & Jones B J, *Eur J Pharmacol,* 68 (1980) 381.
11. Cowen P J, Green A R, Nutt D J & Martin I L, *Nature,* 290 (1981) 54.
12. Dorow R, Horowski R, Paschelke G. Amin M & Braestrup C, *Lancett, ii* (1983) 98.
13. Hunkeler W, Mohler H, Pieri L, Bonett E P, Cumin R, Schaffner R & Haefely W, *Nature,* 290 (1981) 515.
14. Haefely W, Kyburz E, Gerecke M & Mohler M, *Adv Drug Res,* 14 (1985) 165.
15. Braestrup C, Honore T, Nielsen M, Petersen E N & Jensen L H, *Biochem Pharmac,* 33 (1984) 889.
16. Haefely W, *Clin Neuropharmac,* 7 (suppl. 1) (1984) 670.
17. Heninger G & Gallager D W, *Neuropharmacology,* 27 (1988) 1073.
18. Bonetti E P, Pieri L, Cumin R, Schaffner R, Pieri M, Gamzu E R, Muller R K M & Haefely W, *Psychopharmacology,* 78 (1982) 8.
19. Mohler H & Richards J G, *Nature,* 294 (1981) 763.
20. Chan C Y & Farb D H, *J Neurosci,* 5 (1985) 2365.
21. Corda M G, Costa E & Guidotti A, *Neuropharmacology,* 21 (1982) 91.
22. Velluci S V & Webster R A, *Eur J Pharmacol,* 90 (1983) 263.
23. Miller L G, Greenblatt D J, Barnhill J G & Shader R I, *J Pharmac Exp Ther,* 246 (1988a) 170.
24. Miller L G, Greenblatt D J, Roy R B, Summer W R & Shader R I, *J Pharmac Exp Ther,* 246 (1988b) 177.
25. Kulkarni S K & Ticku M K, *Brain Res Bull,* 22 (1989b) 575.
26. Olsen R W, *J Neurochem,* 37 (1981) 1.
27. Ticku M K, *Neuropharmacology,* 22 (1983) 1459.

Paper Published In:
I.J.E.B. (Vol. 28, December 1990, pp. 1149-1159)

10

Benzodiazepine inverse agonist, DMCM- and peripheral agonist, Ro 5-4864-induced convulsions in mice: Effect of adenosinergic agents

S.N. THORAT & S.K. KULKARNI
Pharmacology Division, Department of Pharmaceutical Sciences.
Panjab University. Chandigarh 160 014, India

Adenosinergic agents such as adenosine, 2-chloroadenosine, N^6-cyclohexyladenosine produced dose-dependent protective effect against DMCM- and Ro 5-4864-induced convulsions and mortality. N^6-cyclohexyladenosine produced most significant protective effect against Ro 5-4864-induced convulsions whereas 2-chloroadenosine was more effective than N^6-cyclohexyladenosine in antagonising DMCM-induced convulsions. Pretreatment of animals with subprotective doses of adenosine and dipyridamole significantly prolonged the latencies for the onset of myoclonic jerks and convulsions due to both DMCM and Ro 5-4864. DMCM and Ro 5-4864-induced mortality rate was also significantly reduced by pretreatment with subprotective doses of adenosine and dipyridamole. Similarly, subprotective doses of adenosine and diazepam further delayed the latencies for myoclonic jerks and convulsions due to DMCM and Ro 5-4864 treatment. The results suggest that adenosine and adenosine receptor agonists, 2-chloroadenosine and N^6-cyclohexyladenosine are protective against both DMCM- and Ro 5-4864-induced convulsions. It is suggested that adenosinergic agents via activation of central A_1 adenosine receptors may modulate the convulsant effects mediated by DMCM and Ro 5-4864. This study further supports the notion that adenosinergic mechanisms mediate neuroprotective effects in the central nervous system.

Recent evidence has indicated that certain benzodiazepine receptor ligands designated as inverse agonists[1,2] such as the β-carboline derivatives by reducing GABA-ergic inhibition via an allosteric interaction with the $GABA_A$ receptor produce anxiogenic, proconvulsant and convulsant effects[3,4]. DMCM has been shown to produce convulsions in rodents[4-7]. Recently, Ro 5-4864 (p-chlorodiazepam) a 'peripheral type' benzodiazepine receptor ligand has also been suggested to possess anxiogenic and convulsant properties at high doses in rodents[6-8]. Ro 5-4864 has been shown to interact with GABA-benzodiazepine receptor complex in the CNS possibly due to its ability to bind at high concentrations to the picrotoxinin domain on this complex[9,10].

Recently, it has been suggested that β-carbolines may share some of the psychopharmacological properties of adenosine antagonists such as caffeine and theophylline, in addition to any actions at the GABA-benzodiazepine receptor complex[11]. Ro 5-4864 has also been reported to possess the ability to both antagonise and potentiate the actions of a putative neurotransmitter neuromodulator adenosine[12]. Recent experimental evidence has suggested that adenosine receptor-coupled processes might be the possible substrates for the pathology underlying certain syndromes of epilepsy, and in addition these processes may contribute significantly to the homeostatic regulation of CNS excitability[13,14]. At cellular level, adenosine and its stable analogues have been shown to inhibit both spontaneous and evoked neuronal firing through activation of specific receptors at pre- and post-synaptic domains throughout the CNS[15,16]. Adenosine has been reported to be an endogenous anticonvulsant[17] and neuroprotective agent[18,19]. However, the exact mechanisms and the CNS sites of action subserving the modulation by adenosine of seizure susceptibility have not been fully established. Moreover, compared to the electrophysiological and biochemical evidence on the role of adenosine, in the brain, relatively little is known concerning the CNS effects of adenosine and adenosine analogues in the intact animals[20,21]. Therefore, the present study was undertaken to investigate the effects of adenosinergic agents against benzodiazepine inverse agonist DMCM- and peripheral agonist Ro 5-4864-induced convulsions in mice.

Materials and Methods

Wistar mice of either sex (20-25 g) (from the CAH, Panjab University, Chandigarh) were used. The animals were maintained at room temperature (25°±2°C) and under 12 hr light/dark cycle. They were allowed free access to food and water except during experiments. Animals were divided into different groups at random, each comprising a minimum of 5 animals. All experiments were carried out between 08.00 and 14.00 hrs.

Animals were challenged with DMCM (25 mg/kg) or Ro 5-4864 (60 mg/kg) for inducing convulsions. These doses were selected on the basis of preliminary experiments or based on the earlier reports from our laboratory. The latencies for the onset of jerks and full body convulsions were recorded. In cases in which tonic convulsions were observed (which were almost invariably fatal in mice), time of onset was recorded as well. Animals that did not convulse within 30 min were considered not convulsing.

Drugs: DMCM (Methyl-6, 7-dimethoxy-beta-carboline-3-carboxylate, Schering, Berlin), Ro 5-4864 (p-chlorodiazepam, Hoffmann-La Roche, Nutley), diazepam (Ranbaxy, New Delhi, India), and adenosine (Sigma, USA) were uniformly suspended using Tween 80 (1 to 2 drops/10 ml) in distilled water. 2-Chloroadenosine (Sigma), N^6-cyclohexyl adenosine (Sigma) were dissolved in distilled water. Dipyridamole (German Remedies, Bombay, India) solution was prepared in distilled water with a few drops of dilute HCI (0.1 N). All drugs were administered (ip), in a constant volume of 10 ml/kg. In all cases, adenosinergic agents and diazepam were administered 25 min before the convulsant challenge. Theophylline was administered 15 min prior to agonists.

Statistical analysis was done using Student's t test.

Results

DMCM- and Ro 5-4864-induced convulsions: DMCM (25 mg/kg) produced myoclonic jerks, intermittent clonic convulsions with a loss of righting reflex followed by continuous tonic convulsions within 4 min. Ro 5-4864 (60 mg/kg) produced myoclonic jerks followed by tonic-clonic convulsions within 6 min. The Ro 5-4864-induced convulsions also consisted of rotational movements, profuse salivation, loss of righting reflex and chewing of the forelimbs.

Effect of adenosinergic agents and diazepam on DMCM-induced convulsions: Pretreatment of animals with adenosine (100 and 200 mg/kg) dose-dependently prolonged the latencies for the onset of myoclonic jerks and convulsions due to DMCM challenge. The tonic extensor phase and mortality was completely blocked by a high dose of adenosine (200 mg/kg). Potent adenosine receptor agonists such as 2-chloroadenosine and N^6-cyclohexyladenosine also significantly prolonged in a dose-dependent manner the latencies for the onset of myoclonic jerks and convulsions (Table 1). Pretreatment of animals with 2-chloroadenosine and N^6-cyclohexyladenosine completely blocked the tonic extensor phase. 2-Chloroadenosine and N^6-cyclohexyladenosine also reversed the mortality due to DMCM treatment. Dipyridamole (5 mg/kg) an adenosine uptake inhibitor, did not produce any significant protective effect against DMCM-induced convulsions. Pretreatment of animals with diazepam (2 mg/kg) completely blocked DMCM induced convulsions and mortality (Table 1).

Table 1. Effect of adenosinergic agents and diazepam on DMCM-induced convulsions and mortality in mice

Treatment	Dose (mg/kg)	n	Latency in min (mean ± SE)			Death (n/n)
			Jerks	Convulsions	Tonic extensor	
DMCM	25	21	2.50±0.09	3.27±0.14	14.01±0.49	20/21
Adenosine	100	5	3.55±0.26	4.28±0.30	32.12±2.50**	3/5
+ DMCM	25					
Adenosine	200	5	6.57±0.38**	8.20±0.53**	-	0/5
+ DMCM	2.5					
2-Chloroadenosine	0.5	5	2.23±0.17	3.34±0.20	18.21 ±0.67*	4/5
+ DMCM	25					
2-Chloroadenosine	1.0	5	7.39±1.08**	8.54±0.81 **	-	0/5
+ DMCM	25					
2-Chloroadenosine	2.0	5	9.07±0.17**	16.34±0.64**	-	0/5
+ DMCM	25					
N^6-Cyclohexyladenosine	0.5	5	4.24±0.10*	5.36±0.45*	-	3/5
+ DMCM	25					
N^6-Cyclohexyladenosine	1.0	5	6.60±0.91**	7.54±0.76**	-	1/5
+ DMCM	25					
N^6-Cyclohexyladcnosine	2.0	5	7.14±1.08**	8.02±1.01**	-	0/5
+ DMCM	25					
Dipyridamole	5.0	5	3.58±0.19	4.05±0.43	13.30± 1.73	2/5
+ DMCM	25					
Diazepam	0.5	5	3.60±0.51	4.05±0.52	29.23±1.37**	4/5
+ DMCM	25					
Diazepam	1.0	5	4.33±0.41*	5.40±0.44*	-	2/5
+ DMCM	25					
Diazepam	5.0	5	-	-	-	0/5
+ DMCM	25					

*P<0.05; **P<0.001 when compared with respective control groups.

Effects of combined pretreatment with subprotective doses of adenosine, dipyridamole and diazepam on DMCM-induced convulsions: Combined pretreatrnent of animals with subprotective doses of adenosine (100 mg/kg) and dipyridamole (5 mg/kg) significantly prolonged the latencies for the onset of myoclonic jerks as well as convulsions due to DMCM challenge. The tonic extensor phase was also completely blocked due to this treatment. Mortality rate was also significantly reduced (Table 2). Pretreatment of animals with subprotective doses of adenosine (100 mg/kg) and diazepam (0.5 mg/kg) significantly prolonged the latencies for onset of myoclonic jerks and convulsions. Thirty-three percent of animals (2/6) were fully protected and the tonic extensor phase was completely blocked due to this combination and mortality rate was also significantly reduced (Table 2).

Table 2. Effect of combined pretreatment with subprotective doses of adenosine, dipyridamole and diazepam on DMCM-induced convulsions and mortality in mice

Treatment	Dose (mg/kg)	n	Latency in min (mean ± SE)			Death (n/n)
			Jerks	Convulsions	Tonic extensor	
DMCM	25	16	2.32±0.03	3.03±0.10	11.35±0.87	16/16
Adenosine	100	5	3.55±0.26	4.28±0.26	32.12±2.50**	3/5
+ DMCM	25					
Dipyridamole	5.0	5	3.58±0.19	4.05±0.43	13.30± 1.73	2/5
+ DMCM	25					
Diazepam	0.5	5	3.60±0.51	4.05±0.52	29.23±1.37**	4/5
+ DMCM	25					
Adenosine	100	6	6.17±0.22*	8.17±0.60**	-	1/6
+Dipyridamole	5					
+ DMCM	25					
Adenosine	100	6	8.53±0.39**	10.38±1.41**	-	1/6
+Diazepam	0.5					
+ DMCM	25					

*P<0.05; **P<0.001 when compared with respective control values.

Effects of adenosinergic agents and diazepam on Ro 5-4864-induced convulsions: Pretreatment of animals with various doses of adenosinergic agents offered significant dose-dependent protective effect against Ro 5-4864-induced convulsions in mice (Table 3). N^6-cyclohexyladenosine, a selective A_1-adenosine receptor agonists produced more potent dose-dependent protective effect compared to other adenosinergic agents. The tonic extensor phase was completely blocked by N^6-cyclohexyladenosine pretreatment (Table 3). Diazepam (5 mg/kg) fully antagonised the convulsant effects due to Ro 5-4864 challenge.

Table 3. Effects of adenosinergic agents and diazepam on Ro 5-4864-induced convulsions in mice

Treatment	Dose (mg/kg)	n	Latency in min (mean ± SE)			Death (n/n)
			Jerks	Convulsions	Tonic extensor	
Ro 5-4864	60	14	4.44±023	5.14±0.31	11.04±0.72	14/14
Adenosine	100	5	4.52±0.39	5.09±1.20	11.09±1.84	5/5
+ Ro 5-4864	60					
Adenosine	200	5	6.17±0.22*	6.51±0.15*	17.21±0.81**	5/5
+ Ro 5-4864	60					
2-chloroadenosine	1.0	5	5.18±0.23	6.26±0.52*	13.5±1.01	5/5
+ Ro 5-4864	60					
2-chloroadenosine	2.0	5	6.20±0.03*	7.36±0.38*	14.05±0.38*	3/5
+ Ro 5-4864	60					
N^6-cyclohexyladenosine	1.0	5	10.06±1.33**	13.20±1.74**	-	0/5
+ Ro 5-4864	60					
N^6-cyclohexyladenosine	2.0	5	14.31±1.58**	16.49±1.53**	-	0/5
+ Ro 5-4864	60					
Dipyridamole	5.0	5	5.55±0.18	6.60±025	14.08±0.96*	5/5
+ Ro 5-4864	60					
Diazepam	0.5	5	4.20±0.30	6.15±0.27	13.35±0.44	5/5
+ Ro 5-4864	60					
Diazepam	1.0	5	6.18±0.14*	8.32±0.33*	-	3/5
+ Ro 5-4864	60					
Diazepam	5.0	5	-	-	-	0/5
+ Ro 5-4864	60					

* $P < 0.05$; ** $P < 0.001$ when compared with control groups

Effect of combined pretreatment with subprotective doses of adenosine, dipyridamole and diazepam on Ro 5-4864-induced convulsions– Combined pretreatment of animals with subprotective doses of adenosine and dipyridamole significantly prolonged the latency for the onset of myoclonic jerks, convulsions and tonic extensor phase (Table 4). However, all the animals tested produced fully body convulsions followed by death. Pretreatment of animals with subprotective doses of adenosine and dipyridamole significantly prolonged the latencies for the onset of myoclonic jerks, convulsions and tonic extensor phase. Mortality rate was also reduced due to this combination.

Table 4. Effect of combined pretreatment with subprotective doses of adenosine, dipyridamole and diazepam on Ro 5-4864-induced convulsions in mice

Treatment	Dose (mg/kg)	n	Latency in min (mean ± SE)			Death (n/n)
			Jerks	Convulsions	Tonic extensor	
Ro 5-4864	60	10	4.34±0.15	5.33±0.30	11.30±0.78	10/10
Adenosine	100	5	4.52±0.39	5.09±1.20	11.09±1.84	5/5
+ Ro 5-4864	60					
Dipyridamole	5.0	5	5.55±0.18	6.60±025	14.08±0.96*	5/5
+ Ro 5-4864	60					
Diazepam	0.5	5	4.20±0.30	5.15±0.27	13.35±0.44	5/5
+ Ro 5-4864	60					
Adenosine	100	5	8.11±1.12**	9.44±1.06**	18.21±0.24**	5/5
+ dipyridamole	5.0					
+ Ro 5-4864	60					
Adenosine	100	5	12.10±0.60**	18.37±2.10**	31.13±0.51**	2/5
+ diazepam	0.5					
+ Ro 5-4864	60					

* $P < 0.05$; ** $P < 0.001$ when compared with control groups

Discussion

In the present study, the benzodiazepine inverse agonist, DMCM produced myoclonic jerks, intermittent clonic convulsions followed by repeated tonic convulsions in mice. On the other hand, Ro 5-4864 produced myoclonic jerks followed by severe tonic-clonic convulsions consisting of rotational movements, profuse salivation, loss of righting reflex and chewing of the forelimbs. Pretreatment of animals with adenosinergic agents offered significant dose-dependent prolongation in the latencies for the onset of myoclonic jerks and convulsions due to both DMCM and Ro 5-4864 treatment. The stable analogues of adenosine such as 2-chloroadenosine and N^6-cyclonexyladenosine offered more pronounced delay in the latencies for the onset of myoclonic jerks and convulsions. N^6-cyclohexyladenosine, a selective A_1-adenosine receptor agonist offered most significant effect against Ro 5-4864-induced convulsions as it has not only prolonged the latencies for the onset of myoclonic jerks and convulsions and completely blocked the tonic extensor phase but also completely reversed the Ro 5-4864-induced mortality. Pretreatment of animals with subprotective doses of adenosine and dipyridamole produced significant prolongation in the latencies for the onset of myoclonic jerks and convulsions due to both DMCM and Ro 5-4864. Similarly, subprotective doses of adenosine and diazepam further delayed the latencies for the onset of myoclonic jerks and convulsions due to Ro 5-4864. The tonic extensor phase was completely blocked by pretreatment with subprotective doses of adenosine and dipyridamole as well as adenosine and diazepam against DMCM-induced convulsions.

It has been suggested that β-carbolines produce the anxiogenic and convulsant effects via negative allosteric modulation of $GABA_A$ receptors, thus reducing the GABA mediated chloride conductance[3,4]. DMCM-induced convulsions observed in the present study may be due to DMCM-induced, reduction in the chloride conductance mediated via GABA-benzodiazepine receptor ionophore complex. Diazepam pretreatment antagonised the convulsant effect of DMCM.

However, the dose-dependent protective effect offered by adenosinergic agents suggest that adenosinergic system may also possibly play a modulatory role against DMCM-induced convulsions. Moreover, subprotective doses of adenosine and diazepam produced enhanced protective effect. Diazepam has been shown to block the uptake of adenosine[22]. It is also possible that DMCM may possess antagonistic properties at the brain adenosine receptors in addition to any actions at the GABA-benzodiazepine receptor complex. The evidence for such adenosine-antagonistic properties of some β-carbolines has been recently presented[11]. It has been suggested that activation of adenosine receptors has modulatory effects on calcium channels which may stabilise the CNS neurones as well as cause cerebral vasodilation thereby improving the cerebral circulation[23]. Such effects may contribute to the observed adenosinergic protective effect.

Ro 5-4864 has been suggested to bind at high concentration to the picrotoxinin domain on the GABA-benzodiazepine receptor ionophore complex leading to convulsant effects[8-10]. Recently, it has been suggested that Ro 5-4864 interacts with brain adenosine system[12]. In the present study, Ro, 5-4864-induced convulsions were antagonised by adenosinergic agents. Moreover, subprotective doses of adenosine and dipyridamole as well as adenosine and diazepam produced significantly enhanced protective effect indicating the involvement of adenosinergic system. It has been suggested that adenosine receptor-coupled processes may be possible substrates for the mechanisms underlying some of the syndromes of epilepsy and these processes may contribute significantly to the homeostatic regulation of CNS excitability[13-14]. The observed protective effect of adenosine and adenosine analogues may be due to the inhibition of both spontaneous and evoked neuronal firing via activation of brain adenosine receptors[15,16]. Moreover, adenosine has been shown to modulate the release of several neurotransmitters in the brain[24,25].

The present results suggest that adenosine and adenosine receptor agonists, 2-chloroadenosine and N^6-cyclohexyladenosine are protective against both DMCM- and Ro 5-4864-induced convulsions. It is suggested that adenosinergic agents possibly modulate the convulsant effects of benzodiazepine inverse agonist DMCM- and peripheral agonist Ro 5-4864 via activation of central adenosine receptors in mice. This study further supports the notion that adenosinergic mechanisms mediate the neuroprotective effects.

REFERENCES

1. Hunkeler W, Mohler H, Pieri L, Polc P, Bonetti E P, Cumin R, Schaffner R & Haefely W, *Nature,* 290 (1981) 514.
2. Ehlert F J, *Trends Pharmacol Sci,* 7 (1986) 28.
3. Braestrup C, Nielsen M, Honore T, Jensen L H & Petersen E N, *J Neuropharmacology,* 22 (1983) 1451.
4. Petersen E N, *Eur J Pharmacol,* 94 (1983) 117.
5. Braestrup C, Schmiechen R, Neef G, Nielsen M & Petersen E N, *Science,* 216 (1982) 1241.
6. Kunchandy J & Kulkarni S K, *Indian J Exp Biol,* 26 (1988) 625.
7. Massotti M, Lucantoni D, Caporali M G, Mele L & Gatta F, *J Pharmacol Exp Ther,* 234 (1985) 274.
8. Pillow S & File S E, *Neurosci Biobehav Rev,* 8 (1984) 405.
9. Ticku M K & Ramanjaneyulu R, *Life Sci,* 34 (1984) 631.
10. Kunchandy J & Kulkarni S K, *Psychopharmacology,* 93 (1987) 113.
11. Phillis J W & O'Regan M H, *Prog Neuropsychopharmacol Biol Psychiatry,* 12 (1988) 389.
12. Phillis J W, O'Regan M H & Stair R E, *Brain Res,* 416 (1987) 171.
13. Murray T F, Sylvester D, Schutz C S & Szot P, *Neuropharmacology* 24 (1985) 761.
14. Franklin P H, Tripp E D, Zhang G, Gale K & Murray T F, *Eur J Pharmacol,* 150 (1988) 207.
15. Fredholm B B & Hedqvist P, *Biochem Pharmacol,* 29 (1980) 1635.

16. Phillis J W & Wu P H, *Prog Neurobiol,* 16 (1981) 187.

17. Dragunow M, *Trends Pharmacol Sci,* 7 (1986) 128.

18. Dragunow M & Faull R L M, *Trends Pharmacol Sci,* 9 (1988) 193.

19. Thorat S N & Kulkarni S K, *Meth Find Exp Clin Pharmacol,* 12 (1990) 17.

20. Williams M, *Annu Rev Pharmacol Toxicol,* 27 (1987) 315.

21. Deckert J & Gleiter C H, *Trends Pharmacol Sci,* 10 (1989) 99.

22. Phillis J W, *Can J Physiol Pharmacol,* 57 (1979) 432.

23. Kuroda Y in *Adenosine: Receptors and modulation* of *cell function* edited by Stefanovich V. Rudolphi K & Schubert P (IRL Press, Oxford) 1985, 233.

24. Snyder S H, *Annu Rev Neurosci,* 8 (1985) 103.

25. Fredholm B B & Dunwiddie T V, *Trends Pharmacol Sci,* 9 (1988) 130.

Paper Published In:
I.J.E.B. (Vol. 28, December 1990, pp. 1160-1165)

11

Effect of NMDA-receptor ligands on neocortical and hippocampal EEG activity of rat brain

AVADHESH C SHARMA & S.K. KULKARNI
Pharmacology Division, Department of Pharmaceutical Sciences,
Panjab University, Chandigarh 160 014, India
and **USHA NAYAR**
Department of Physiology, All India Institute of Medical Sciences,
New Delhi 110 029, India

Neocortex and hippocampus play important role in motor activity, neuronal plasticity and learning and memory mechanisms. Electroencephalographic (EEG) activity of neocortex and hippocampus of rat following NMDA-receptor agonist, N-methyl-D-aspartate (NMDA), 0.25-2 nmol in 10 µl, ICV and noncompetitive NMDA-receptor antagonists, MK 801 (0.025-0.1 mg/kg, ip) and ketamine (10-50 mg/kg, ip) at 0H, ½H, 4H, 8H and 24H was recorded. The electrodes were implanted stereotaxically in hippocampus and neocortex respectively. NMDA (0.25 and 1 nmol) showed longer lasting decrease in amplitude in hippocampus and in frequency in cortical neurons while 2 nmol produced epileptogenic neurotoxicity. Opposite effect i.e. increase in amplitude in both, hippocampus and neocortex was observed with MK 801 and ketamine and these agents also showed longer lasting influence. Administration of MK 801 (0.05 mg/kg) and ketamine (50 mg/kg) prior to NMDA 2 nmol protected 40% animals from NMDA-induced neurotoxicity and blockade of NMDA-induced long term influence. The EEG effect of NMDA agonist and NMDA-induced neurotoxicity at higher dose and its modification by NMDA-antagonist, MK 801 and ketamine suggest that beside NMDA agonists (NMDA), its antagonists may, also affect long lasting changes in hippocampus and cortex. These antagonists reverse NMDA-mediated long term influence in these brain areas.

Excitatory amino acids (EAA), neurotransmitters, glutamate and aspartate participate in normal synaptic transmission in the brain through well characterized EAA-receptor system(s). A significant advancement in EAA-receptor pharmacology has been made and the NMDA-receptor(s) have been described to play a role in the synaptic plasticity, cognitive performance and memory mechanisms[1,2]. Electrophysiological and radioligand binding studies employing fairly selective agonist (e.g. L(^{3}H) glutamate) and antagonist, D-2-amino-5-phosphopentanoic acid suggested wide spread distribution of NMDA-receptor(s) in neocortical and hippocampal brain areas which are well in association with motor and memory functions[3-6]. Recent studies have demonstrated that activation of NMDA-receptors causes the induction of long term potentiation (LTP) in CA1 region of hippocampus and neocortex brain areas and this phenomenon is thought to be an attractive mechanism for information storage and learning and memory mechanisms[2]. Various competitive (AP5) and noncompetitive antagonists, including dizocilpine (MK 801), of NMDA receptors blocked the induction of LTP and reported to disrupt acquisition and produce attentional deficits in several psychobehavioural studies[7-10]. MK 801 produced acquisition deficits in passive avoidance step-down task paradigm in mice[11]. Sagrettela and coworkers reported that MK 801 and other NMDA-antagonists produced cortical desynchronisation and typical cortical complexes[12]. Presence of atropine sensitive and resistant hippocampal EEG activity with low doses of MK 801 have also been demonstrated by Whinshaw and Auer[13].

In the present study EEG changes in rat cortex and hippocampal brain areas due to NMDA and its modification by non-competitive NMDA-receptor antagonists, MK 801 and ketamine, were investigated to understand long lasting effect of these agents, if any.

Materials and Methods

Male wistar albino rats (Central Animal House, AIIMS, New Delhi) weighing 200-250 g were used in the study. The rats were housed and maintained on 12 hr light/dark cycle and fed with food and water *ad libitum*. Under pentobarbitone anaesthesia (40 mg/kg, ip) iron electrodes were implanted in hippocampus (2.7 mm posterior to bregma, 3 mm lateral to midline and 3.5 mm ventral to the surface of skull) and neocortex (2 mm posterior to bregma, 2 mm lateral to midline and 1.5 mm ventral to surface of skull)[14]. A polyethylene canula (2 mm posterior to bregma, 2 mm lateral to midline and 4 mm ventral to the surface of skull), for intracerebroventricular administration of NMDA, was also implanted with dental cement taking all necessary aseptic precautions. The animals were kept individually in cages for three days to provide recovery from surgical trauma. Each animal was acclimatized to recording room for 24H preceding experiment. EEG recordings were carried out on Grass Model 7D polygraph (Grass Instruments Co., Quincy, Mass, USA). The changes in EEG were recorded simultaneously for cortex and hippocampus 30 min before and after 30 min, 4H, 8H and 24H of administration of testing drug. In case of NMDA, EEG changes were also recorded immediately after icv administration. Each animal served its own control and mean % change at each time point was calculated from EEG recorded 30 min prior drug administration (control).

Drugs: The drugs used as pharmacological interventions were NMDA, 0.25-2 nmol in 10 μl (Sigma, USA); MK 801, 0.025-0.1 mg/kg (MSD, England); ketamine, 10-50 mg/kg (Themis Chemical Ltd, India) and pentobarbitone sodium (John Baker Inc.; USA). All drugs were dissolved in distilled water and administered intraperitoneally, except NMDA, which was administered by icv route in a volume of 10 μl.

Statistical analysis: The data was analysed by one way analysis of variance (ANOVA) amongst the groups. Further application of least significant difference procedure was performed for testing significance of each group. $P < 0.05$ was considered as significant[15].

Results

I. Effect of NMDA-receptor ligands on cortical EEG activity of rat brain

(a) NMDA: ICV administration of NMDA at lower doses (0.25-1 nmol/rat) showed significant decrease in frequency, the effect lasting up to 24 hr (Table 1). However, the effect on the amplitude was not unidirectional and hence found statistically insignificant (Table 2, Fig. la). NMDA (2 nmol) produced severe convulsions and death within few seconds of NMDA administration (Tables 1, 2 and Fig. 1 b).

(b) MK 801 and ketamine: NMDA antagonists, MK 801 (0.025 mg/kg) and ketamine (10-25 mg/kg) produced significant decrease in frequency of cortical impulses. Higher dose of ketamine (50 mg/kg) produced significant increase in frequency, the effect lasting up to 24 hrs. However, MK 801 (0.10 mg/kg) showed increase in frequency but found statistically insignificant (Table1).

Table 1. Effect of NMDA-receptor ligands on neocortical EEG activity (% change in frequency) of rat brain [Five animals were used in each group]

Treatment Dose & Route		Frequency 0H	½H	4H	8H	24H	*P<0.05 F-ratio
NMDA (icv)	0.25 nmol	↓25.76	↓16.27	↓15.30	↓9.12	↓22.03	*
	1.00 nmol	↓29.33	↓46.94	↓11.09	↓6.66	↓10.71	***
	2.00 nmol		Severe convulsion and death				5.794
MK 801 (ip)	0.025 mg/kg		↓17.46	↓15.34	↓20.70	↓21.76	*
	0.05 mg/kg		↑2.97	↓2.11	↑7.01	↑10.73	*
	0.10 mg/kg		↓19.80	↓15.63	↓26.20	↓21.60	NS
							44.217
Ketamine (ip)	10 mg/kg		↓16.27	↓14.38	↓14.28	NR	*
	25 mg/kg		↓9.47	↓13.18	↓17.09	NR	*
	50 mg/kg		↑29.09	↑30.91	↑37.47	↑30.84	*
							246.22
MK 801 (ip)	0.5 mg/kg	↓33.11	↓11.29	↓12.22	-		NS
	+						
NMDA (icv)	2 nmol						6.855
Ketamine (ip)	50 mg/kg	↓35.23	↓15.85	↓10.76	↑0.97	↑2.74	NS
	+						
NMDA (icv)	2 nmol						2.874

MK 801 (0.025-0.1 mg/kg) showed significant increase in amplitude which lasted up to 24 hr (Table 2), associated with muscular incoordination (data not shown). Typical cortical EEG pattern, after administration of MK 801 (0.05 mg/kg) is illustrated in Fig. 2. Ketamine (25 and 50 mg/kg) though showed an initial increase in amplitude (0.5 decreased the same afterwards and found statistically insignificant.

(c) NMDA and MK 801 or ketamine: Administration of MK 801 (0.05 mg/kg) or ketamine (50 mg/kg) followed by NMDA (2 nmol, icv) protected, 2 out of 5 animals (data not shown in table) from NMDA-induced convulsions and death. The change in amplitude and frequency was not found statistically significant, however, showed a decrease in amplitude and frequency immediately after administration of NMDA (Tables 1 and 2; Fig.3).

II. Effect of NMDA-receptor ligands on hippocampal EEG activity of rat brain

(a) NMDA: ICV administration of NMDA (0.25-1 nmol) did not show unidirectional effect on percent frequency of hippocampal neurons and hence found statistically insignificant (Table 3). However, NMDA (1 nmol) significantly decreased the amplitude even up to 24 hr (Table 4). EEG pattern obtained from hippocampal neurons is illustrated in Fig. 4a. NMDA (2 nmol, icv) produced severe convulsions and death (Tables 3, 4 and Fig.4b).

Table 2. Effect of NMDA-receptor ligand on neocortical EEG activity (% change in amplitude) of rat brain [Five animals were used in each group]

Treatment Dose & Route		Frequency					*P<0.05* F-ratio
		0H	½H	4H	8H	24H	
NMDA (icv)	0.25 nmol	↓18.98	↓13.92	↓26.58	↑2.28	↓0.52	NS
	1.00 nmol	↑9.68	↓23.38	↑77.41	↓35.48	↓39.51	NS
	2.00 nmol	Severe convulsion and death					0.205
MK 801 (ip)	0.025 mg/kg		↑341.58	↑355.16	↑470.60	↑409.50	*
	0.05 mg/kg		↑132.80	↑122.09	↑257.74	↑106.83	*
	0.10 mg/kg		↑269.30	↑269.72	↑622.79	↑272.09	*
							10.711
Ketamine (ip)	10 mg/kg		↓30.77	↓23.08	↓61.54	NR	NS
	25 mg/kg		↑51.06	↓36.17	↓29.78	NR	NS
	50 mg/kg		↑51.32	↓10.53	↓44.74	↓40.79	NS
							8.821
MK 801 (ip)	0.5 mg/kg +	↓6.25	↑68.75	↑56.25		NS	
NMDA (icv)	2 nmol						3.046
Ketamine (ip)	50 mg/kg +	↓47.5	↓30.0	↑15.0	↑15.0	↓30.0	NS
NMDA (icv)	2 nmol						1.454

Table 3. Effect of NMDA-receptor ligands on hippocampal EEG activity (% change in frequency) of rat brain [Five animals were used in each group]

Treatment Dose & Route		Frequency					*P<0.05* F-ratio
		0H	½H	4H	8H	24H	
NMDA (icv)	0.25 nmol	↓13.53	↓5.09	↓2.45	↑7.31	↓7.35	NS
	1.00 nmol	↓4.05	↓14.00	↓2.91	↑8.58	↓0.32	NS
	2.00 nmol	Severe convulsion and death					0.537
MK 801 (ip)	0.025 mg/kg		↓31.06	↓22.52	↓18.64	↓25.09	*
	0.05 mg/kg		↑6.10	↓5.66	↑4.94	↑19.64	NS
	0.10 mg/kg		↓13.25	↓22.09	↓19.12	↓21.98	*
							14.397
Ketamine (ip)	10 mg/kg		↓6.77	↓13.36	↑11.07	NR	NS
	25 mg/kg		↓9.04	↓12.56	↓8.60	NR	*
	50 mg/kg		↑20.17	↑33.86	↑41.11	↑19.08	*
							15.765
MK 801 (ip)	0.05 mg/kg +	↓18.51	↓6.02	↓23.18	-	-	*
NMDA (icv)	2 nmol						8.178
Ketamine (ip)	50 mg/kg +	↓34.87	↓0.61	↓2.58	↓23.59	↓9.36	NS
NMDA (icv)	2 nmol						4.699

(b) MK 801 and ketamine: Administration of MK 801 (0.025 and 0.10 mg/kg) showed significant larger lasting decrease in frequency (Table 3). Ketamine (25 mg/kg) also showed significant decrease in frequency while higher dose (50 mg/kg) showed an increase in frequency (Table 3). Significant increase in amplitude was observed with MK 801 (0.05 and 0.1 mg/kg) and ketamine (50 mg/kg). However, ketamine (10 and 25 mg) did not show significant change in amplitude (Table 4). Typical EEG pattern from hippocampal brain area of rats after adminstration of MK 801 (0.05 mg/kg) is shown in Fig. 5.

(c) NMDA and MK 801 or ketamine: Administration of MK 801 (0.05 mg/kg) or ketamine (50 mg/kg) followed by NMDA (2 nmol, icv) protected, 2 out of 5, rats from NMDA-induced convulsions and death (data not shown in table). No significant change in hippocampal EEG activity was observed, however MK 801 (0.05 mg/kg) showed significant decrease in amplitude only (Tables 3 & 4). EEG pattern obtained after MK 801 (0.05) administration 30 min prior NMDA (2 nmol), is shown in Fig. 6.

Table 4. Effect of NMDA-receptor ligands on hippocampal EEG activity (% change in amplitude) of rat brain [Five Animals Were Used In Each Group]

Treatment Dose & Route		Frequency					**P<0.05* F-ratio
		0H	½H	4H	8H	24H	
NMDA (icv)	0.25 nmol	↓19.40	↓9.70	↓7.46	↑30.59	↓1.75	NS
	1.00 nmol	↓14.68	↓15.40	↓36.50	↓52.38	↓48.41	*
	2.00 nmol	Severe convulsion and death					7.868
MK 801 (ip)	0.025 mg/kg		↓10.52	↑28.05	↑17.10	↓2.63	NS
	0.050 mg/kg		↑161.31	↑201.09	↑175.90	↑57.66	*
	0.10 mg/kg		↑436.11	↑830.55	↑410.27	↑205.55	*
							10.686
Ketamine (ip)	10 mg/kg		↑57.45	↓31.91	↓42.55	NR	NS
	25 mg/kg		↑4.61	↓38.46	↓35.38	NR	NS
	50 mg/kg		↑134.38	↑50.0	↑25.0	↑30.21	*
							3.207
MK 801 (ip)	0.05 mg/kg +	↓7.08	↓73.45	↓60.18	-	-	NS
NMDA (icv)	2 nmol						8.178
Ketamine (ip)	50 mg/kg +	↓25.80	↓26.66	↑30.0	↑33.33	↓6.66	NS
NMDA (icv)	2 nmol						0.004

Discussion

The involvement of EAA-receptor system(s) particularly NMDA-receptors in synaptic plasticity, cognitive performance and memory mechanisms has been amply described[1,2]. Induction of LTP in hippocampal and neocortical synapses has been suggested as an attractive mechanism for learning and memory[2]. Collingridge and workers have demonstrated the activation of NMDA receptors in CA1 area of hippocampus as an absolute requirement for induction of LTP which was blocked by antagonist AP5 and noncompetitive antagonist MK 801[16]. Increase in second messenger Ca^{2+} is found to be an essential component of NMDA-receptor activation and LTP induction in neuronal synapses [17]. Moreover, numerous psychobehavioural studies strongly supported the requirement of NMDA-receptor dependent induction in LTP in hippocampus[2,7].

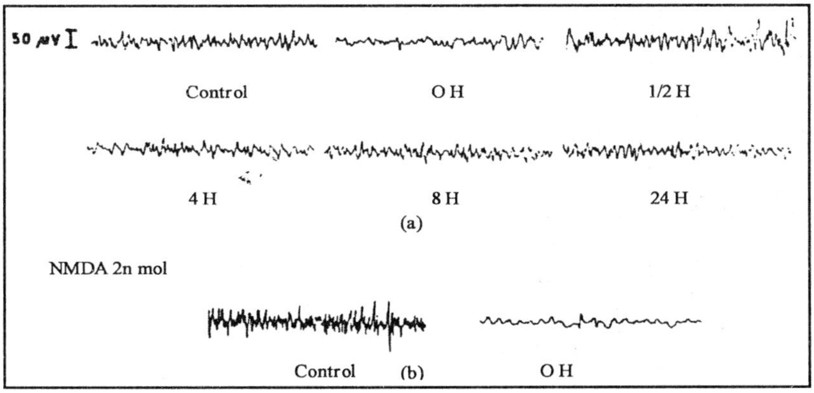

Fig. 1. Neocortical EEG activity recorded at different time intervals in rat brain after icv administration of NMDA 1 nmol (a) and 2 nmol (b)

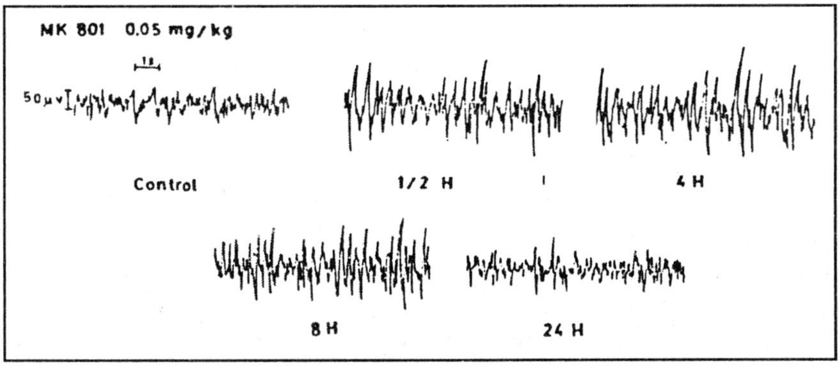

Fig. 2. Neocortical EEG activity recorded at different time intervals in rat brain after administration of MK 801 (0.05 mg/kg, ip)

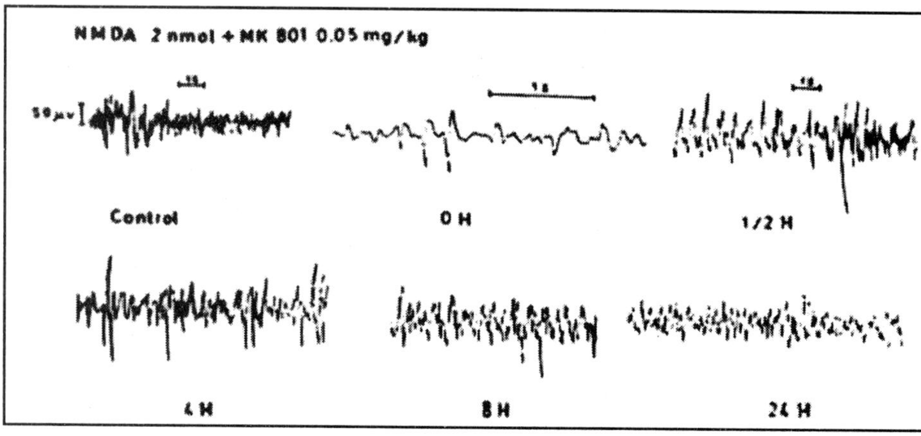

Fig. 3. Neocortical EEG activity recorded at different time intervals in rat brain after administration of MK 801 (0.05 mg/kg, ip) followed by NMDA (2 mol, icv)

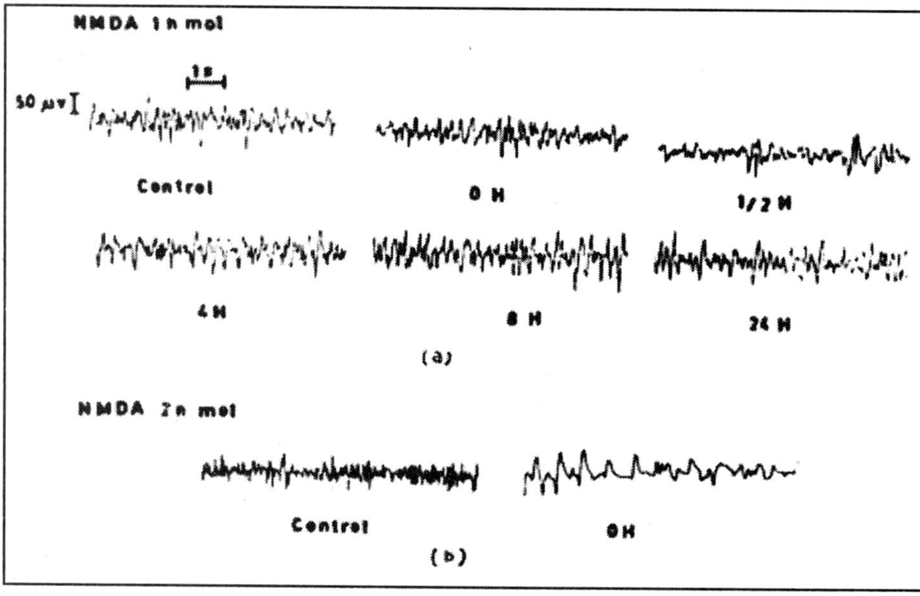

Fig. 4. Hippocampal EEG activity recorded at different time intervals in rat brain after administration of NMDA (a) 1nmol, icv and (b) 2 nmol, icv

The present study revealed that NMDA (0.25 and 1 nmol) significantly decreased frequency in cortical neurons for 24 hr. However, changes in amplitude were not unidirectional. In case of hippocampus, where there was no significant change in frequency observed, NMDA (1 nmol) showed significant decrease in amplitude, suggesting longer lasting influence of NMDA. However, the

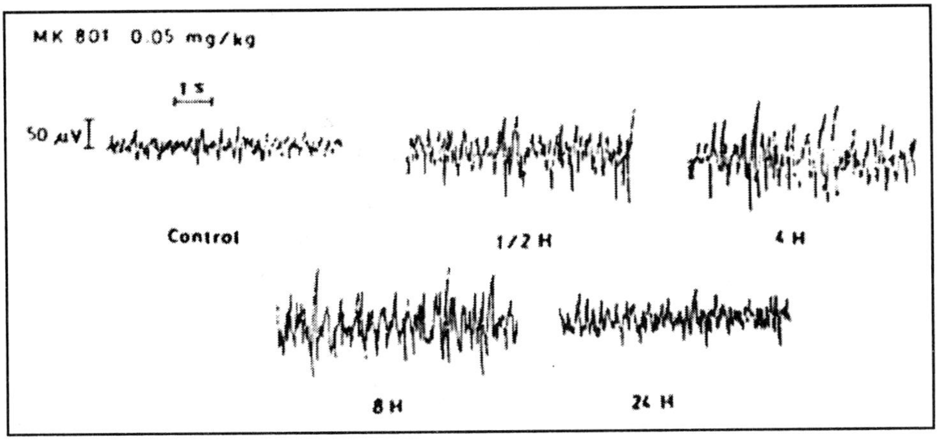

Fig. 5. Hippocampal EEG activity recorded at different time intervals in rat brain after administration of MK 801 (0.05 mg/kg, ip)

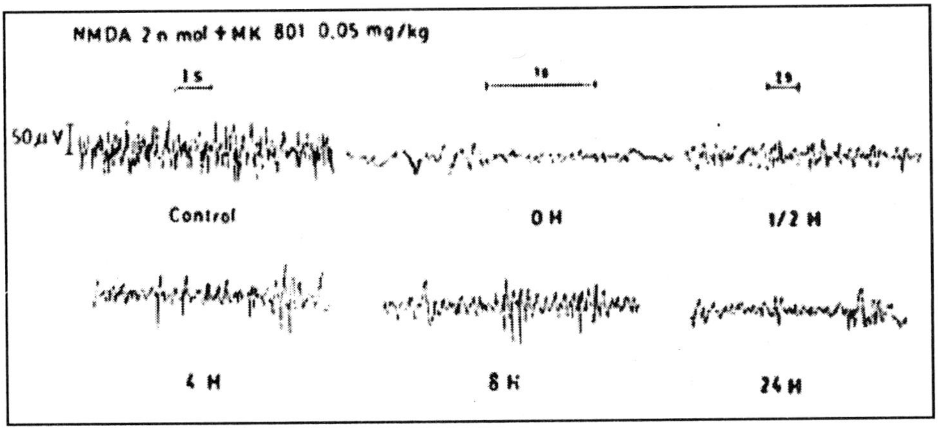

Fig. 6. Hippocampal EEG activity recorded at different time intervals in rat brain after administration of MK 801 (0.05 mg/kg, ip) followed by NMDA (2 nmol, icv)

inconsistency in changes in both areas can't be overlooked but it may be because of neurophysiological functional differences of both areas. Larger dose of NMDA (2 nmol) produced epileptogenic neurotoxicity and death in all animals. Noncompetitive NMDA-receptor antagonists, MK 801 and ketamine also influence neocortical and hippocampal EEG activity. MK 801 showed increase in neocortical and hippocampal EEG amplitude and decreased frequency where ketamine (50 mg/kg) significantly increased frequency up to 24 hrs, suggesting longer lasting effect of these agents, an opposite effect that was recorded with NMDA.

In combination studies NMDA-induced neurotoxicity was reversed by prior administration of both MK 801 (0.05 mg/kg) and ketamine (50 mg/kg). The major EEG changes were not found statistically significant in these brain areas suggesting the reversal of NMDA-induced EEG changes in the animals that survived.

The results provide an evidence for long term influence of NMDA-receptor in neocortical and hippocampal brain areas and suggest that it is not only restricted to NMDA-receptor agonist but NMDA-receptor antagonist may also affect the NMDA-receptor mediated neurotransmission. These observations support the contention that NMDA receptors are involved in synaptic plasticity and memory mechaisms.

REFERENCES

1. Monaghan D T, Bridges R J & Cotman C W, *Annu Rev Pharmacol Toxicol*, 29 (1989) 365.
2. Collingridge G L & Singer W, *TIPS*, 11 (1990) 290.
3. Fagg G E, *TIPS*, 8 (1985) 207.
4. Foster A C & Fagg G E, *Eur J Pharmacol*, 133 (1987) 291.
5. Cowburn R, Hardy J, Roberts P & Briggs R, *Brain Res*, 452 (1988) 403.
6. Young A B & Fagg G E, *TIPS*, 11 (1990) 126.
7. Staubli U, Thibault O, Dilorenzo M & Lynch G, *Behav Neurosci*, 103 (1989) 54.
8. Herberg L J & Rose I C, *Psychopharmacology*, 99 (1989) 87.
9. Butelman E R, *Pharmacol Biochem Behav*, 35 (1990) 533.
10. Upchurch M & Wehner J M, *Psychopharmacology*, 100 (1990) 200.
11. Sharma A C & Kulkarni S K, *Meth Find Exp Clin Pharmacol*, 13 (1991) 155.
12. Sagratella S, Benedetti M, Pezzola A & Scotti DeCarolis A, *Neuropharmacology*, 28 (1989) 57.
13. Whinshaw I Q & Auer R N, *Psychopharmacology*, 98 (1989) 500.
14. Paxinos G & Watson C, *The brain in stereotaxic coordinates* (Academic Press, Sydney) 1982.
15. Rudolph L K & Ciminara J L, *Remington's Pharmaceutical Sciences*, edited by Gennaro A R, 17th Ed (Mack Publishers, USA) 1985, 104.

16. Collingridge G L, Kehl S J & Mclennan H, *J Physiol,* 334 (1983) 33.

17. Mayer M L & Miller R J, *TIPS,* 11 (1990) 254

18. Venable N & Kelly P H, *Psychopharmacology,* 100 (1990) 215.

Paper Published In:
I.J.E.B. (Vol. 29, August 1991, pp. 744-750)

12

On the convulsant action of DMCM and Ro 5-4864 in Mice

JOSEPH KUNCHANDY & S.K. KULKARNI
Pharmacology Division. Department of Pharmaceutical Sciences,
Panjab University, Chandigarh 160 014, India

The difference in the mechanism of convulsant action of the benzodiazepine (BZ) inverse agonist DMCM and the peripheral type BZ receptor agonist Ro 5-4864 were elucidated in mice. DMCM and Ro 5-4864 produced clonic-tonic convulsions in mice at 25 and 60 mg/kg dose, respectively. Activation of central $alpha_2$ adrenoceptors by clonidine significantly delayed the onset of Ro 5-4864-induced convulsions while no significant effect was seen in DMCM-induced seizures mice. Pretreatment with Ro 15-1788 failed to antagonise the convulsant effect of Ro 5-4864. On the other hand, DMCM induced seizures were fully antagonized by the BZ receptor antagonist Ro 15-1788. The possible difference in the convulsive mechanism of DMCM and Ro 5-4864 is discussed.

Benzodiazepine (BZ) receptor is the site of action of three classes of pharmacologically distinct agents. They are agonists, inverse agonist and competitive antagonist[1]. DMCM is a BZ inverse agonist with anxiogenic and convulsant properties[2-4]. It is demonstrated that the inverse agonist reduces GABAergic effects[5] leading to anxiety and convulsion. Ro 5-4864 is also a BZ receptor ligand preferring the peripheral type BZ receptors, with anxiogenic and convulsant properties[6,7]. The centrally located $alpha_2$ adrenoceptors are shown to have a modulatory role on diazepam and Ro 5-4864-induced GABAergic responses[8-11].

In the present study, the differences in the mechanisms of the convulsive actions of BZ inverse agonist, DMCM and BZ peripheral receptor agonist, Ro 5-4864 are elucidated, and also the protective effect of $alpha_2$ adrenoceptor agonists when studied as we have extensively reported about diazepam-like and anticonvulsant actions of clonidine, a prototype $alpha_2$-adrenoceptor agonist.

Materials and Methods

Wistar mice of either sex (25-30g) from the CAH, Panjab University, Chandigarh, were used. Food and water were withdrawn 1 hr prior to the experiments.

Convulsions were induced by DMCM (25 mg/kg, ip) or Ro 5-4864 (60 mg/kg, ip). These doses were selected on the basis of preliminary study or based on the earlier report from our laboratory. The latencies of jerk and full body convulsions were noted as described by Dunwiddie and Worth[12]. Doses of clonidine, guanfacine, B-HT 920 and ICI 106270 were given 15 min prior to the convulsant agent. Antagonists were given 10-15 min prior to the agonists.

Drugs: DMCM (methyl-6,7-dimethoxy-beta-carboline-3-carboxylate, Schering, Berlin), Ro 5-4864 (p-Chlorodiazepam, Hoffmann-La Roche, Nutley), Ro 15-1788 (flumazenil, F. Hoffmann-La Roche, Basel), clonidine (Boehringer, Ingelheim, FRG), guanfacine (Sandoz, Switzerland), B-HT 920 (6-allyl-2-amino-5, 6, 7, 8-tetrahydro-4H-thiazolo [4,5-d] azepine dihydrochloride, Boehringer, Ingelheim, FRG), ICI 106270 (6-aryl-2,3,6,7-tetrahydro-5H-pyrrolo [1, 2-a]-imidazole, Imperial Chemical Industries, U.K.), Idazoxan (Reckitt and Colman, Hull) were used in the present study. DMCM, Ro 5-4864 and Ro 15-1788 were uniformaly dispersed in distilled water with a few drops of Tween 80. Injection volume of 10 ml/kg was kept constant. All drugs were administered ip.

Statistical analysis: The data were analysed using Student's t test.

Results

Convulsant effect of Ro 5-4864 and DMCM: Ro 5-4864 (60 mg/kg) produced violent clonic-tonic convulsion within 7 min. DMCM (25 mg/kg)-induced convulsions were of intermittent clonics followed by multiple tonic convulsion.

Effect of $alpha_2$ adrenoceptor agonists and Ro 15-1788 on Ro 5-4864-induced convulsions: Various doses of clonidine (0.1-1 mg/kg) shared dose-dependent increase in latency for jerk and convulsion. Other alpha$_2$ adrenoceptor agonists such as guanfacine, ICI 106270 and B-HT 920 also delayed the latency for jerk and convulsion (Table 1). Pretreatment with BZ receptor antagonist, Ro 15-1788 (10 mg/kg, ip) failed to modify the latency of jerk or convulsion due to Ro 5-4864 (Table 1).

Effect of pretreatment with idazoxan on clonidine and ICI-106270-induced protection– Pretreatment with the specific alpha$_2$ adrenoceptor antagonist, idazoxan, reversed the protective effect of clonidine and ICI 106270 against Ro 5-4864-induced convulsion. Idazoxan (1 mg/kg) was devoid of any *per se* effect (Table 1).

Effect of clonidine, diazepam and Ro 15-1788 *on DMCM-induced convulsions in* mice– Treatment with varying doses of clonidine (0.1-1 mg/kg) failed to protect the animals against DMCM-induced convulsions. The latencies for jerk and convulsion were unchanged compared to control values. However, pretreatment with BZ antagonist, Ro 15-1788 and diazepam reversed the convulsant effect of DMCM (Table 2).

Table 1. Effect of Various Doses of Clonidine, Guanfacine, B-HT 920, ICI 106270 and Ro 15-1788 on Ro 5-4864-Induced Seizures in Mice: Modification of Clonidine and ICI 106270 Effects by Idazoxan [Values are mean ± SE]

Sl No	Treatment (mg/kg, ip)	n	Latency (min)	
			Jerk	Convulsion
1	Control-R$_0$5-4864(60)	13	6.05 ±0.27	7.37±0.47
2	Clonidine(0.1)	5	6.30±0.19	8.22±0.28
3	Clonidine (0.2)	5	7.07 ± 0.28	9.20 ± 1.00
4	Clonidine(0.5)	6	10.04±0.40	18.01 ± 1.27
5	Clonidine (1)	8	14.3 ± 0.62	28.3 ± 0.68
6	Guanfacine(0.5)	6	6.45±0.56	9.38±0.53*
7	B-HT 920 (0.5)	6	6.41 ± 1.19	9.37±0.49*
8	ICI 106270 (0.5)	5	7.02±0.21**	13.33±0.53**
9	Ro 15-1788(10)	5	4.06 ±0.28	5.3±0.31
10	Idazoxan + Clonidine (1) (0.5)	6	6.04 ±0.51	10.5 ± 1.12
11	Idazoxan +ICI 106270 (1) (0.5)	5	5.40 ±0.33	9.15 ± 1.31
12	Idazoxan (1)	5	5.49±0.42	8.1 ± 1.38

*P<0.05; ** P< 0.001 when compared with control. P<0.001 when compared between groups 1&4; 1&5; 2&4; 2&5; 3&4; 3&5; 4&5 using ANOVA test.

Table 2. Effect of Various Doses of Clonidine, Diazepam and Ro 15-1788 on DMCM-induced Seizures in Mice [Values are mean ± SE]

Sl No.	Treatment (mg/kg, ip)	n	Latency (min)	
			Jerk	Convulsion
1	Control (DMCM) (25)	10	3.20±0.15	3.27 ± 1.44
2	Clonidine (0.1)	6	4.0 ±0.33	4.37±0.40
3	Clonidine(0.25)	6	3.56±0.60	4.20±0.31
4	Clonidine(0.5)	5	3.20±0.20	3.54±0.22
5	Clonidine (1)	6	3.06 ±0.45	3.30 ±0.32
6	Diazepam (5)	5	-	-
7	Ro 15-1788 (10)	6	-	-

Discussion

The peripheral BZ receptor agonist, Ro 5-4864 produced severe clonic-tonic convulsions. The myoclonic jerks were, followed by severe convulsion characterised by rotational movements, violent abdominal writhing, chewing response and profused salivation. On the other hand, the BZ inverse agonist, DMCM convulsions were of intermittent clonic type of jerks followed by tonic convulsion. Pretreatment with $alpha_2$ adrenoceptor agonists shared significant protective effect as the latencies for jerk and convulsion are concerned. Similar treatment with the potent $alpha_2$ adrenoceptor agonist, clonidine, failed to exhibit any protective effect in DMCM-induced convulsions. However the benzodiazepine receptor antagonist, Ro 15-1788, antagonized the convulsant action of DMCM but not that induced by Ro 5-4864.

Ro 5-4864, chlorodiazepam, is a selective ligand for GABA independent peripheral and micromolar binding sites[13,14] but the pharmacological relevance of these sites is still not clearly defined. However, convincing evidences suggest a regulator role of Ca- channel function by these BZ sites[15]. PK 11195, the peripheral BZ receptor antagonist, reversed the anxiogenic and the convulsant actions of Ro 5-4864[16,17]. The involvement of micromolar BZ site in Ro-4864 was ruled out since phenytoin which has high affinity for the micromolar BZ site[18] failed to protect the animals from Ro 5-4864-induced seizures[10]. But the electrophysiological evidences suggest the involvement of GABA BZ chloride ionophore complex in Ro 5-4864 actions. Ticku and Ramanjaneyulu[19] have shown that Ro 5-4864 can displace ^{35}S-TBPT from the picrotoxinin domain of GABA BZ complex. Similar conclusion of the involvement of picrotoxinan site was also reported[10]. Hence, in the light of the pharmacological, electrophysiological and radioligand studies, it may be concluded that the convulsant action of Ro 5-4864 is mediated through the picrotoxinin site in the GABA BZ complex.

Apart from the picrotoxinin site, another convulsant site has been demonstrated in GABA BZ complex. The BZ receptors are speculated to contain recognition sites for three types of high affinity exogenous ligands with different pharmacological profile. The agonists, anxiolytics and anticontulsants are the positive allosteric modulators of $GABA_A$ receptors thus enhancing GABA mediated chloride conductance. The inverse agonists, anxiogenic and convulsant, are the negative allosteric modulators of $GABA_A$ receptors, thus reducing GABA mediated chloride conductance. The competitive antagonists are practically inactive *per se* but abolish BZ receptor-mediated pharmacological effects of agonists and inverse agonists[1]. Thus the BZ receptor probably contains a convulsant site and an anticonvulsant site which modulates GABA mediated chloride flux.

Ro 5-4864-induced seizures are not antagonized by BZ receptor antagonist, Ro 15-1788, indicating that the convulsant site of BZ receptor is not involved while the convulsant action of DMCM is fully antagonised by Ro 15-1788.

Clonidine is reported to have anticonvulsant effect against electro- and chemoconvulsions[11,20,21]. In the present study also clonidine and other $alpha_2$ adrenoceptor agonists shared significant anticonvulsant effect against Ro 5-4864-induced seizures. Similar activation of $alpha_2$ adrenoceptors failed to show any protection against DMCM-induced seizures. But the basic mechanism of DMCM- and Ro 5-4864-induced seizures are known to be due to reduction in GABA mediated chloride conductance[5,22]. However, the pathways or sites involved in modulating GABAergic chloride conductance by Ro 5-4864 and DMCM appears to be different since the anticonvulsant profile of $alpha_2$ agonists were different in Ro 5-4864- and DMCM-induced seizures. $Alpha_2$ adrenoceptor have a modulatory effect on the pathway or site of Ro 5-4864 seizures while no such effect could be seen in DMCM seizures. However, the differences in the site of action of these agents as well as the pharmacokinetic possibilities cannot be ruled out. The present study shows that $alpha_2$ adrenoceptors can modulate picrotoxinin site mediated GABAergic effects while BZ inverse agonist mediated GABAergic effects remain unaffected.

REFERENCES

1. Richards J G, Schoch P, Mohler H & Haefely W, *Experientia*, 42 (1986) 121.
2. Braestrup C, Schmiechen R, Neef G, Nielsen M & Petersen E N, *Science*, 216 (1982) 1241.
3. Petersen E N, *Eur J Pharmacol*, 94 (1983) 117.
4. Skovgaard Jensen M S & Lambert J D C, *Neurosci Lett*, 40 (1983) 175.
5. Barker J L, Gratz E, Owen D G & Study R E, in *Actions and interactions of GABA and benzodiazepines*, edited by NG Bowery (Raven Press, New York) 1984, 203.
6. File S E & Lister R G, *Neurosci Lett*, 35 (1983) 93.
7. Weissman B A. Cott J, Paul S M & Skolnick P, *Eur J Pharmacol*, 90 (1983) 149.
8. Kunchandy J & Kulkarni S K, *Psychopharmacology*, 90 (1986) 198
9. Kunchandy J & Kulkarni S K, *Indian J Exp Biol*, 25 (1987) 115.
10. Kunchandy J & Kulkarni S K, *Psychopharmacology*, 93 (1987)113.
11. Kulkarni S K. *Arch Int Pharmacodyn*, 252 (1981) 124.
12. Dunwiddie T V & Worth T, *J Pharmacol Exp Ther*, 220 (1982)70.
13. Braestrup C & Squires R F, *Proc Natl Acad Sci USA*, 74 (1977) 3805.
14. DeLorenzo R J, Burdette S & Holderness J, *Science*, 213 (1981)546.
15. Rampe D & Triggle D J, *Eur J Pharmacol*, 134 (1987) 189.
16. File S E & Pellow S, *Psychopharmacology*, 80 (1983) 166.
17. File S E & Pellow S, *Brain Res*, 278 (1983) 370.
18. Bowling A C & DeLorenzo R J, *Science*, 216 (1982) 1247.
19. Tieku M K & Ramanjaneyulu R, *Life Sci*, 34 (1984) 631.
20. Kulkarni S K & Mehta A K, *Physchopharmacology*, 79 (1983) 287.
21. Kulkarni S K & Nagrath A, *Clin Exp Pharmacol Physiol*, 10 (1983) 125.
22. MacNeil D A, D'Amico J A, Horst W D, O'Brien R A & Spirit N, *Soc Neurosci Abstr*, 9 (1983) 412.

Paper Published In:
I.J.E.B. (Vol. 26, August 1988, pp. 625-627)

13

Autonomic hyperactivity on diazepam withdrawal in rats

JOSEPH KUNCHANDY & S.K. KULKARNI
Pharmacology Division, Department of Pharmaceutical Sciences, Panjab University, Chandigarh 160014, India
and **V.K. SHUKLA**
Department of Pharmacology, Postgraduate Institute of Medical Education and Research, Chandigarh 160012, India

Brain biogenic amines such as noradrenaline, dopamine, 5-hydroxytryptamine and its metabolite 5-hydroxyindoleacetic acid were estimated on 3rd day of chronic diazepam withdrawal as hyperactivity was noticed on the same day. The hyperfunction of adrenergic system in diazepam abstinence was indexed by monitoring the heart rate also. Significant increase in brain noradrenaline content and, locomotion and heart rate indicated a state of adrenergic hyperfunction in diazepam withdrawal. Clonidine (100 mg/kg, ip, twice daily) attenuated this observed hyperactivity. Involvement of adrenergic system in diazepam abstinence syndrome is discussed.

Like other hypnotics and narcotics, benzodiazepines have the pharmacological potential to produce dependence and thereby withdrawal symptoms in experimental animals and human beings[1-4]. Biochemical studies have shown that chronic diazepam treatment caused a selective subsensitivity to GABA in serotonergic dorsal raphae nucleus in rats which can be correlated with the abstinence syndromes[5]. However, Gonsalves and Gallager[6] reported that GABAergic and 5-HT mechanisms in dorsal raphae are not directly responsible for CNS hyperexcitability in diazepam abstinence. An adrenergic hyperactivity in diazepam withdrawal has been demonstrated[4]. The possibility of such a non-GABAergic mechanism has already been suggested[7,8].

Recent studies have shown that central catecholamine release plays an important role in the initiation and maintenance of opiate withdrawal symptoms[9,10]. Measurement of autonomic changes associated with abstinence syndrome is more sensitive index than behavioral signs[11].

In the present study, changes in heart rate and locomotion as diazepam withdrawal symptoms have been measured and an attempt has been made to correlate these activities with brain monoamines in rats.

Materials and Methods

Male albino Wistar rats (200-250 g) bred in Departments animal colony were provided with rat chow (Hindustan Lever) and had free access to water.

Diazepam treatment: Diazepam (20 mg/kg, ip) was administered every day at 9.00 a.m. for 3 weeks. Control rats received a proportional quantity of 1% carboxymethylcellulose as vehicle. On completion of 3 weeks of diazepam treatment, the drug was withdrawn and the animals were divided into different groups consisting of minimum of six animals in each.

One group served as withdrawal control, the second group was treated with clonidine (100 mg/kg, ip, twice a day at 12 hr interval). Clonidine treatment was started on the day of diazepam withdrawal and continued till the 3rd day of withdrawal. The other groups were used for brain monoamine estimation and for the measurement of heart rate and locomotion.

Brain amines: On 3rd day of diazepam withdrawal the animals were sacrificed by decapitation, the whole-brain was isolated and homogenized in cold acidified butanol. The DA, NA, 5-HT and 5-HIAA contents in the whole brain were estimated fluorometrically according to the method of Cox and Perhach[12]. The following different groups were processed (1) animals on 3rd day of chronic diazepam withdrawal, (2) animals on 3rd day of clonidine therapy after the termination of chronic diazepam, (3) animals on chronic diazepam treatment, and (4) control animals which are non-diazepam and non-drug treated.

Hyperlocomotion and heart rate: The change in basal heart rate as an index of hyperfunction of adrenergic system was recorded using an electrocardiograph. The study was done on 3rd day of chronic diazepam withdrawal. The locomotor activity of the animals was measured using a photoactometer[13]. A cut off period of 10 min was fixed for each animal.

Drugs: Diazepam (Ranbaxy, New Delhi) was uniformly suspended in 1 % carboxymethylcellulose. Clonidine (Boehringer Ingelheim, New York) was dissolved in distilled water. Noradrenaline (NA), dopamine (DA), 5-hydroytryptamine (5-HT) and 5-hydroxyindoleacetic acid (5-HIAA) [Sigma, USA] were used as standards. All reagents used in the assay were of recommended analytical grade.

Statistical analysis was done using Student's t test.

Results

Brain amine content- Chronic diazepam treatment resulted in reduction of NA, 5-HT and 5-HIAA contents in the whole brain while an increase in DA content was noted. On abrupt termination of chronic diazepam, NA, 5-HT and 5-HIAA levels increased while DA level was reduced. On 3rd day of clonidine treatment, no significant changes were observed in NA and DA contents while 5-HT and 5-HIAA levels were altered when compared with diazepam-withdrawn group (Table1).

Withdrawal-induced hyperlocomotion and heart rate - A significant increase in heart rate was seen on 3rd day of chronic diazepam termination when compared with controls ($P< 0.001$ when absolute values were compared) indicating autonomic hyperfunction in diazepam abstinence in rats. Similarly a significant increase in motor activity of the rats was also observed on 3rd day of diazepam withdrawal ($P<0.001$ when absolute values were compared) (Table2).

Discussion

Incidence of diazepam withdrawal hyperactivity in rats has been reported earlier[4]. An adrenergic hyperactivity is documented in diazepam abstinence since $alpha_2$ adrenoceptor agonists such as clonidine, guanfacine and B-HT 920 were shown to be effective[4]. It was also noticed that the peak withdrawal symptoms occurred on 3rd day of diazepam withdrawal.

In the present study, the heart rate as well as locomotion was monitored since the measurement of autonomic changes is shown to

Table 1. Changes in Brain Monoamines, Noradrenaline (NA), Dopamine (DA) and 5-hydroxytryptamine (5-HT) and its metabolite, 5-hydroxyindoleacetic acid (5-HIAA) on Chronic Diazepam (3 weeks) Treatment in Rats: Modification by Clonidine
[Values are mean ± SE]

Sr. No.	Treatment (Dose)	No. of animals	Brain Tissue ng/g			
			NA	DA	5-HT	5-HIAA
1.	Control	8	522.3 ± 6.000	1203.2 ± 55.8	1293.7 ± 107.4	601.6 ± 12.9
2.	On chronic diazepam (20 mg/kg, ip)	6	389.9 ± 24.6[a]	2018.0 ± 280[c]	796.3 ± 95.0[b]	485.3 ± 18.6[a]
3.	Diazepam withdrawn (third day)	6	687.03 ± 27.8[b]	1080.0 ± 92.3	1338.8 ± 113.3	644.4 ± 35.3
4.	Diazepam withdrawn + Clonidine (100 µg/kg, ip twice daily)	6	606.5 ± 49.85	1378.5 ± 184	2155.75 ± 93.5[a]	337.2 ± 55.5[a]

[a]P<0.001 when compared with 2:1,4: 1; [b]P<0.01 when compared with 2:1,3: 1; [c]P<0.02 when compared with 2: 1.

Table 2. Change in Locomotion and Heart Rate on 3rd day of Chronic Diazepam Withdrawal in Rats: Modification by Clonidine
[Values are mean ± SE]

Sr. No.	Treatment	No. of animals	% change	
			Locomotion	Heart rate
1.	Control	12	00.0 ±0.0	00.0 ± 0.0
2.	Chronic diazepam (20 mg/kg, ip/day/3 weeks)	6	- 74.5 ± 12.8	- 12.0 ± 2.8
3	Diazepam withdrawn (third day)	11	+ 262.5 ± 14.2	+ 18.0 ± 1.5
4.	Diazepam withdrawn + Clonidine (100µg/kg, ip twice daily)	5	- 51.5 ± 16.3	–

+= increase in activity; -= decrease in activity.

be more sensitive index than behavioral signs where an adrenergic hyperactivity exists[11]. A significant increase in heart rate was seen on 3rd day of diazepam withdrawal when compared with control group. Similarly, a withdrawal hyperactivity was observed in the photoactometer studies on 3rd day of diazepam termination. This supports our previous findings, indicating an adrenergic hyperactivity on diazepam withdrawal.

An increase in NA and 5-HT brain levels was seen in diazepam withdrawn rats when compared with control and with rats on chronic diazepam treatment indicating higher level of central autonomic function. The change in DA content could not be correlated with the activity (Table 1). Clonidine treatment did not influence NA level while DA and 5-HT levels were increased. The withdrawal induced hyperlocomotion was checked by clonidine treatment (Table 2). Clonidine as such is reported to lower the adrenergic activity through central mechanism[14,15]. Hence the above observations support the fact of an increased noradrenergic function in diazepam abstinence in rats.

REFERENCES

1. Hallstrom C & Lader W, *Int Pharmacopsych,* 16 (1981) 235.
2. Tyrer P, Rutherford D & Huggett T, *Lancet,* 1 (1983) 520.
3. Murphy S M, Owen R T & Tyrer P J, *Lancet,* 2 (1984) 1389.
4. Kunchandy J & Kulkarni S K, *Psychopharmacology,* (1986) 90 (1986) 198.
5. Martin W R, McNicholas L F & Cherian S, *Life Sci,* 31(1982) 721.
6. Gonsalves S F & Gallager D W, *EurJ Pharmacol,* 110 (1985) 163.
7. Cowen P J & Nutt D J, *Lancet,* 2 (1982) 360.
8. Fariello R W & Ticku M K, *Life Sci,* 33 (1983) 1629.
9. Aghajanian G K, *Nature,* 276 (1978) 186.
10. Swann A C, Elsworth J D, Charney DS, Jablons J W, Roth RH, Redmond D E & Mass J W, *Eur J Pharmacol,* 86 (1983) 167.
11. Buccafusco J J, Marshall D C & Turner R M, *Life Sci,* **35** (1984) 1401.
12. Cox Jr R H & Perhach Jr J L, *J Neurochem,* 20 (1973) 1777.
13. Dews P B, *Br J Pharmacol Chemothr,* 8 (1953) 46.
14. Kobinger W & Walland A, *Eur J Pharmacol,* 2 (1967) 155.
15. Kobinger W & Pilcher L, *Eur J Pharmacol,* 27 (1974) 151.

Paper Published In:
I.J.E.B. (Vol. 25, February 1987, pp. 115-117)

14

Central nervous system depressant activities of melatonin in rats and mice

A.V. SHAJI & S.K. KULKARNI
Pharmacology Division, University Institute of Pharmaceutical Sciences,
Panjab University, Chandigarh 160014, India

Melatonin (10 and 20 mg/kg) potentiated pentobarbitone (45 mg/kg) induced hypnosis; it (50 and 100 mg/kg) decreased both total and ambulatory activity; produced (10, 25 and 50 mg/kg) hypothermia and possessed (10-400 mg/kg) significant analgesic property both in tail-flick and acetic acid-induced writhing tests. Melatonin in low dose (10 mg/kg) significantly reduced the forced-swimming induced immobility period *per se* and also reserpine induced immobility. While the antinociceptive effect of melatonin was sensitive to reversal by naloxone (2 mg/kg), other CNS depressant profile resembled the effects of benzodiazepines.

The pineal indoleamine melatonin plays an important role in the central nervous system not only in the modulation of biological time clóck but also in neuroendocrine and behavioural processes in man and animals. One of the earliest observations in man was a sleep-inducing effect of melatonin[1,2]. During the night its levels are high and therefore, it facilitated sleep[3]. Although melatonin is reported to decrease spontaneous activity in animals[4] there are conflicting reports regarding its effects in animal studies[5,6]. Moreover, some of the behavioural responses of melatonin have been reported to resemble those of benzodiazepines[4], the well known CNS depressant drugs. Therefore the present study has been undertaken to investigate the central nervous system depressant actions of melatonin in various animal models and the effect was compared with standard drugs.

Attempts have also been made to understand the possible mechanism of action and CNS profile of melatonin.

Materials and Methods

Animals: Wistar rats (150-200 g) and albino mice (Laka strain) (15-25 g) of either sex bred in the Central Animal House facility of the Panjab University were used. The animals were housed under standard laboratory conditions and were acclimatized to the laboratory conditions prior to experimentation and maintained at 12 hr day/night cycle. All the experiments were carried out between 10.00 and 17.00 hrs. The animals were randomly selected for each study.

Drugs: Melatonin (Morepen Laboratories, Parwanoo, HP, India) was prepared for injection by dispersion in 0.9% w/v NaCl (saline) - Tween 80 (0.3%) immediately before use; pentobarbitone sodium (John Bake Inc, USA); naloxone (Endo Laboratories, NY, USA); desipramine (Ciba Geigy, Bombay, India); fluoxetine (Torrent Lab, Ahmedabad, India) were dissolved in distilled water. Reserpine (Loba Chemicals, Bombay, India) was dissolved in a few drops of glacial acetic acid and the volume was made up with distilled water. The drug solutions were prepared afresh at beginning of each experiment.

Central nervous system depressant activity of melatonin

(a) Potentiation of barbiturate induced hypnosis in mice:

Treatment schedule– Laka mice receiving pentobarbitone sodium (45 mg/kg) served as control[7]. Melatonin (10 and 20 mg/kg) was injected 30 min prior to pentobarbitone administration for acute treatment. In chronic study, melatonin (10 mg/kg) was injected once daily for 8 days and on 8th day after 30 min of melatonin injection pentobarbitone was administered. All the drugs were injected intraperitoneally. The time of onset of sleep (loss of righting reflex) and its duration (recovery of righting reflex) in minutes were recorded.

(b) Effect of melatonin on locomotor activity:

Measurement of locomotor (ambulatory) and behavioural (total) activities was done using computerised animal activity meter (Opto Varimex Mini, Columbia Instruments, Ohio, USA). An array of 15 infrared emitter/detector pairs, spaced at 2.5 cm intervals measured the animal activity. The animals were placed individually in a transparent plastic cage (29 x 22 x 22 cm) for 5 min after giving 1 min extra before for exploration and the ambulatory and total activities recorded. After 30 min of melatonin (50 and 100 mg/kg) administration, activity was recorded for 5 min. The effect was compared with control.

(c) Effect of melatonin on body temperature:

Variation in the rectal temperature was recorded using a telethermometer (Yellow Springs Instrument Co., Inc. USA) by inserting the thermister probe to a depth of 5 cm into the rectum of rat. The rectal temperature of each animal was recorded just before drug administration and at 30, 60, and 120 min after administration, respectively. The temperature of each animal was recorded for 1 min. The ambient temperature was 20° ± 2°C, and rectal temperature recorded at 0 time served as control for each animal in addition to a separate control group being included in the study. Melatonin was administered at different doses and rectal temperature was noted at different intervals.

(d) Effect of melatonin on nociceptive response in mice:

(i) *Tail flick method:* Antinociceptive response was assessed by measuring tail flick latency to radiant heat as described by D'Amour and Smith[8] (1941) and modified by Kulkarni[9] (1980). Baseline latencies to tail - flick withdrawal from the radiant heat source (3-4 sec) were established. A cut off time of 10 sec was observed to prevent any injury to the tail. A minimum of three trials were recorded for each animal. Melatonin (50 mg/kg, 100 mg/kg, 200 mg/kg, 400 mg/kg) was injected intraperitoneally 30 min before the measurement after noting the basal time in each group. Naloxone (2 mg/kg) was administered intraperitoneally 15 min before the analgesic test in combination study with melatonin (100 mg/kg).

(ii) *Acetic acid-induced writhing:* The mice were injected, ip 1% acetic acid and placed individually in glass chamber for observation. The parameters noted were onset of writhing, number of abdominal contractions, trunk twist response and extension of hind limbs. The number of such responses were noted during 10 min period following acetic acid administration. Melatonin (75, 150 and 300 mg/kg) injected, ip 30 min before the measurement after noting the basal time in each group. Naloxone (1 and 2 mg/kg) was administered, ip 15 min before the analgesic test in combination studies with melatonin (150 and 300 mg/kg).

(e) Effect of melatonin on forced swimming induced immobility in mice

The mice (Laka strain weighing 20-25g) were forced to swim individually in a glass jar (25 x25 x 12 cm) containing fresh water at room temperature. The height of water level was adjusted to 15 cm, and kept constant throughout the experiments. After an initial period of vigorous activity, each animal assumed a typical immobile posture. The total duration of immobility was measured during a total period of 6 min[10]. Mice were judged to be immobile, when they ceased struggling and made minimal movements of their limbs to keep the head above the water level. The changes in immobility duration were recorded after administering various drugs. In combination studies, after 3 1/2 hr and 23 1/2 hr of reserpine treatment, melatonin and desipramine were administered in both the cases. In combination studies with melatonin and desipramine or with melatonin and fluoxetine, the drugs were administered together 30 min prior to the immobility test.

Statistical analysis: The data expressed as mean (mean ± SEM) were compared with respective control groups. The difference in the response was assessed by employing ANOVA followed by Student's t test. $P<0.05$ was considered statistically significant.

Results

Central nervous system depressant activity of melatonin

(a) Potentiation of barbiturate-induced hypnosis in mice

Acute treatment with melatonin (10 and 20 mg/kg) dose-dependently decreased the onset of sleep (loss of righting reflex) and increased the duration of sleep (recovery of righting reflex) due to pentobarbitone (45 mg/kg). (Fig 1.).

Chronic administration of melatonin (10 mg/kg x 8 days) followed by pentobarbitone administration, even though decreased the onset of sleep, it failed to increase the duration of sleep. (Fig. 2.).

(b) Effect of melatonin on locomotor activity in mice

Melatonin (50 and 100 mg/kg) dose-dependently decreased the total and ambulatory activities in mice significantly ($P<0.001$; Fig. 3.).

(c) Effect of melatonin on body temperature in rats

In lower doses (10 and 25 mg/kg), melatonin produced a dose-dependent hypothermia which was significant after 120 min ($P < 0.05$,

< 0.01) when compared with control. At a dose of 50 mg/kg melatonin failed to produce any significant change in body temperature as compared to its previous dose.

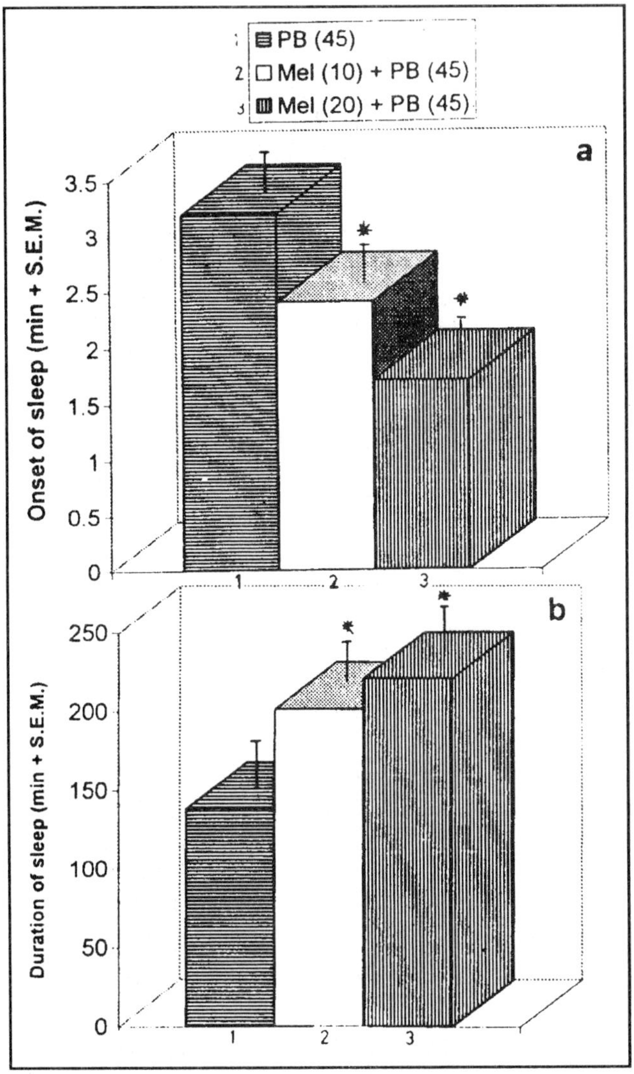

Fig. 1. Effect of acute treatment of melatonin (Mel, 10 and 20 mg/kg) on pentobarbitone(PB, 45 mg/kg)-induced (a) onset of sleep (b) duration of sleep in mice(n=5) *P<0.05 as compared to acute pentobarbitone treated group.

Melatonin at a dose of 100 mg/kg produced a quick onset of hypothermia (as early as 30 min) and the peak effect was observed at 60 min. (Fig. 4).

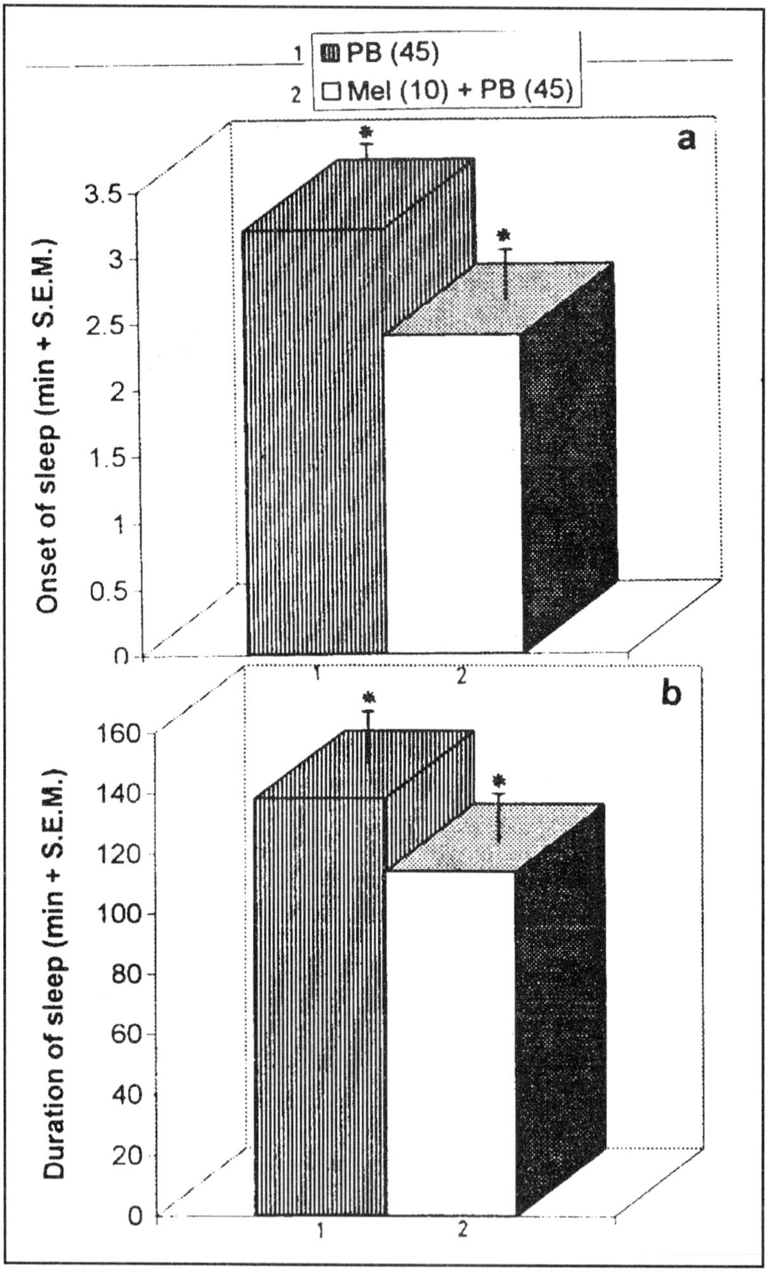

Fig. 2. Effect of chronic treatment (x8 days) of melatonin (Mel, 10 mg/kg) on pentobarbitone (PB, 45 mg/kg)-induced (a) onset of sleep (b) duration of sleep in mice (n=5). *P<0.05 as compared to acute pentobarbitone (PB) treated group.

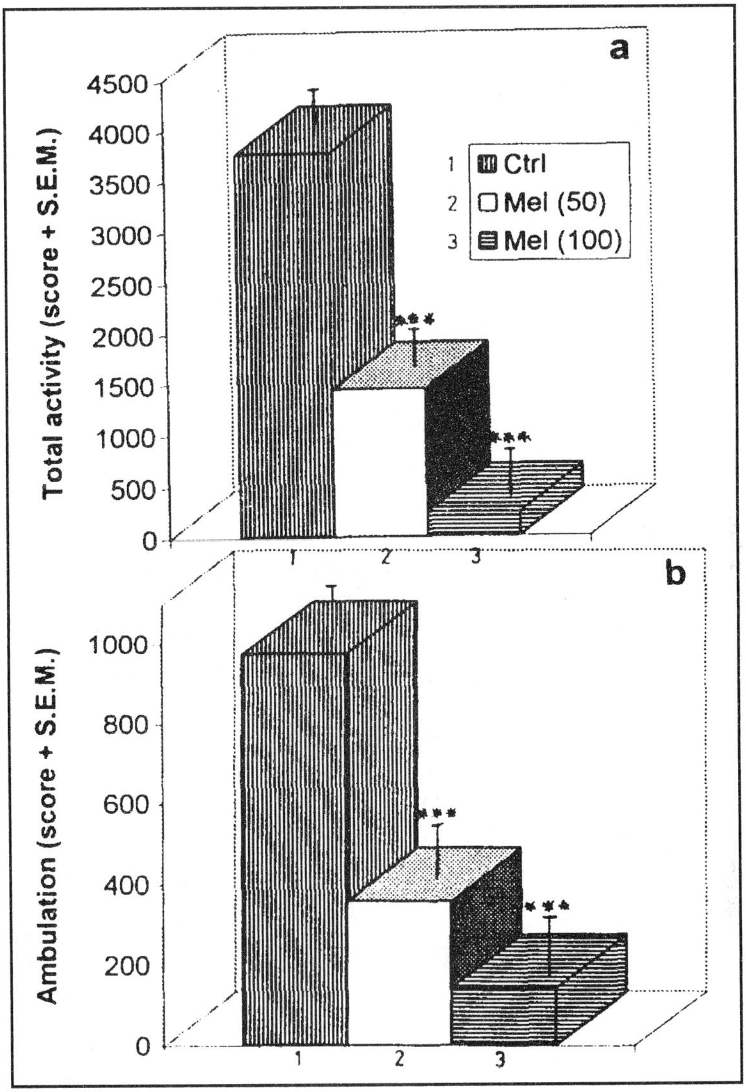

Fig. 3. Effect of melatonin (Mel, 50 and 100 mg/kg) on locomotor activity in mice (a) total score (b) ambulation (n=5). ***P<0.001 as compared to control (Ctrl) group.

(d) Effect of melatonin on nociceptive responce in mice

Melatonin dose-dependently (50, 100, 200, 400 mg/kg) delayed the tail-flick response to radiant heat (analgesia) with a maximum significance at higher dose (P<0.001) when compared with control group (Fig. 5). Naloxone (2 mg/kg) significantly reversed the tail-flick response due to melatonin (100 mg/kg) (P<0.05) (Fig. 6).

Melatonin dose-dependently (75, 150, 300 mg/kg) delayed the onset of acetic acid-induced writhing and decreased the number of writhings when compared with control (acetic acid treated group) (P<0.001). Naloxone (1 mg/kg) when given in combination with melatonin (150 mg/kg), significantly decreased the onset of writhing but could not significantly reduce the number of wriths as compared to melatonin *per se*. When a high dose of naloxone (2 mg/kg) was combined with melatonin (300 mg/kg), it significantly decreased the onset and number of wriths when compared with *per se* melatonin effect (Fig. 7).

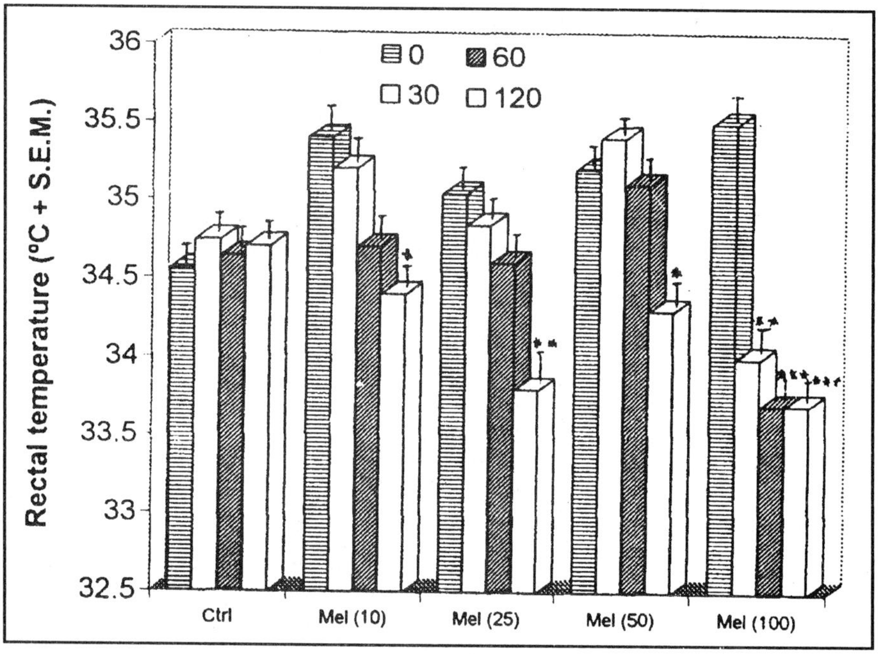

Fig. 4. Effect of melatonin (Mel, 10, 25, 50 and 100 mg/kg) on rectal temperature at different intervals (0, 30, 60 and 120 min) measured in rats (n=5). *P<0.05, **P<0.01 and ***P<0.001 as compared to corresponding control (Ctrl) group.

Effect of melatonin on forced swimming-induced immobility in mice

Both desipramine and melatonin (10 mg/kg) significantly reduced the duration of immobility in mice. But higher doses of melatonin (20 and 50 mg/kg) failed to show any significant difference in immobility duration when compared with control (Table 1).

Melatonin (10 mg/kg) when combined with reserpine (2 mg/kg), significantly reversed reserpine - induced immobility duration after 4 hr (P<0.05). But melatonin in higher doses (20 and 50 mg/kg) could not produce any significant effect on reserpine response (Table 1).

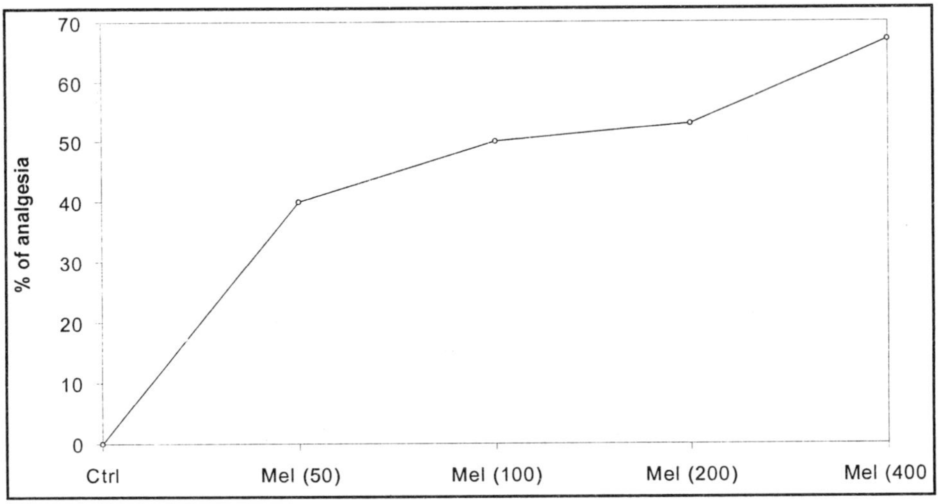

Fig. 5. Effect of melatonin (Mel, 50, 100, 200 and 400 mg/kg) on percentage analgesia as observed by tail-flick method in mice.

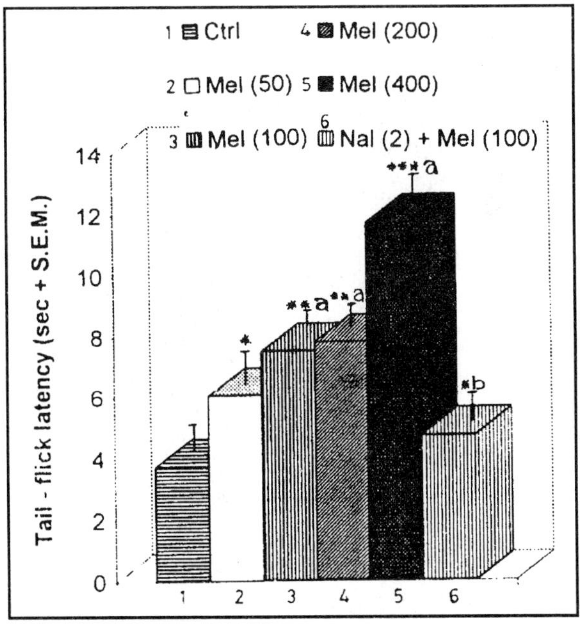

Fig. 6. Effect of melatonin (Mel, 50, 100, 200 and 400 mg/kg) and naloxone (Nal, 2 mg/kg) reversal on tail-flick latency measured in mice (n=5). *P<0.05, **P<0.01 and *** P<0.001 as compared to (a) control group (b) melatonin (100 mg/kg) treatment groups.

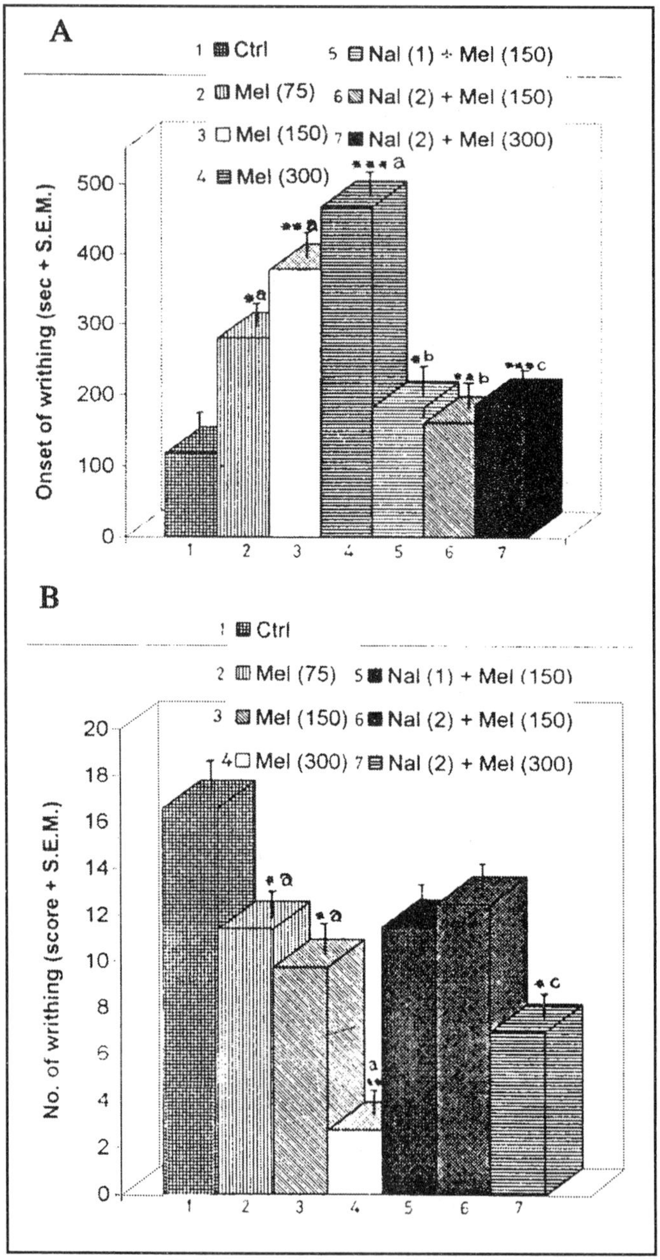

Fig. 7. Effect of melatonin (Mel, 75, 150 and 300 mg/kg) and naloxone (Nal, 1 and 2 mg/kg) reversal of melatonin analgesia in acetic acid-induced writhing in mice (A) onset of writhing (B) No. of writhing (n=5). *P<0.05, **P<0.01 and ***P<0.001 as compared to (a) control (Ctrl) group (b) melatonin (Mel, 150 mg/kg) (c) melatonin (Mel, 300 mg/kg) treatment groups.

When the animals were tested 24 hr after reserpine administration (2 mg/kg), desipramine (10 mg/kg) or melatonin (10 mg/kg) treatment significantly reversed reserpine-induced increase in immobility period (P<0.05). On the other hand, melatonin in higher doses (20 and 50 mg/kg) significantly potentiated the reserpine-induced immobility period in a dose-dependent manner (P<0.01; <0.001) (Table 2).

On co-administration of desipramine (10 mg/kg) and melatonin (10 mg/kg) produced a significant reduction in reserpine-induced immobility period when compared with reserpine *per se* after 24 hr (P < 0.05) (Table 2).

Fluoxetine (10 mg/kg) produced a significant decrease in immobility when compared with control (P<0.05). Co-administration of melatonin (10 mg/kg) with desipramine produced a significant reduction in immobility period when compared with desipramine response *per se* (P<0.05), but with fluoxetine (10 mg/kg), it failed to observe any significant difference in immobility as compared to fluoxetine *per se* (Table 2).

Table 1. Effect of melatonin, desipramine and reserpine on forced swimming-induced immobility in mice (6 min test)
[Values are mean±SE of 5 animals in each group]

Group	Treatment (mg/kg, ip)	Duration of immobility (sec)
1	Control	139.6 ± 10.9
2	Desipramine (10)	87.4 ± 6.61**a
3	Melatonin (10)	20.8 ± 4.2***a
4	Melatonin (20)	144 ± 9.5
5	Melatonin (50)	160.8±8.3
6	Reserpine (2) (Acute, 4 hr)	137.6 ± 7.6
7	Reserpine (2) + Desipramine (10)	132 ± 6.5
8	Reserpine (2) + Melatonin (10)	96.8 ± 7.5*b
9	Reserpine (2) + Melatonin (20)	153 ± 7.48
10	Reserpine(2) + Melatonin (50)	198.2 ± 12.2**b
11	Reserpine (2) + Desipramine (10) + Melatonin (10)	164 ± 6.7

P values; * <0.05, ** <0.01, *** <0.001 as compared between treatment. (a) control group; (b) reserpine (2 mg/kg) after 4 hr group.

Discussion

Melatonin in nervous system depressant studies demonstrated dose-dependent increase in duration of barbiturate hypnosis and decreased onset time in acute treatment. But on chronic administration, it failed to potentiate the duration of pentobarbitone induced sleep. Melatonin, like benzodiazepines is reported to enhance $GABA_A$ binding and the CNS profile of action of melatonin was comparable to agents that positively modulated brain GABA benzodiazepine receptors[11,12]. Therefore, melatonin, probably through this receptor system modulation produced tolerance on chronic administration. The present findings demonstrated a decrease in locomotor activity by melatonin. Melatonin produced significant hypothermia when measured at different intervals. In higher dose (100 mg/kg), it produced an early hypothermia, i.e., quick onset when compared to lower doses. Non-neuronal melatonin receptors in cerebral and caudal arteries may be involved in the cardiovascular functions and temperature[13]. Acute suppression of core body temperature by melatonin may be an integral part of its phase-shifting mechanisms. Further that melatonin sends signals to the preoptic area of anterior hypothalamus where it adjusts the set point of body temperature consistent with the metabolic rate of animal[14].

Table 2- Effect of melatonin, desipramine and reserpine on forced swimming-induced immobility in mice (6 min test)
[Values are mean±SE of 5 animals in each group]

Group	Treatment (mg/kg, ip)	Duration of immobility (sec)
12	Reserpine (2)-4hr	182.6±11.9*a
13	Reserpine (2) + Desipramine (10)	128.4±13.6*c
14	Reserpine (2) + Melatonin (10)	122.4±10.2*c
15	Reserpine (2) + Melatonin (20)	223.2±10.0**c
16	Reserpine (2) + Melatonin (50)	292±5.4***c
17	Reserpine (2) + Desipramine(10) + Melatonin (10)	140.8±5.3*c
18	Desipramine (10) + Melatonin (10)	50±3.9*d
19	Fluoxetine (10)	96.6±5.7*a
20	Fluoxetine (10) + Melatonin (10)	114.8±6.3

P values; * <0.05, ** <0.01, *** <0.001 as compared between treatment. (a) control group; (c) reserpine (2 mg/kg) after 24 hr group; (d) desipramine (10 mg/kg) group.

In the present study, a dose-dependent analgesic response of melatonin was observed in both tail-flick test and acetic-acid induced writhing. Reports suggest a role of endogenous opioids in the regulation of pineal synapse and it has been suggested that at least one opioid function may be involved in the modulation of nocturnal rise of pineal melatonin[15]. The pineal gland and melatonin are also involved in modulating the diurnal rhythms of analgesia and in influencing the age related changes in opioid responses in mice[16]. Analgesia induced by morphine lasts longer during the scotophase, but this diurnal variation is absent in pinealectomized mice. Melatonin may act by releasing endogenous peptides which perform at opioid receptors that induce analgesia[17]. The analgesic response in both tail-flick test and acetic acid induced writhing were sensitive to naloxone reversibility thereby confirming the possible opiatergic mechanism in the action of melatonin.

Melatonin at a lower dose (10 mg/kg) in behavioural despair test possessed a significant antidepressant effect and it reversed reserpine-induced increase in duration of immobility both after 4 and 24 hr. At the same dose of melatonin, it potentiated the effect of desipramine (10 mg/kg). But higher doses of melatonin (20 and 50 mg/kg), significantly enhanced the reserpine-induced immobility period. Combination of melatonin with fluoxetine, a specific 5-HT uptake blocker, could not reduce the immobility duration. It suggested that the observed antidepressant action of melatonin may not be due to increase in the serotonin level. This can be further clarified by the report that fluoxetine treatment produced a significant decrease in melatonin secretion and this effect was different from tricyclics and fluvoxamine, both of which increase melatonin secretion[18]. Porsolt *et al.*[19] argued that serotoninergic component of reserpine may be masking the effect on despair behaviour. But others have reported serotoninergic involvement in despair and antidespair action of drugs[20,21]. Studies suggested that GABA is an essential modulator of dopamine related functions with the striatal and limbic system[22]. As melatonin inhibition of dopamine release is reported,[23,24] it can be suggested that there is an increase in cerebral noradrenergic transmission which ultimately may be responsible for bringing about the antidepressant activity. This is quite evident[25], that GABA and GABA-ergic agents at higher concentrations do not exhibit their antidepressant effect in this model. At this dose, the specificity or the locus of drug action may be different.

Melatonin, a possible GABA-ergic modulator has also shown a similar biphasic response in the present study, that at still higher doses

(20 and 50 mg/kg) it significantly increased the immobility wher measured after both 4 and 24 hr. These observations not only stres the involvement of GABA-ergic receptor system in the actions o antidepressant drugs but also, resolve to some extent, the mysteriou decrease in melatonin levels in depression and its therapy in affectiv disorders.

Acknowledgement

The study was supported by the financial assistance from UGC New Delhi in the form of JRF.

REFERENCES

1. Lerner A B & Nordlund J J, in *frontiers of pineal physiology,* edited by M.D Altschule (MIT Press, Cambridge, MA), 1975, 42.
2. Marczynski T J, Yamaguchi N, Ling G M & Gordzinka L, *Experientia,* 2((1964) 435.
3. Cagnacci A, Elliot, J A & Yen S S C, *J Clin Endocri and Metab,* 75 (1992) 447
4. Sugden D, *J Pharm Exp Ther,* 227 (1983) 587.
5. Redman J, Armstrong S & Ng K T, *Science,* 219 (1983) 1089.
6. Rodriguez M, Sosa J & Hernandez G, *Experientia,* 40 (1984) 397.
7. Kulkarni S K, *Handbook of Experimental Pharmacology* (Vallabh Prakashan New Delhi), 1993, 41.
8. D'Amour F E & Smith D L, *J Pharm Exp Ther,* 72 (1941) 74.
9. Kulkarni S K, *Life Sci,* 27 (1980) 185.
10. Kulkarni S K & Mehta A K, *Psychopharmacology,* 85 (1985) 460.
11. Holmes S W & Sugden D, *Br J Pharmacol,* 76 (1982) 95.
12. Coloma F M & Niles L P, *Biochem Pharmacol,* 37 (1988) 271.
13. Dubocovich M L, *Trends Pharmacol Sci,* 16 (1995) 50.
14. Saarela Seppo Reiter R J, *Life Sci,* 54 (1994) 295.
15. Lowenstein P R, Pereyra E N, Solveyra C G & Cardinali D P, *Eur J Pharmacol* 98 (1984) 261.
16. Kavalsiers M, Hirst M & Teskey G C, *Life Sci,* 32 (1983) 2279.
17. Erlich S S & Apuzzo L J M, *J Neurosurg,* 63 (1985) 321.
18. Childs P A, Rodin I, Martin N J, Allen N H P, Plaskett L, Symthe P J & Thompson C, *Br J Psychiat,* 166 (1995) 196.

19. Porsolt R D, Bertin A, Blaret N, Daniel M & Jalfre M, *Eur J Pharmacol*, 57 (1979) 201.
20. Borsini F & Meli A,.*Psychopharmacology*, 94 (1988) 147.
21. Malinge M, Bourin M, Colombel M C & Larousse C, *Psychopharmacology*, 96 (1988) 104.
22. DiChiara G & Gessa L, *Adv. Biochem Psychopharmacol*, 30 (1981) 129.
23. Exposito Inmaculada Mora F & Oaknin S, *Neuroreport*, 6 (1995) 661.
24. Iuvone Michael P & Gan J, *J Neurosci*, 15 (1995) 2179.
25. Aley K O & Kulkarni S K, *Naunyn Schmiedeberg's Arch Pharmacol*, 339 (1989) 306.

Paper Published In:

I.J.E.B. (Vol. 36, March 1988, pp. 257-263)

15

Reversal of diazepam withdrawal induced hyperactivity in mice by BR 16-A (Mentat®), a herbal preparation

S.K. KULKARNI & ALOK SHARMA
Pharmacology Division, Department of Pharmaceutical Sciences,
Panjab University, Chandigarh 160 014, India

Abrupt cessation of chronic treatment of diazepam (20 mg/kg/day for 21 days) produced withdrawal reactions. BR 16-A, a multicomponent herbal preparation shown to reverse the withdrawal reactions to opiates was studied against diazepam induced withdrawal reactions in mice. Acute dose of diazepam (20 mg/kg) produced a decrease in the ambulatory and total activity. However, chronic administration for 21 days produced tolerance and no significant change in the ambulatory and total activity. On abrupt termination of diazepam treatment after 21 days, the animals showed anxiety and excitement as there was an increase in ambulatory and total activity. The withdrawal excitement was highest at 72 hr of the last dose of diazepam. Concomittant administration of BR 16-A (100 and 500 mg/kg) reversed the acute effect of diazepam in a dose dependent manner. Similarly, chronic administration of BR 16-A (100 and 500 mg/kg/day for 21 days) with diazepam (20 mg/kg/day for 21 days) also reversed the withdrawal induced hyperambulation and total activity. Chronic administration of BR 16-A *per se* had no significant effect on the ambulatory and total activity, however, in acute doses, BR 16-A (100 and 500 mg/kg) produced a dose dependent increase in the ambulatory and total activity. BR 16-A with its CNS profile of activity could be a useful preparation in the management of substances of abuse.

BR 16-A, a multicomponent herbal psychotropic preparation possesses a number of effects on the central nervous system. It is reported to be effective in cases of cerebral deficit, behavioural disturbances following post-natal organic lesions of the central nervous system and in cases having organic loss of bladder function (personal communication). It has also been shown to possess anticonvulsant effect in animals (personal observations) and, clinically effective in improving memory and learning tasks in mentally retarded children. The experimental studies in animals have extensively demonstrated a GABA-mediated action of BR 16-A[1]. The efficacy of BR 16-A on preventing the development of tolerance and withdrawal symptoms against opiates and alcohol has also been reported earlier[2,3]. The present study is an attempt to find out whether the preparation (BR 16-A) also prevents the withdrawal reactions to chronic treatment with diazepam in mice.

Materials and Methods

Animals: Laka mice of either sex bred in the Central Animal House facility of the Panjab University were used. The animals were housed under standard laboratory conditions and were provided with food and water *ad libitum.*

Treatment schedule: Diazepam (20 mg/kg) was administered, ip, once daily for 21 days. BR 16-A (100 and 500 mg/kg) was administered, po, for 21 days. Similarly, in combination studies, BR 16-A and diazepam were administered concurrently for 21 days. All administrations were done between 0900 and 1000 hrs daily. The control animals were treated with the vehicle alone. The body weight of the animals were recorded on a weekly basis.

Measurement of locomotor (ambulatory) and behavioural (total) activity: The ambulatory and total activity was measured using Computerized Animal Activity Meter (Opto Varimex Mini, Columbus Instruments, Ohio USA). An array of 15 infrared emitter/detector pairs, spaced at 2.5 cm intervals, measured the animal activity along a single axis of motion, the digital data being displayed on the front panel meters as ambulatory activity and total activity. The animals were placed individually in a transparent plastic cage (29 cm x 22 cm x 22 cm) for 5 min and the ambulatory and total activities recorded. The measurement of the animal activity was performed between 0900 and 1300 hrs.

Drugs: Diazepam (Ranbaxy, New Delhi) was wetted using a few drops of Tween 80 and uniformly dispersed in distilled water. BR 16-

A (Mentat, Himalaya Drug Company, Bombay) was suspended uniformly in distilled water. The suspensions were made afresh and administered in a constant volume of 1 ml/ 100g of body weight.

Statistical analysis: The data expressed as mean ±SD were analysed by one way ANOVA followed by Dunnett's post hoc test and P values < 0.05 were considered statistically significant.

Results

Effect of diazepam on ambulatory and total activity: An acute dose of diazepam (20 mg/kg) caused a reduction in the ambulatory and total activity (Fig. 1A and B). Chronic administration, however, produced tolerance to the sedative effect and no significant change in ambulatory and total activity was observed as compared to control group (Table 1). On abrupt termination of diazepam after 21 day administration, the animals showed severe anxiety response as evidenced by a significant increase in ambulatory and total activities (Fig. 2A and B). The maximum withdrawal hyperactivity was observed after 72 hr of the last dose of diazepam.

Effect of BR 16-A on withdrawal induced ambulatory and total activities: Acute doses of BR 16-A (100 and 500 mg/kg) showed a dose-dependent increase in ambulatory and total activities, higher dose showing a significant effect (Fig. 1 A and B). However, chronic administration of BR 16-A (100 and 500 mg/kg) did not produce any significant change in the ambulatory and total activities (Table 1), as compared to the control group.

Table 1. Ambulatory and total activity scores in vehicle, diazepam, BR 16-A and their combination after 21 days of treatment [Values are mean ± SD]

S.No.	Treatment (mg/kg)	N	Ambulatory activity	Total activity
1.	Control	10	319.1±111.2	482.7±139.8
2.	Diazepam (20)	11	393.0±165.3	595.2±217.2
3.	BR 16-A (100)	10	329.6±75.0	510.7±89.2
4.	BR 16-A (500)	10	377.3±46.0	554.9±54.2
5.	Diazepam (20) + BR 16-A (100)	11	393.7±128.9	554.9±177.9
6.	Diazepam (20) + BR 16-A (500)	10	455.0±117.9	616.3±145.6

Concomittant administration of BR 16-A alongwith diazepam produced a dose-dependent reversal of the acute effect of diazepam, higher dose producing a significant reversal (Fig. 1A and B). Chronic administration of BR 16-A alongwith diazepam had no significant effect *perse* (Table 1), but significantly reversed the withdrawal induced hyper ambulation and total activities (Fig. 2A and B).

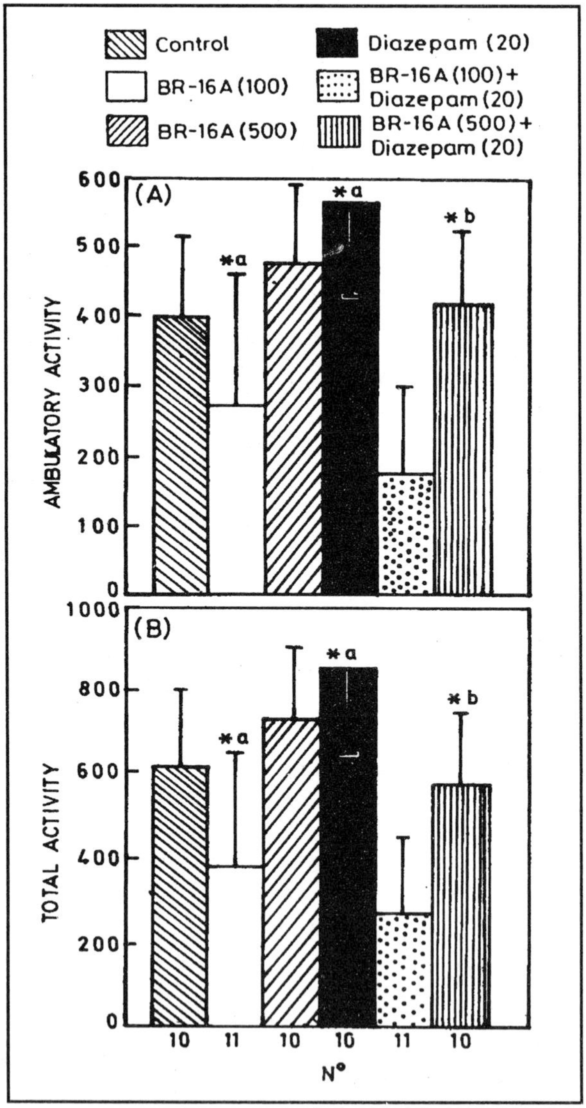

Fig. 1. Modification of **(A)** ambulatory, and **(B)** total activity by acute treatment with diazepam, BR 16-A or their combination in mice [Values are mean ± SD. *P < 0.05 as compared to (a) control and (b) diazepam treated group]

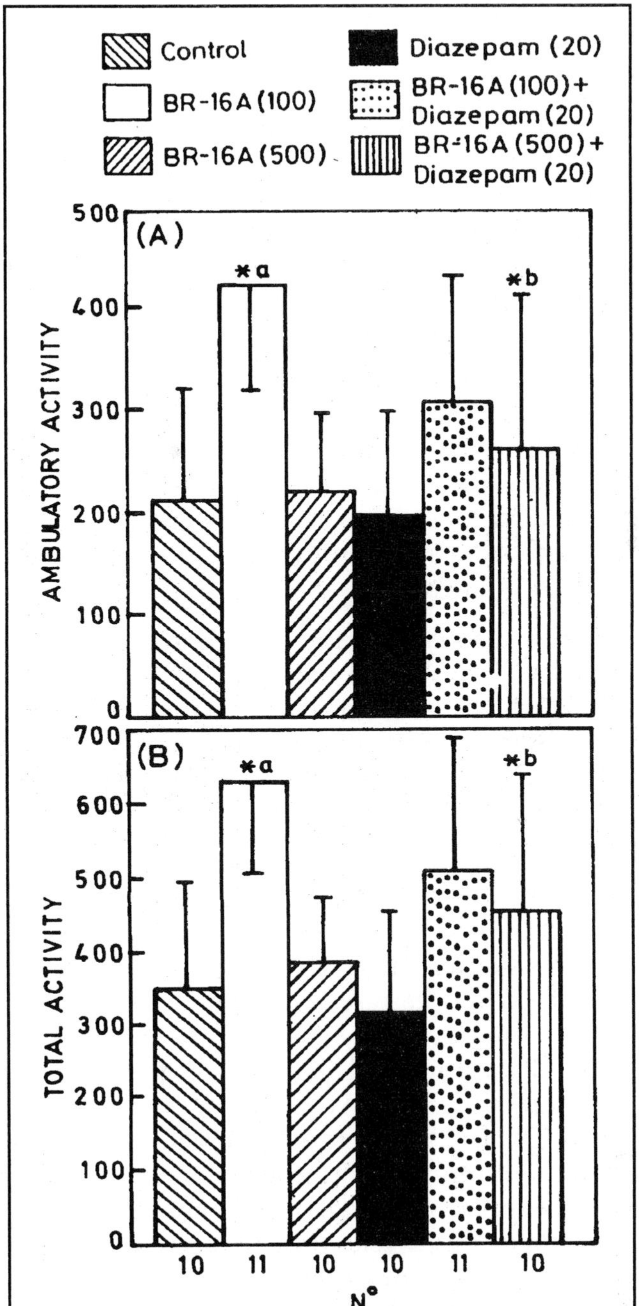

Fig. 2. Modification by BR 16-A of withdrawal (72 hr)-induced hyperambulation (A) and increase in total activity (B) due to diazepam in mice [Values are mean ± SD. *$P < 0.05$ as compared to (a) control and (b) diazepam treated group]

Discussion

Benzodiazepines are one of the most widely used class of drugs in the management of anxiety, insomnia, muscle spasms, convulsions and alcohol withdrawal. However, their indiscriminate use has shown that these agents have a potential for producing physiological and psychological dependence[4,5]. Benzodiazepines produce drug dependence and withdrawal reactions on abrupt termination[6]. These reactions involved both GABA/BZ receptor system and noradrenergic hyperfunction in the brain[6,7].

BR 16-A (Mentat®), a herbal psychotropic preparation containing several indigenous ingredients such as brahmi *(Hydrocotyl asiatica)*, shaṭavari *(Asparagus racemosus)*, buchh *(Acorus calamus)*, aswagandha *(Withania somnifera)*, giloi *(Tinospora cardifolia)*, amla *(Embelica officinalis)*, shankpushpi *(Evolvulus alsinoides)*, kuth *(Saussurea lappa)* and triphala, is reputed to be useful in nervous disorders and reported to be a safe preparation[1]. It is also reported to prevent the development of tolerance and dependence to opiates and alcohol[2,3].

Abrupt termination of chronic diazepam treatment produced anxiety response and increased ambulatory (horizontal) and total activity. The onset of withdrawal reaction was evident after 24 hr of the last dose of diazepam and showed maximum manifestation at 72 hr. Earlier studies in rats have shown a similar profile of withdrawal reactions[6].

Involvement of GABAergic and non-GABAergic mechanisms in withdrawal reactions are well documented. Diazepam withdrawal is reported to activate the inverse agonistic site on the GABA/BZ receptor complex[8]. BR 16-A significantly prevented the development of severe-withdrawal to diazepam, the response being more pronounced at 72 hr of withdrawal. BR 16-A acted by GABAergic mechanism in its effect[9]. It has also been reported that one of the active, ingredients, *Withania somnifera* modulated GABA receptors in a positive way[10]. It appears that through its CNS profile, BR 16-A could provide a useful therapy in the prevention of withdrawal reactions to diazepam and in deaddiction therapy of various drugs of abuse. Being safe with no major side effect reported (personal communication) it has an added advantage in the management of drug addiction.

Acknowledgement

The study was supported by the financial assistance of Himalaya Drug Company, Bangalore.

REFERENCES

1. Kulkarni S K & Verma A, *Indian Drugs,* 30 (1993) 97.
2. Kulkarni S K & Verma A, *Indian J Exp Biol,* 30 (1992) 885.
3. Kulkarni S K & Verma A, *Indian J Exp Biol,* 31 (1993) 435.
4. Petursson H & Lader M H, *Br Med J,* 283 (1981) 643.
5. Tyrer P, Rutherford D & Hugget T, *Lancet, i* (1983) 520.
6. Kunchandy J & Kulkarni S K, *Psychopharmacology,* 90 (1986) 198.
7. Kunchandy J & Kulkarni S K, *Indian J Exp Biol,* 25 (1987) 115.
8. Kulkarni S K & Ticku M K, *Brain Res,* 519 (1990) 6.
9. Aley K O & Kulkarni S K, *Indian J Exp Biol,* 28 (1990) 1149.
10. Kulkarni S K, Sharma A, Verma A & Ticku M K, *Indian Drugs,* 30 (1993) 305.

Paper Published In:
I.J.E.B. (Vol. 32, December 1994, pp. 886-888)

16

Protective effect of BR-16A (Mentat®), a herbal preparation on alcohol abstinence-induced anxiety and convulsions

S.K. KULKARNI & ANITA VERMA
Pharmacology Division, Department of Pharmaceutical Sciences,
Panjab University, Chandigarh 160 014, India

Chronic administration of ethanol (2-5 g/ kg, po) on days 1 to 6 and its withdrawal produced anxiogenic reaction in mice and rats as assessed on the elevated plus-maze. Daily administration of BR-16A (100 mg/kg) prior to ethanol intoxication for 6 days prevented withdrawal induced anxiety in both rats and mice. However, acute administration of a single dose of BR-16A, to animals withdrawn from ethanol, i.e. on the 7th day, showed significant anxiogenic response. Ethanol withdrawal also sensitized the convulsogenic reaction to pentylenetetrazole (PTZ). A non-convulsive dose (40 or 60 mg/kg) of PTZ produced full blown convulsions and increased mortality in ethanol withdrawn rats and mice, respectively. Both acute and chronic administration of BR-16A (100 mg/kg) exhibited significant protection against ethanol withdrawal-induced reduction in PTZ threshold in rats and mice. The results suggest the usefulness of this safe herbal psychotropic preparation in the management of ethanol withdrawal reactions.

Physical dependence on ethanol is defined by the presence of an ethanol withdrawal syndrome that becomes apparent following cessation of ethanol intake and elimination of ethanol from the system. The withdrawal syndrome, well characterized in humans and in animal models[1,2], consists of an early (tremor, diaphoresis, hallucinations, convulsions) and delayed (delirium, tremors, increased autonomic activity, profound sweating, and profound disorientation) reaction. Alcoholism and withdrawal of its chronic intake are grave social and medical problems. There is no single drug therapy that helps patients in overcoming alcoholism[3].

BR-16A (Mentat®), a herbal psychotropic preparation, contains the following indigenous ingredients reputed in the ancient system of Ayurvedic medicine to be useful in the management of nervous disorders: brahmi *(Hydrocotyl asiatica)*, shatavari *(Asparagus racemosus)*, bach *(Acorus calamus)*, aswagandha *(Withania somnifera)*, giloi *(Tinospora cardifolia)*, amla *(Embelica officinalis)*, shankhpushpi *(Evolulus alsinoides)*, kuth *(Saussurea lappa)* and triphala. Preliminary toxicity studies have shown it to be a safe preparation and no adverse effect ensued its chronic use (unpublished data). Recent studies have demonstrated effectiveness of BR-16A in preventing the development of tolerance and dependence to morphine in mice[4]. The present study has been undertaken to evaluate the de-addiction liability of this herbal preparation against alcohol. Alcohol withdrawal reactions are determined as reduction in pentylenetetrazole (PTZ) threshold (convulsions) and increase in anxiety response as measured on elevated plus-maze.

Materials and Methods

Effectiveness of BR-16A in suppressing the symptoms of ethanol withdrawal was investigated in rats and mice. Balb'c strain, albino mice weighing 20-25 g and porton rats weighing 150-200 g of either sex, bred in Central Animal House facility of the University were used. The animals were housed under standard light/dark cycle with food and water *ad libitum*. The experiments were performed between 0900 and 1700 hrs.

Treatment schedule: In acute studies, animals received ethanol (2 g/kg of 10% ethanol in mice and 5 g/kg of 20% ethanol in rats), intragastrically. After 30 min its effect on elevated plus-maze was studied. In chronic studies, mice received 2 g/kg of 10% w/v ethanol, intragastrically, twice a day on 1st day and once daily on the successive days for a total of 6 days. In rats, 5 g/kg of ethanol (20% w/v) was administered intragastrically, three times a day for 6 days. On 7th day i.e. 24 hr after the last dose of ethanol rats/mice were tested for withdrawal reaction. The other treatment groups included (pretreatment: treatment): (i) saline:saline (ii) saline:ethanol, and (iii) BR-16A (100 mg/kg):ethanol. Control experiments were performed on day 7 to determine whether BR-16A prevented the development of withdrawal syndrome or it simply altered the behavioural expression of the withdrawal symptoms. On this day, the treatments were reversed so that the animals that had received BR-16A followed, 30 min later, by ethanol on days 1 through 6 were challenged with saline. Similarly, the animals which received saline followed, 30 min later, by ethanol received only BR-16A. The group chronically treated with saline received the same (saline only). The withdrawal reaction was assessed by studying the anxiogenic reaction on elevated plus-maze or decreased threshold to pentylenetetrazole (PTZ; convulsive response to an otherwise non-convulsive dose in naive animals).

Elevated plus-maze measurement of anxiety: The elevated plus-maze used for rats and mice was same as described earlier[5,6]. Briefly, the apparatus for mice consisted of two open arms (16 x 5 cm) and two enclosed arms (16 x 5 x 12 cm) and for rats consisted of two open arms (50 x 10 cm) and two enclosed arms (50 x 10 x 40 cm). The maze was elevated to a height of 25 cm for mice and 50 cm for rats[7,8]. During 5 min test session the following parameters were noted: (1) number of entries the animal made in open and enclosed arms, (ii) the total time spent in each arm, and (iii) choice of open/enclosed arm as first entry. Animals were put individually at the centre of the plus-maze facing towards an open arm at the beginning of the test. An anxiogenic response was defined as decreased number of entries and time spent in open arm. There was reduction in percent preference for the open arm in anxiogenic animals.

PTZ-threshold: The onset of body jerks, clonic convulsions followed by tonic convulsions and death were recorded following PTZ challenge in naive and ethanol withdrawn animals. Each animal was observed individually for 2 hr for acute response. Reduction in the dose of PTZ to produce full blown convulsions in ethanol withdrawn animals was considered as withdrawal-induced reduction in the convulsive threshold. The protective effect of BR-16A following acute and chronic treatment was noted in rats and mice.

Drugs: The drugs used were BR-16A (Mentat®; Himalaya Drug Co., Bombay, India), pentylenetetrazole (Sigma, USA) and ethanol (Bengal Chemicals & Pharmaceuticals Ltd, Calcutta, India).

PTZ and ethanol were prepared in distilled water. BR-16A (100 mg/kg) powder was suspended uniformly in distilled water. Ethanol (2 g/kg of 10% w/v in mice and 5 g/kg of 20% w/v in rats) and BR-

16A were administered orally while PTZ (40-80 mg/kg) was injected ip. All the drugs except ethanol were administered in a constant volume of 1 ml/100 g of body weight. PTZ was administered 24 hr after the last dose of ethanol (withdrawal animals) and BR-16A was given 30 min prior to ethanol.

Statistical analysis– The data expressed as mean± SE were analysed by Student's *t* test. Probability levels < 5% were considered significant.

Results

Effect of BR-16A on ethanol withdrawal-induced anxiety: Acute administration of ethanol (2 g/kg; 10% w/v) in mice produced significant increase in the duration in open arms as compared with the vehicle treated control mice (Table 1). Similarly, in rats ethanol (5 g/kg; 20% w/v) produced significant decrease in the number of entries in closed arms and increase in the time spent in open arms (Table 2). Percent preference for closed arm entry was also reduced following acute treatment with ethanol as compared with the vehicle-treated group in rats and mice.

On the other hand, mice withdrawn from chronic ethanol treatment showed greater preference for closed arm entry and significant reduction in the duration of time spent in open arms as compared with the vehicle-treated control group (Table 1). Rats withdrawn from chronic ethanol treatment also exhibited increase in percent preference for closed arms and the duration in closed arms as compared with the vehicle treated control. The duration and the number of entries in open arms was also reduced significantly (Table2).

Mice receiving chronic treatment with BR-16A (100 mg/kg) followed by ethanol failed to show any withdrawal-induced anxiety. There was a significant decrease in the duration in closed arms. The duration and the number of entries in open arms increased significantly as compared with the ethanol withdrawn group (Table 1). Daily administration of BR-16A (100 mg/kg) prior to ethanol intoxication for 6 days in rats completely abolished entry into open arms. Duration and number of entries in closed arm were same as those in ethanol-withdrawn group (Table 2).

Mice treated repeated with saline followed by ethanol for 6 days and then challenged with BR-16A on 7th day displayed significant increase in preference for closed arm entry and time spent in closed arms. The duration in open arms reduced significantly as compared with the vehicle treated control (Table 1). Acute administration of BR-16A (100 mg/kg) in ethanol withdrawn rats failed to exhibit any entry in to the open arm. The duration in closed arm displayed significant decrease. The duration in closed arms was not significantly different from the vehicle-treated control group (Table 2).

Table 1. Effect of BR-16A on ethanol (EtOH) withdrawal-induced anxiety in mice [Values are mean±SE]

Group	Treatment	n	% Preference for closed arm entry	Closed arm		Open arm	
				Duration (sec)	Entries (mean)	Duration (sec)	Entries (mean)
1	Vehicle	8	50	177.50± 21.33	8.25 1.93	34.25± 8.03	3.75± 0.63
2	EtOH, 10% (2 g/kg; Acute)	6	20	150± 17.73	10.00± 1.78	87.75± 16.11*	4.00± 0.74
3	EtOH, 10% (2 g/kg; Chronic) W/D	10	80	199.50± 10.96	10.90± 1.62	15.20± 1.09*	1.90± 0.55
4	EtOH, 10% (2 g/kg; Chronic) W/D +BR-16A (100 mg/kg; Acute)	7	100	243.28± 16.10†	7.00± 0.72†	7.00± 1.32†	1.14± 0.45
5	EtOH, 10% (2 g/kg; Chronic) W/D +BR-16A (100 mg/kg; Chronic)	7	50	158.43± 11.35†	9.86± 1.37	46.28± 6.30†	4.14± 0.74†

P values: * < 0.05 as compared with the vehicle-treated control †<0.05 as compared with the ethanol (EtOH)-withdrawal (W/D) group.

Table 2. Effect of BR-16A on ethanol (EtOH) withdrawal-induced anxiety in rats [Values are mean± SE]

Group	Treatment	n	% Preference for closed arm entry	Closed arm		Open arm	
				Duration (sec)	Entries (mean)	Duration (sec)	Entries (mean)
1	Vehicle	7	50	167± 8.25	7.82± 0.64	42.51 3.50	5.20± 0.64
2	EtOH, 20% (5 g/kg; Acute)	5	20	154.80± 17.81	3.33± 0.75*	112± 14.90*	4.16± 0.58
3	EtOH, 20% (5g/kg; Chronic) W/D	6	66.6	272± 9.56*	1.00± 0.25*	22.40± 6.95*	0.80± 0.20*
4	EtOH, 20% (5 g/kg; Chronic) W/D + BR-16A (100 mg/kg Acute)	5	100	262.75± 27.62	1.25± 0.25	-	-
5	EtOH, 20% (5 g/kg; Chronic) W/D + BR-16A (100 mg/kg; Chronic) W/D	5	80	155.33± 6.76*a	1.00± 0.33	-	-

P values: < 0.05 as compared with *vehicle-treated control group; *aethanol (EtOH)-withdrawal (W/D) group.

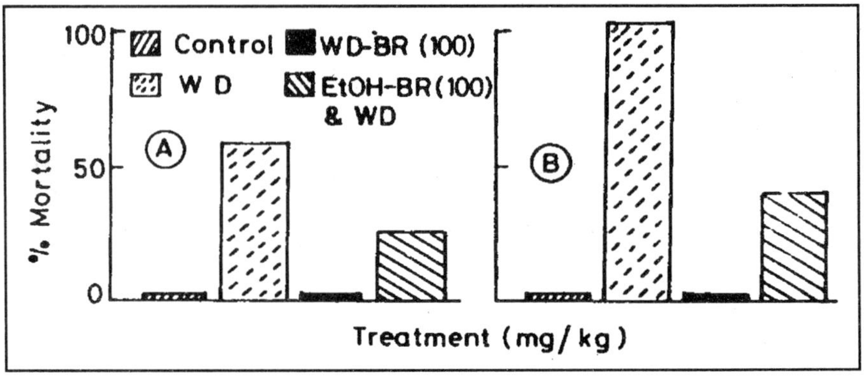

Fig. 1. Modification of pentylenetetrazole (PTZ)-induced convulsions by BR-16A (BR) in ethanol (EtOH) withdrawal groups of mice (A) and rats (B)

Effect of BR-16A on PTZ threshold in ethanol withdrawn animals: PTZ (80 mg/ kg) induced severe clonic-tonic seizures followed by 100% mortality in naive mice. A lower dose (60 mg/kg) induced mild clonic-tonic seizures with no mortality (Fig. IA), whereas a still lower dose failed to cause any observable behavioural change in naive mice or rats. However, in ethanol-withdrawn mice PTZ (60 mg/kg) produced severe clonic-tonic seizures (Fig. 2A) and 60% mortality (Fig. 1A). Acute administration of BR-16A (100 mg/kg) to ethanol withdrawn mice showed protection against PTZ (60mg/kg) convulsions. Animal showed only mild clonic convulsions followed by recovery (Fig. 2A). Chronic administration of BR-16A (100 mg/kg) followed by ethanol for 6 days exhibited only mild clonic seizures with delayed onset and 25% mortality following administration of PTZ (60 mg/kg) on day 7 in mice (Fig. 1 and 2).

In ethanol-withdrawn rats, severe tonic seizures (Fig. 2B) and 100% mortality (Fig. 1B) were observed following administration of PTZ (40 mg/kg). Acute administration of BR-16A (100 mg/kg) to ethanol withdrawn rats produced complete protection against PTZ convulsions (Fig. I B). Mild jerks and clonus with delayed onset were observed following administration of PTZ (40 mg/kg; Fig. 2B). Withdrawal of chronic treatment with BR-16A (100 mg/kg) followed by ethanol over 6 days in rats also produced mild clonic-tonic convulsions with delayed onset following PTZ (40 mg/kg) administration (Fig. 2B). There was only 40% mortality in this group (Fig. 1 B). In addition to ethanol withdrawal-induced anxiety and convulsions, both animals generally exhibited various other abstinence signs such as body tremors, escape attempts, jumping and increased locomotor activity which were suppressed by prior treatment with BR-16A.

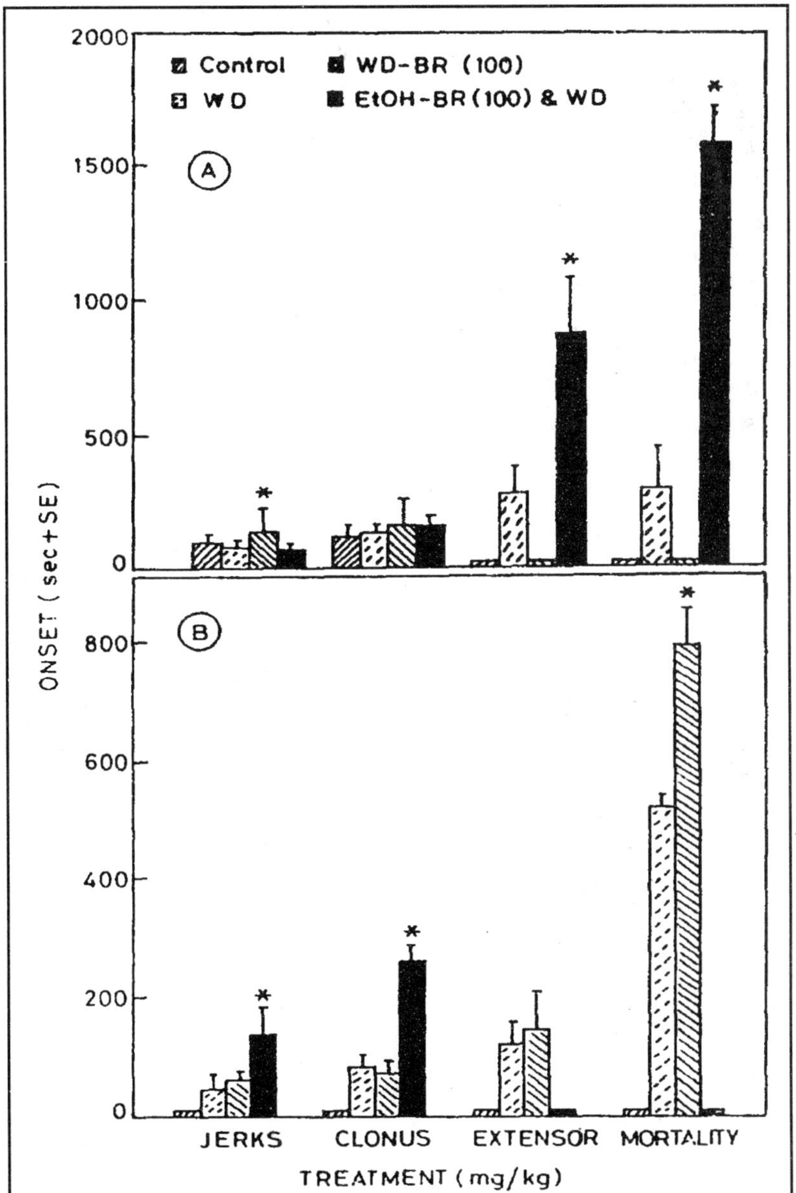

Fig. 2. Effect of BR-16A (BR) on pentylenetetrazole (PTZ)-induced convulsions in ethanol (EtOH) withdrawal groups of mice (A) and rats (B). *$P<0.05$ as compared with respective control groups.

Discussion

Chronic ethanol administration is known to produce behavioural and biochemical changes in humans and animals. Withdrawal from chronic intake of ethanol is also known to produce withdrawal reactions which range from craving behaviour to severe seizures[2]. Although the exact cellular and biochemical mechanism of development of tolerance and dependence to ethanol is not fully understood, recent studies have, however, focussed attention to the involvement of inhibitory neurotransmitter γ-aminobutyric acid (GABA) in the action of ethanol. At pharmacologically active concentrations ethanol produces some of its pharmacological effects through GABAergic transmission[9-11]. In the present study, acute administration of ethanol produced a significant increase in the time spent in open arms, thereby suggesting an anxiolytic profile of ethanol in rats and mice. Biochemical studies have provided evidence that enhancement of GABA-mediated neuronal chloride fluxes may contribute to the sedative and anxiolytic profile of ethanol[11-13]. The observed anxiogenic action following ethanol withdrawal would, therefore, be consistent with the notion that GABAergic system is down regulated during withdrawal. The animals treated chronically with BR-16A followed by ethanol for 6 days displayed significant reversal of withdrawal-induced anxiety on 7th day. Acute administration of BR-16A on 7th day to ethanol withdrawn animals also displayed considerable anxiety on 7th day. The anxiety reaction in ethanol withdrawn animals may be attributed to the anxiogenic action of BR-16A *per se*[14] or to an acute interaction between BR- I6A and ethanol. Reversal of anxiogenic response following substitution of BR-16A with saline in ethanol withdrawn animals suggests that BR-16A need not be present during testing to observe anxiety in chronically BR-16A treated animals.

PTZ, a chemoconvulsant, is reported to induce seizures by depressing chloride channel function by binding to picrotoxin site on the GABA receptor complex. In ethanol withdrawn animals lower doses of PTZ as compared to control animals was required so as to exhibit severe tonic seizures and mortality. Sensitization of inverse agonistic site on GABA-benzodiazepine receptor complex following ethanol withdrawal has been shown to be responsible for decrease in convulsive threshold to PTZ in ethanol withdrawn animals[15]. BR-16A significantly inhibited PTZ convulsions in these animals when given repeatedly for 6 days. Acute BR-16A administration following ethanol withdrawal also produced significant attenuation of PTZ convulsions. The reversal of ethanol withdrawal sensitized convulsant response to PTZ suggests the effectiveness of this herbal preparation in suppressing ethanol withdrawal syndrome whether given acutely or chronically. The above data suggests that the anticonvulsant effect of BR-16A alone or its acute interaction with ethanol is unlikely to account for its de - addiction potential.

BR-16A is a safe preparation having no apparent response *per se* on reward system. Concurrent administration of this multicomponent herbal preparation may help in preventing the development of tolerance and dependence to ethanol and other psychotropic drugs[3]. The preparation is also effective in combating withdrawal reactions to chronic administration of ethanol. The present study provides yet another evidence for the de-addiction potential of acute as well as chronic administration of BR-16A against ethanol.

Acknowledgement

This work was supported by grant from Himalaya Drug Co., Bombay, India.

REFERENCES

1. Tabakoff B & Rothstein J D, *Medical and social aspects of alcohol abuse,* edited by B Tabakoff; P B Sutker & C L Randall (Plenum Press, New York), 1983, 187.
2. Parale M P & Kulkarni S K, *Psychopharmacology,* 88 (1986) 237.
3. Kulkarni S K, *Drugs Today,* 24 (1988) 411.
4. Kulkarni S K & Verma A, *Indian J Exp Biol,* (1992) 885.
5. Pellow S, Chopin P, File S E & Briley M, *J Neurosci Meth,* 14 (1985) 149.
6. Lister R G, *Psychopharmcology,* 92 (1987) 1980.
7. Sharma A C & Kulkarni S K, *Drug Der Res.* 22 (1991) 251.
8. Kulkarni S K, Sharma A C & Verma *A, Ann Natl Acad Med Sci (India),* 27 (1991) 61.
9. Hunt W A, *Neurosci Biobehav Res,* 7 (1983) 87.
10. Ticku M K & Kulkarni S K, *Pharmacol Biochem Behav,* 30 (1988) 501.
11. Suzdak P,Glowa J R, Crawley J N, Schwartz R D, Skolnick P & Paul S M, *Science,* 234 (1986) 1243.

12. Allan A M & Harris R A, *Pharmacol Biochem Behar,* 27 (1987) 665.
13. Mehta A K & Ticku M K, *J Pharmacol Exp Ther,* 246 (1988) 558.
14. Verma A & Kulkarni S K, *Indian J Exp Biol,* 29 (1991) 1120.
15. Mehta A K & Ticku M K, *Brain Res.* 489 (1989) 93.

Paper Published In:
I.J.E.B. (Vol. 31, May 1993, pp. 435-439)

17

Alprazolam modifies animal behaviour on elevated plus-maze

S.K. KULKARNI & KOMAL SHARMA
Pharmacology Division, Department of Pharmaceutical Sciences,
Panjab University, Chandigarh 160 014, India

Exposure to elevated plus-maze is known to evoke approach-avoidance conflict behaviour and anxiety related movements in mice. Alprazolam (0.1 to 1 mg/kg, ip) produced dose dependant increase in antianxiety response, 100% first preference to open arm, open arm entries and exploratory behaviour. This effect was not only comparable to diazepam but also sensitive to reversal by flumazenil, a benzodiazepine receptor antagonist. Withdrawal of alprazolam (2 mg/kg/day for 14 days) and diazepam (20 mg/kg/day for 14 days) from chronic treatment produced typical anxiety response in animals. When tested for transfer latency, a parameter for learning and memory, both diazepam and alprazolam interfered with cognitive behaviour. Besides these actions, alprazolam also possesses anti-depressant property which makes it an atypical benzodiazepine for anxiety, panic disorder and endogenous depression.

Extensive progress made in the field of GABA/benzodiazepine receptor pharmacology has not only helped in better understanding of biological psychiatry of anxiety and related disorders but also led to the development of newer antianxiety agents with target specific actions[1]. Most of the benzodiazepines though relieve anxiety, fail to overcome the other associated depression, panic and phobic disorders. However, alprazolam, a triazolobenzodiazepine has been claimed to alleviate panic and phobic disorders and also to possess some degree of antidepressant properties[2,3]. In the present study the effect of alprazolam on anxiety responses in elevated plus-maze, development of dependence to drug and its effect on learning have been investigated in mice. The behavioural profile of alprazolam has been compared with a classical benzodiazepine, diazepam.

Materials and Methods

Animals: Albino mice (BALB'C and LAKA strain) weighing 20-25 g obtained from the Central Animal House facility of the University, were used. The animals were maintained under standard 12 hr dark and light cycle with food and water provided *ad libitum.* All experiments were carried out between 0800 and 1200 hrs.

Procedure: The method to measure anxiety response in mice using elevated plus-maze was essentially same as validated by Pellow *et al.*[4,5] and described by Sharma and Kulkarni[6]. The anxiety parameters recorded were (a) preference of the animal for the first entry, (b) number of entries the animal made in open and enclosed arms, (c) average time each animal spent in open and enclosed arms, and (d) total number of entries made by the animal in both open and enclosed arms. The animals were placed individually at the centre of the plus-maze with head facing towards open arm at the beginning of the test.

For measuring the effect of the drug on working (short term) memory, transfer latency of animals on elevated plus maze was measured[7]. The animals were placed individually at the end of either of the open arms and the time interval animal took to move from open to enclosed arm (transfer latency, TL) was noted on the first day. The animals were allowed to explore the apparatus for 20 sec. After 24 hr of first exposure, TL was again noted (second day TL). Each animal was used only once.

Drug treatment: For antianxiety studies, alprazolam (0.1, 0.25, 0.5 and 1 mg/kg) and diazepam (1 and 2 mg/kg) were administered 30 min prior to test. Flumazenil (4 mg/kg) was administered 5 min prior to the administration of alprazolam or diazepam. The control animals received only the vehicle, water or saline.

In chronic study, diazepam (20 mg/kg) and alprazolam (2 mg/kg) were administered once daily between 0900 and 1000 hrs for 14 days. The control animals received only the vehicle and were tested on day 1 and 14. The animals in different groups were tested on day 1, 14 of treatment and 24, 48 and 72 hr after the last dose for chronic and withdrawal induced anxiety, respectively.

For studying short-term memory, alprazolam (0.5, 1 and 2 mg/kg) and diazepam (1, 2 and 4 mg/kg) were administered either immediately after the first day trial to study the effect of drugs on retention of memory or 30 min prior to first day trial to study the effect of drugs on learning or acquisition.

Each group consisted minimum 5 animals and all drug administrations were done intraperitoneally. The results are expressed as mean ± SEM and the statistical analysis was done using Student's *t* test. $P < 0.05$ was considered as statistically significant.

Results

Effect on anxiety response in mice using elevated plus-maze: Control mice showed only 13.3% preference for first entry into open arm and they also showed increased number of total entries and time spent in closed arm as compared to open arm (Table 1).

Alprazolam and diazepam significantly and dose-dependently increased the percent preference for open arm and the open arm entries as compared to control group. At 0.5 and 1 mg/kg dose alprazolam exhibited 100% preference for first entry into open arm, while at 2 mg/kg dose diazepam exhibited 83% preference for first entry into open arm. Flumazenil did not show any effect *per se* but it significantly antagonized the anti-anxiety response of both alprazolam and diazepam on all the parameters (Table 1).

In rats also similar profile of antianxiety effect by alprazolam was obtained (data not included).

Effect of chronic treatment and its withdrawal on anxiety response in mice: Withdrawal of diazepam (20 mg/kg) from chronic treatment produced severe withdrawal-induced anxiety in mice. The anxiety response was more pronounced 48 hr after diazepam withdrawal and it even persisted at 72 hr post-withdrawal. Chronic treatment for 14 days had produced significant antianxiety response (Table 2).

Chronic treatment with alprzolam for 14 days produced significant antianxiety response but the percent preference for open arm was less as compared to its acute effect. However, 24 hr after the withdrawal the animals showed anxiety response as the percent preference, number of entries and duration spent in open arm were significantly less as compared to acute treatment with alprazolam (Table 2).

Table 1. Effect of diazepam and alprazolam treatment on various parameters on elevated plus-maze apparatus and their modification by flumazenil in mice [Values are mean ± SE]

Treatment (mg/kg)	n	Preference to open arm (%)	Open arm		Closed arm		Both arms
			Number of entires	Average time spent (See)	Number of entries	Average time spent (Sec)	Number of total entries
Control	15	13.3	2.46±0.52	5.60±2.03	6.2±0.75	46.21±7.83	7.91±1.51
Diazepam (1)	6	50.0	5.1±0.79**	5.42± 1.0	7.0±0.8	19.43±2.81**	12.66± 1.28*
Diazepam (2)	6	83.3	8.1±0.86**	5.70± 1.52	9.4±1.75	17.58±6.23**	17.6±2.5**
Alprazolam (0.1)	6	33.3	5.66±0.41†	4.17±0.47	11.66± 1.03†	15.3± 1.52†	17.33±0.74†
Alprazolam (0.25)	6	83.3	13.0±2.7†	4.18±0.35	19.1±1.60†	5.43±0.42†	35.5±2.1†
Alprazolam (0.5)	5	100	14.2±1.4†	7.7±1.1	19.0±4.4**	6.9± 1.3†	35.8±3.2†
Alprazolam (1.0)	6	100	3.83±0.39	36.66±3.75†	2.33±0.41**	40.96±4.87	6.16±0.58
Flumazenil (4)	6	16.6	5.83±1.0	9.33±0.88	10.16±0.22	13.73±1.71†	16.0±1.0†
Flumazenil (4) + Diazepam (2)	5	0	1.5±0.93**[a]	1.08±0.57**[a]	6.5±0.55	34.44±2.9*	8.0± 1.38**[a]
Flumazenil (4) + Alprazolam (0.5)	6	20.0	2.8±0.86†[b]	4.98±1.3	3.8±0.37†[b]	55.61±5.7†[b]	6.6±0.98†[b]

P values: * < 0.05; ** < 0.01; † < 0.001 as compared to Control. [a]as compared to the effect of diazepam (2 mg/kg), [b]as compared to the effect of alprazolam (0.5 mg/kg)

Effect of post-trial administration of alprazolam and diazepam on transfer latency: Alprazolam (0.5 to 2 mg/kg) significantly increased the 2nd day shortened transfer latency, while diazepam (2 to 4 mg/kg) did not significantly affect the 2nd day shortened transfer latency, when compared to control animals (Table 3).

Effect of pre-trial administration of alprazolam and diazepam on transfer latency: Alprazolam (0.5-2 mg/kg) and diazepam (1-4 mg/kg) when administered 30 min before 1st day trial significantly delayed the TL of mice. Both the drugs also significantly delayed the 2nd day shortened transfer latency, diazepam being more potent in inducing acquisition deficit (Table 4).

Discussion

Most of the animal models of anxiety are based on the pharmacological profile of benzodiazepines, particularly diazepam. Anticonflict, amnesic, sedative and myorelaxant properties, though dose dependent, constitute as total antianxiety activity of diazepam. No single test procedure adequately describes all these properties. However, recently, elevated plus-maze apparatus has been developed as a novel test procedure for detecting antianxiety properties of drugs in rodents[4,8] and this procedure has been extensively validated in rats and mice.

Rodents prefer enclosed arms of the elevated plus-maze to open arms and spend greater amount of time in enclosed arms[6,9]. This behavioural paradigm of anxiety is substantiated by the fact that rats entering enclosed arms show higher plasma cortisone levels as compared to those animals in home cages, a biochemical marker of anxiety[9].

Table 2. Effect of acute and chronic treatment of diazepam and alprazolam and their withdrawal on various parameters on elevated plus-maze apparatus in mice [Values are mean ± SE]

Treatment (mg/kg)	n	Preference to open arm (%)	Open arm		Closed arm	
			Number of entries	Average time spent (Sec)	Number of entries	Average time spent (Sec)
Control (acute)	15	13.33	2.46±0.52	5.6±2.03	6.2±0.75	46.21±7.83
Control (chronic)	8	37.5	6.12±0.76	7.35±0.97	7.87±0.69	19.72±3.3
Diazepam (20, acute)	6	16.66	2.48±0.51	6.75±1.6	5.2±0.58	38.2±2.7
Diazepam (20 x 14d, chronic)	6	83.3	$12.8\pm1.7^{\dagger a}$	3.5±0.3	$15.0\pm1.8^{\dagger a}$	$4.9\pm0.03^{\dagger a}$
24 hr diazepam withdrawal	5	50.0	3.6±1.0	1.74±0.27	$13.6\pm 1.02^{\dagger}$	$12.1 \pm 1.51^{\dagger}$
48 hr diazepam withdrawal	6	16.6	$0.5\pm0.33^{**b}$	$0.91\pm0.65^{\dagger b}$	$3.83\pm0.53^{*b}$	$68.1\pm9.5^{*b}$
72 hr diazepam withdrawal	6	16.6	1.33±0.41	1.3±0.29*	6.0±1.36	44.05±8.48
Alprazolam (2 , acute)	6	100	$3.83\pm0.39^{*a}$	$40.96\pm4.87^{\dagger a}$	$2.33\pm0.41^{\dagger a}$	36.66±3.75**
Alprazolam (2 x 14d, chronic)	5	42	$9.00\pm0.8^{\dagger ab}$	$6.76\pm0.4^{\dagger ab}$	$11.0\pm1.5^{\dagger}$	17.9±3.8
24 hr alprazolam withdrawal	5	25	5.2±1.1	$8.48\pm 1.8^{\dagger ab}$	$7.0\pm 1.9^{*ab}$	13.6± 1.9
48 hr alprazolam withdrawal	6	46	5.1±0.2	$12.06\pm1.8^{\dagger ab}$	$6.8\pm0.9^{**ab}$	20.7±2.7

P values: * < 0.05; **< 0.01; †< 0.001 as compared to control, [a]as compared to the effect of diazepam (acute, 20 mg/kg), [b]as compared to the effect of alprazolam (acute, 2 mg/kg)

Table 3. Effect of alprazolam on shortened transfer latency when administered immediately after 1st day trial on elevated plus-maze apparatus in mice [Values are mean ± SE]

Treatment (mg/kg)	n	Transfer latency	
		1st day	2nd day
Control	5	33.61±2.62	11.2±1.85
Diazepam (1.0)	5	30.8±0.9	19.6±5.4
Diazepam (2.0)	5	33.5±4.2	18.1±1.6
Diazepam (4.0)	5	34.2±3.2	15.0±1.0
Alprazolam (0.5)	5	34.16±2.82	29.83±5.0**
Alprazolam (1.0)	5	34.00±2.39	33.8±3.92†
Alprazolam (2.0)	5	32.83±2.12	35.16±2.91†
Alprazolam (2.0) + Flumazenil (4.0)	6	33.33±1.17	29.83±4.65

P values : *<0.05, **<0.01, † <0.001

In the present study alprazolam exhibited a clear-cut antianxiety profile in animals subjected to elevated plus-maze, an effect not only comparable to diazepam but also sensitive to reversal by flumazenil. Further, recently it has been shown that acute alprazolam treatment produced alterations in corticotropin releasing hormone and caused a dose-dependent decrease in plasma ACTH and cortisol secretion in animals[10].

File and Hitchcott[11] have described the elevated plus-maze to study withdrawal anxiety response in rats. It is speculated that the behavioural signs of hyperactivity and increased anxiety seen after abrupt discontinuation of high doses of benzodiazepines could be due to the decreased responsiveness of GABA or activation of negative ligand binding site of benzodiazepine receptor[12,13].

This is considered to be an essential component of phramacologic profile of benzodiazepines. Both diazepam and alprazolam showed withdrawal-induced hyperactivity, the peak effect being seen 48 hr after diazepam and 24 hr after alprazolam, respectively. This could be well correlated with relatively longer half-life (20-70 hr) of diazepam with 96-98% protein binding capacity as compared to the intermediate half-life (7-9 hr) of alprazolam.

Table 4. Effect of alprazolam on transfer latency when administered 30 min before first day trial on elevated plus-maze apparatus in mice [Values are mean ± SE]

Treatment (mg/kg)	n	Transfer latency (sec)	
		1st day	2nd day
Control	7	29.57±3.63	12.0±2.55
Diazepam (1)	5	41.12±8.48	17.66±2.39
Diazepam (2)	5	65.0± 11.38*	30.16±3.66†
Diazepam (4)	5	112±5.16**	46.0± 14.29*
Alprazolam (0.5)	5	89.4 ± 18.1*	50.6 ± 13.01*
Alprazolam (1)	5	102.4± 12.53†	50.2± 12.85*
Alprazolam (2)	5	120±0†	45.6±11.51*

P values : *<0.05, **<0.01, † <0.001

Benzodiazepines are reported to produce amnesia in animals and man. Retrograde amnesic effect of diazepam is considered to be a desirable effect in anaesthesia but it is otherwise [14] a side effect. In the present study, like diazepam, alprazolam affected both learning and acquisition behaviour. Post-trial administration of alprazolam also delayed 2nd day shortened transfer latency. But surprisingly, this effect was not significantly reversed by flumazenil.

Besides the observed antianxiety, amnesic and withdrawal reaction to chronic treatment, alprazolam also possessed antidepressant action (data not shown) when tested in forced swimming-induced despair model in mice. The antidepressant effect was sensitive to reversal by flumazenil thereby substantiating GABA/benzodiazepine receptor involvement in the pathogenesis of depression. This property, clubbed with antianxiety profile widens the therapeutic contention of alprazolam for the treatment of anxiety, panic disorders and endogenous depression.

Acknowledgement

Alprazolam was provided by M/s Torrent Laboratories, Ahmedabad.

REFERENCES

1. Zivkovic B, Perrault G & Sanget D J, in *Target receptors for anxiolytics and hypnotics : From molecular pharmacology to therapeutics,* edited by J Mendlewicz & G Racagni (Karger, Basel) 1992.
2. Fawcett J, Edwards J H, Kravit H M & Jeffriess H, *J Clin Psychopharmacol,* 7 (1987) 295.
3. Schweizer E, Fox I, Case G & Rickets K, *Psychopharmacol Bull,* 24 (1998) 224.
4. Pellow S, Chopin P, File S E & Briley M, *J Neurosci Meth,* 14 (1985) 149.
5. Lister R G, *Psychopharmacology,* 92 (1987) 180.
6. Sharma A C & Kulkarni S K, *Drug Dev Res,* 22 (1991) 251.
7. Sharma A C & Kulkarni S K, *Prog Neuro-Psychopharmacol Biol Psychiat,* 16 (1992) 117.
8. Kulkarni S K & Sharma A C, *Meth Find Exp Clin Pharmacol,* 73 (1991) 573.
9. Harro J, Pold M & Vasar *E, Naunyn Schmiedeberg's Arch Pharmacol,* 341 (1990) 62.
10. Kalogeras K T, Calogero A E, Kuribayashi T, Khan I, Gallucci, W T & King M A, *J Clin Endocrinol Metab,* 70 (1990) 146.
11. File S E & Hitchcott P K, *Psychopharmacology,* 101 (1990) 525.
12. Kulkarni S K & Ticku M K, *Brain Res,* 519 (1990) 6.
13. Miller L G, Greenblatt D J, Baruhill J G & Shaden R I, *J Pharmacol Exp Ther,* 246 (1988) 170.
14. Jensen L H, Stephens D N, Sarter M & Petersen E N, *Brain Res Bull,* 19 (1987) 359.

Paper Published In:

I.J.E.B. (Vol. 31, November 1993, pp. 908-911)

18

Prevention of development of tolerance and dependence to opiate in mice by BR-16A (Mentat®), a herbal psychotropic preparation

S.K. KULKARNI & ANITA VERMA
Pharmacology Division, Department of Pharmaceutical Sciences,
Panjab University, Chandigarh 160 014, India

Chronic treatment with BR-16A (20-500 mg/kg) followed by saline on days 1 to 9 failed to produce any significant change in tail-flick latency from the saline- pretreated group in mice. Repeated administration of BR-16A(20-500 mg/kg) for 9 days however, attenuated the development of tolerance to the analgesic effect of morphine (10 mg/kg). BR-16A (20-500 mg/kg) also suppressed, in a dose-dependent manner, the development of morphine dependence as assessed by naloxone (2 mg/kg) -precipitated withdrawal on day 10 of testing.

BR-16A (Mentat®), a herbal psychotropic preparation, contains the following indigenous ingredients, reputed in the ancient system of Ayurvedic medicine to be useful in the management of nervous disorders: brahmi *(Hydrocotyle asiatica)* shatavari *(Asparagus racemosus)*, buchh *(Acorus calamus)*, ashwagandha *(Withania somnifera)*, giloi *(Tinospora cardifolia)*, amla *(Embelica officinalis)*, shankhpushpi *(Evolvulus alsinoides)*, kuth *(Saussurea lappa)* and triphala[1]. Preliminary toxicity studies have shown it to be a safe preparation and no adverse effect ensued its chronic use (unpublished data).

BR-16A has been reported to be effective in improving learning ability and behavioural disturbances in mentally retarded children. It is also beneficial in cases of cerebral deficit, behavioural disturbances following postnatal organic lesions of the central nervous system and in cases having organic loss of bladder function[2-5]. Recent studies have demonstrated that BR-16A improves passive avoidance acquisition and retention in naive as well as amnesic mice[6,7].

Studies on elevated plus-maze[6] have shown anxiogenic and nootropic action of BR-16A. Since dementia and cognitive dysfunctions are known to occur in narcotic addicts, in the present study an attempt has been made to demonstrate, if any, the effectiveness of this herbal preparation in prevention of development of tolerance and dependence to morphine in mice.

Materials and Methods

Animals: Balb'C strain, albino mice of either sex bred in Central Animal House facility of the University, weighing 20-25g were used. The animals were housed under standard light/dark cycle with food and water provided *ad libitum*. The experiments were performed between 09.00 and 17.00 hrs.

Analgesia: Analgesic response was assessed by tail-flick latency to radiant heat as described by D'Armour and Smith[8] and as modified by Kulkarni[9]. Baseline latencies to tail-flick withrawal from the radiant source (3-4 sec) were established. A cut-off time of 10 sec was observed to prevent any injury to the tail. A minium of three trials were recorded for each animal.

Drugs: The drugs used were BR-16A (Mentat®: Himalaya Drug Co., Bombay, India), morphine (Government Analytical Laboratory, Chandigarh) and naloxone (Endo, New York).

BR-16A powder was suspended uniformly in deionized water and administered orally while the remaining drugs were given, s.c., as aqueous solutions, in a constant volume of 1 ml/100g body weight.

Treatment schedule: In acute studies, the animals received saline or BR-16A (20-500 mg/kg) followed 30 min later by saline or morphine (10 mg/kg). The analgesic response to morphine was assessed by the tail-flick test 60 min after the second injection.

For induction of tolerance to morphine, animals received the opiate injection twice daily (09.00 and 16.00 hrs) for 9 days. On days 1, 3 and 9, analgesic response was assessed by the tail-flick test 60 min after morphine injection. Various treatment groups (pretreatment : treatment) included[10]: (i) saline: saline; (ii) saline : morphine (10 mg/

kg); (iii) BR -16A (20-500 mg/kg): saline; and (iv) BR-16A (20-500 mg/kg): morphine (10 mg/kg). On 10th day treatments were reversed so that the animals that had received BR-16A followed by morphine on days 1 through 9 were challenged with saline followed by morphine. In addition the animals that had been treated with BR-16A followed by saline were challenged with BR-16A followed by morphine. Immediately after the tail-flick test on day 10, the animals were injected with naloxone (2 mg/kg) to precipitate withdrawal. The withdrawal syndrome was assessed by placing each mouse in a 45 cm high plexiglass box and the incidence of escape jumps were recorded for 15 min.

Statistical analysis: The data, expressed as mean ± SE was analysed by one-way analysis of variance (ANOVA) followed by Dunett's t test. Probability levels of less than 5% were considered significant.

Results

Effect of chronic administration of morphine on analgesic response: Animals receiving chronic treatment with morphine (10 mg/kg) displayed maximal analgesia on days 1 and 3 (Fig. 1). In saline treated mice, the analgesic response to morphine displayed rapid development of tolerance, reaching baseline latencies by days 9 and 10 (Fig. 2).

Effect of chronic concomitant treatment with BR-16A and morphine on development of tolerance to morphine: The animals treated repeatedly with BR-16A (20-500 mg/kg) showed significant analgesic response on days 1 and 3 of morphine (10 mg/kg) treatment (Fig. 1). Pretreatment with BR-16A prevented the development of tolerance to the analgesic response of morphine on day 9 of testing (Fig. 2). The animals that had been treated with BR-16A and morphine on days 1 through 9, then given morphine alone on day 10 also displayed considerable analgesia on the 10th day (Fig. 2).

Effect of chronic treatment with BR-16A on analgesic response: Chronic administration of BR-16A (20-500 mg/kg) followed by saline failed to elicit any analgesic response on days 1 and 3 in mice (Fig. 3). Animals treated with BR-16A followed by saline displayed tail-flick latencies no greater than saline-pretreated animals on days 1 through 9 (Fig. 4). Challenging with BR-16A and morphine (10 mg/kg) on day 10 produced significant analgesia; a response comparable to morphine effect on day 1 (Fig. 4).

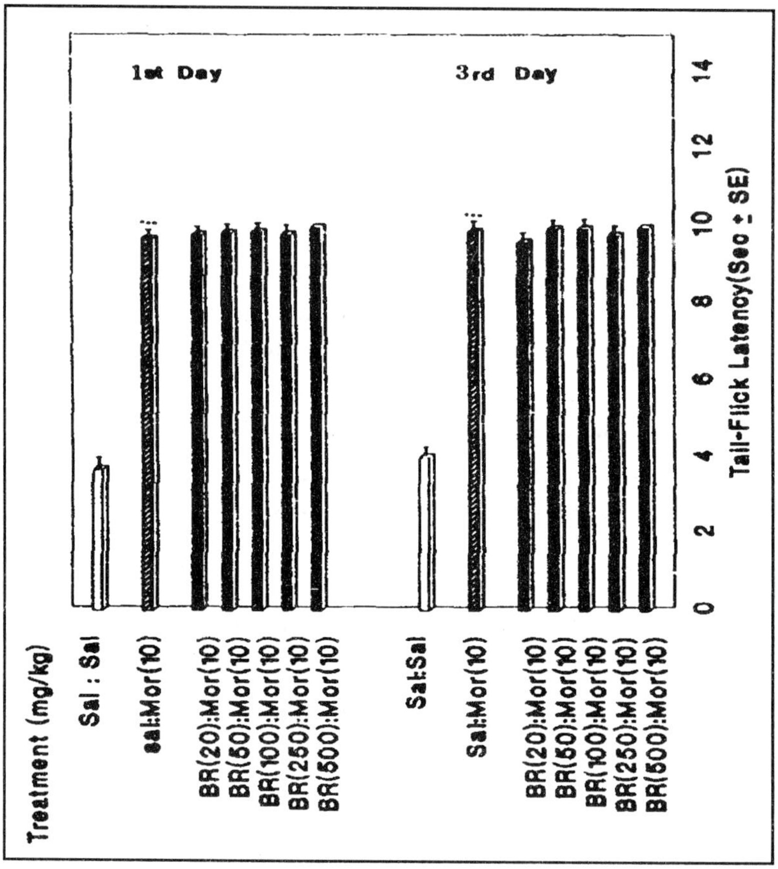

Fig. 1. Effect of various doses of BR-16A on morphine analgesia on day 1 and 3 of the treatment. Values are mean ± SE, n = 10-21. • • • P< 0.001 as compared with sal : sal treated control. Sal- saline; BR- BR-16A; Mor- Morphine.

Effect of chronic treatment with BR-16A and morphine on naloxone-precipitated withdrawal jumps: Animals that had received repeated administration of saline followed by morphine (10 mg/kg) displayed numerous escape jumps in response to an injection of naloxone (2 mg/kg) on day 10. In contrast, the animals treated with BR-16A (20-500 mg/kg) and morphine (10 mg/kg) on days 1 through 9, then with saline and morphine on day 10 displayed significantly fewer jumps after naloxone (2 mg/kg) administration (Fig. 5).

Discussion

Development of physical dependence and tolerance with repeated use is a characteristic feature of all the opioid drugs and entail major

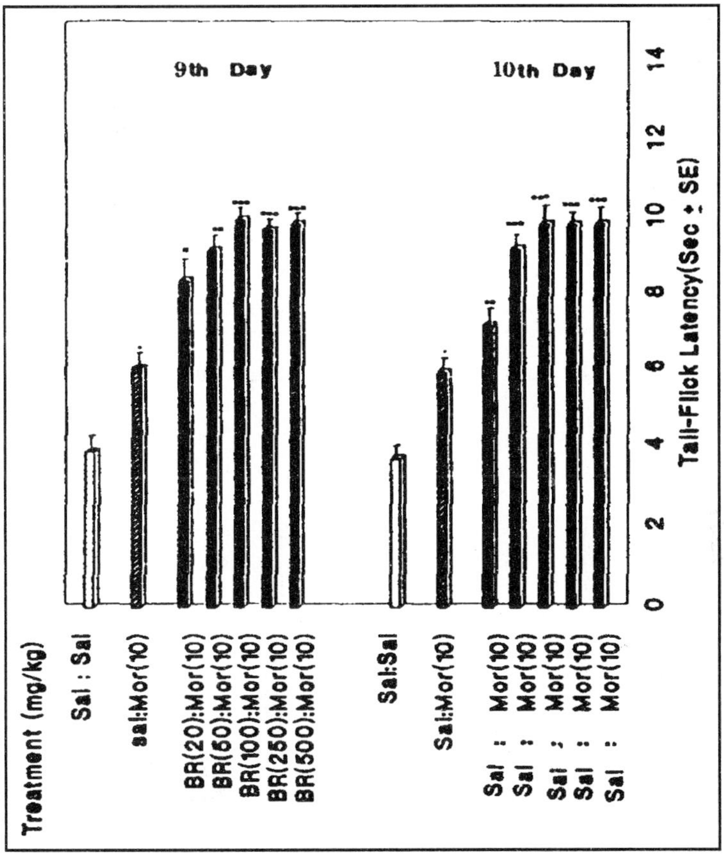

Fig. 2. Effect of various doses of BR-16A on development of tolerance to analgesic effect of morphine on days 9 and 10 of testing. • $P < 0.05$ as compared with sal: sal treated control. • $P < 0.05$, •• $P < 0.01$, ••• $P < 0.001$ as compared with respective sal : Mor- treated groups. [Other details are same as in Fig. 1]

limitation in their clinical use. Thus, a decision to relieve any chronic symptom, especially pain, may be short-sighted and can be disservice to the patient. In the present study potential utility of BR-16A, a herbal psychotropic preparation, has been examined against the development of tolerance and dependence to morphine.

Animals treated with morphine (10 mg/kg) displayed maximal analgesia on days 1 and 3 of treatment. In saline-treated animals the analgesic response to morphine displayed rapid development of tolerance on days 9 and 10. In contrast the animals treated with BR-16A showed less tolerance, maintaining an analgesic response throughout the testing period. The increased analgesia seen in the BR-

16A- treated group was not attributable to an analgesic action of BR-16A alone or to an acute analgesic interaction between BR-16A and morphine. Animals treated acutely with BR-16A (20-500 mg/kg) showed no change in tail-flick latency, demonstrating a lack of effect of BR-16A on pain responsiveness. Further, the animals that were treated with BR-16A and morphine on days 1 through 9, then challenged with saline and morphine on day 10 showed no greater analgesia than that seen the previous day.

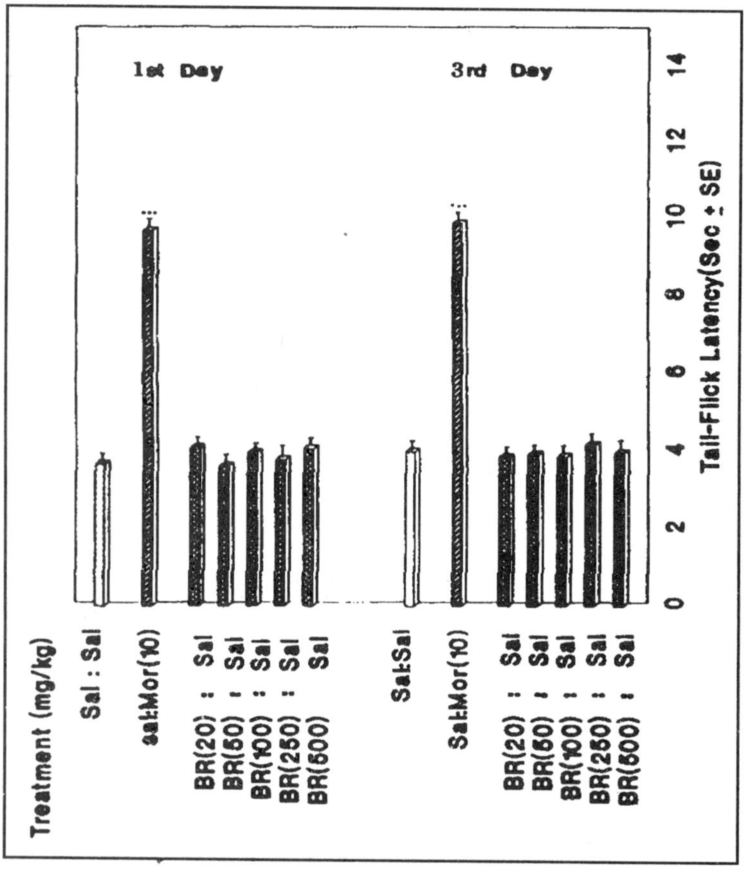

Fig. 3. Effect of morphine and BR-16A alone respectively, on analgesic response on days 1 and 3 of testing. ••• $P < 0.001$ as compared with the Sal : Sal- treated control. [Other details are same as in Fig. 1]

Substitution of saline with morphine on day 10 in the group that had been receiving BR-16A followed by saline on days 1 through 9 produced significant analgesia. This demonstrates that the chronic treatment with BR-16A does not affect the expression of morphine analgesia. Further, the animals receiving chronic-treatment with BR-16A and morphine, then morphine alone on day 10 displayed considerable analgesia on day 10 despite the lack of BR-16A pretreatment on this day. The results suggest that BR-16A need not be present during testing to observe analgesia in chronically BR-16A-treated animals. BR-16A, therefore, inhibits the development of tolerance to the analgesic effect of morphine.

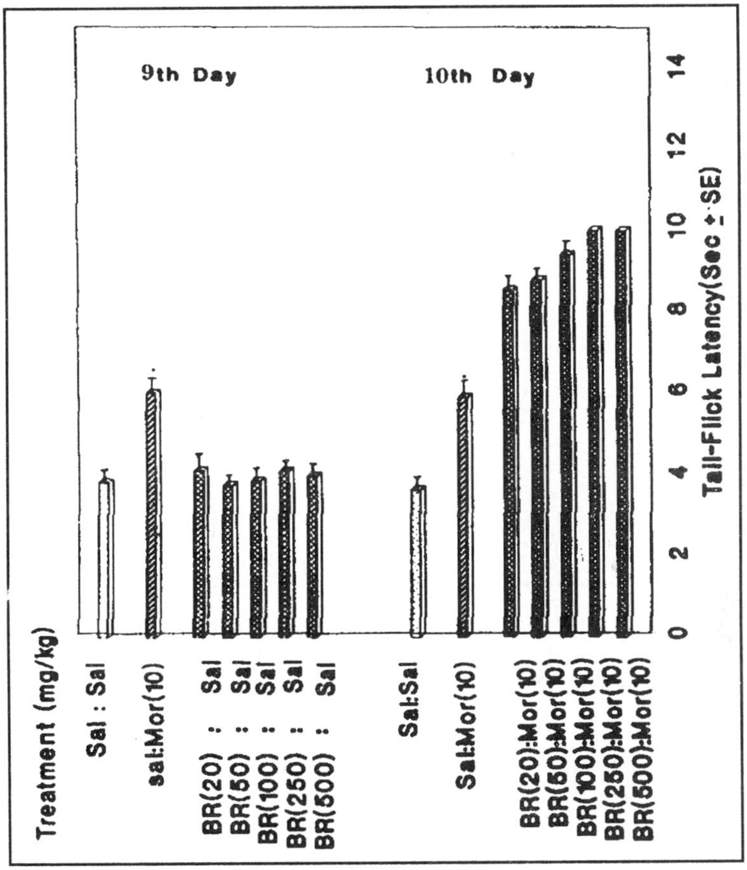

Fig. 4. Effect of various doses of BR- I6A on analgesic response in saline- and morphine-treated mice on days 9 and 10 of testing, respectively. • P < 0.05 as compared with Sal : Sal- treated control. Treatment was reversed on day 10 in BR: Sal group. [Other details are same as in Fig. 1]

In addition to interfering with tolerance, BR-16A pretreatment inhibited naloxone-precipitated abstinence syndrome. Pretreatment with BR-16A (20-500 mg/kg) significantly and in a dose-dependent manner reduced the number of jumps after naloxone administration

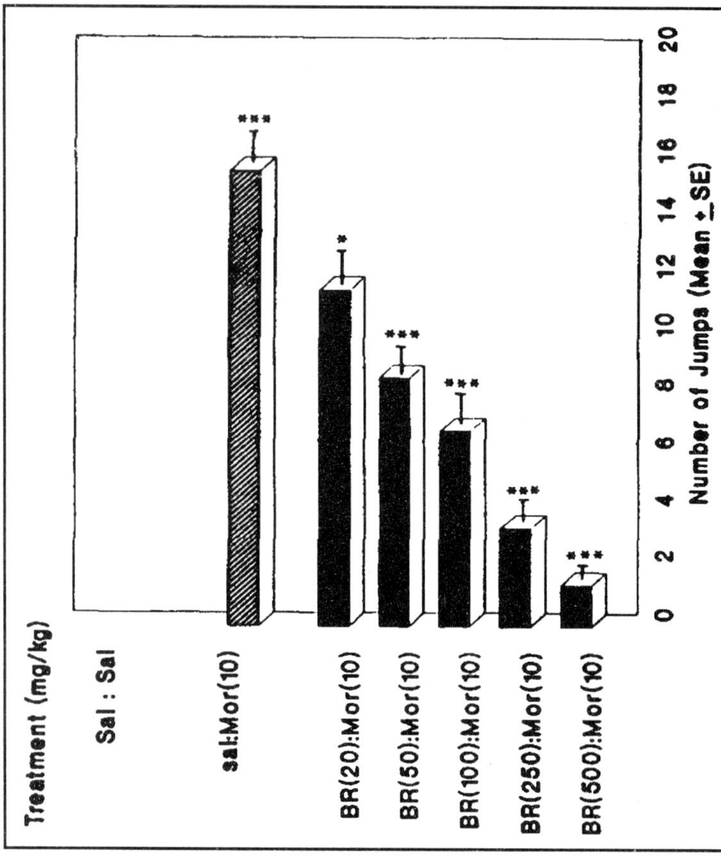

Fig. 5. Effect of various doses of BR-16A on naloxone precipitated morphine-withdrawl. *P < 0.05, *** P < 0.001 as compared with the sal- Mor- treated control. [Other details are same as in Fig. 1].

in groups chornically treated with morphine. As with the above experiments on tolerance, the effect of BR-16A was attributable to the repeated administration of BR-16A with morphine. Animals which received saline and morphine on days 1 through 9 displayed numerous jumps after administration of naloxone (2 mg/kg) on day 10 of testing. Animals that had, received BR-16A and morphine on days 1 through 9 displayed few jumps despite the fact that they did not receive BR-16A on day 10 prior to the naloxone-precipitated withdrawal. Thus, BR-16A administered during repeated treatment with morphine interferes with development of tolerance and dependence to opiates.

In conclusion, BR-16A (Mentat®) is a safe non-analgesic herbal preparation which can be used in the treatment of opiate addiction.

Acknowledgement

The work was supported by the research Grants of Himalaya Drug Co., Bombay, India.

REFERENCES

1. lyengar M A, in *Study of crude drugs,* edited by M A Iyengar (Manipal Power Press, India) 1981.
2. Bai K I & Sastry V N, *Probe,* 30 (1991) 247.
3. D'Souza B D & Cavda K B, *Probe,* 30 (1991) 227.
4. Mehta U R, *Probe,* 30 (1991) 233.
5. Sheth S C, Tibrewala N S, Pal P M, Dube B L & Desai R G, *Probe,* 30 (1991) 222.
6. Verma A & Kulkarni S K, *Indian J Exp Biol,* 29 (1991) 1120
7. Kulkarni S K & Verma A, *Indian J Physiol Pharmacol,* 30 (1992) 29.
8. D'Armour F E & Smith D I, *J Pharmacol Exp Ther,* 72 (1941) 74.
9. Kulkarni S K, *Life Sci,* 27 (1980) 185.
10. Trujillo K A & Huda A, *Science,* 251 (1991) 85.

Paper Published In:

I.J.E.B. (Vol. 30, October 1992, pp. 885-888)

19

Effect of a herbal psychotropic preparation, BR-16A (Mentat), on performance of mice on elevated plus-maze

ANITA VERMA & S.K. KULKARNI
Pharmacology Division, Department of Pharmaceutical Sciences,
Panjab University, Chandigarh 160 014, India

Effect of BR-16A on various parameters of anxiety and transfer latency (TL) was studied in mice using elevated plus-maze. BR- 16A (50-500 mg/kg) reduced the percentage of time spent in open arms and the percent preference of open arms for the first arm entry following acute as well as chronic drug administration. The total number of arm entries and the percentage of open arm entries remained unaffected. In combination with FG 7142 (10 mg/kg), BR-16A (100-500 mg/kg) further reduced the exploration of open arms. BR-16A reversed scopolamine (0.3 mg/kg)-induced delay in TL on 1st day. The reversal effect of BR-16A was enhanced by aniracetam (50 mg/kg). The data suggest anxiogenic and nootropic actions of BR-16A.

BR-16A (Mentat, Himalaya Drug Co.), an ayurvedic preparation, contains the following indigenous ingredients, reputed in the ancient system of Ayurvedic medicine to be of value in the management of nervous disorders: Brahmi *(Hydrocotyl asiatica)*, Shatavari *(Asparagus racemosus)*, Jatamansi *(Nardostachys jatamansi)*, Bidarikand *(Xpomosa digitata)*, Bachh *(Acorus calamus)*, Ashwagandha *(Withania somnifera)*, *Giloi (Tinospora cardifolia)*, Amla *(Embelica officinalis)*, Shankhpushpi *(Evolvulus alsinoides)*, Kuth *(Saussurea lappa)* and Triphala[1].

The recent clinical trials with this drug have shown it to be effective in cases of mental retardation, cerebral deficit, behavioural disorders following postnatal organic lesions of CNS and in cases having organic loss of bladder function (Personal communication). Preliminary toxicity studies have shown it to be a safe preparation. LD_{50} has been reported to be 2400 mg/kg in mice by oral route of administration (Personal communication).

The elevated plus-maze introduced by Pellow *et al.*[2]. for rats and by Lister[3] for mice is based on the apparent natural aversion of rodents to open and high spaces, and is used for the measurement of anxiety[2-4] as well as short-term memory[5]. Because of the disliking for the open arms, the animal spends more time in the enclosed than the open arms and this aversive quality becomes apparent only when the animal enters them[2]. Itoh *et a1.*[5], therefore, speculated that the time in which the animal moves from the open arm to the enclosed arms (transfer latency; TL) might be shortened if the animal had previously experienced entering the open arms. The shortened transfer latency was then related to memory.

In our previous study, BR-16A improved acquisition and memory retrieval in passive avoidance step-down paradigm in mice[6]. Using the above concept and background of elevated plus-maze, an attempt was made to study the effect of BR-16A on anxiety, learning and memory in mice on elevated plus-maze, although this method is not based on positive or negative reinforcers.

Materials and Methods

Animals: Wistar albino mice of either sex (bred in Central Animal House Facility of Panjab University, Chandigarh), weighing 20-25 g were used. They were housed under standard laboratory conditions and allowed free access to food and water. All the experiments were carried out between 9.00 and 17.00 hrs.

Elevated plus-maze: Measurement of anxiety: An elevated plus-maze consisting of two open arms (16 x 5 cm) and two enclosed arms (16 x 5 x 12 cm) was used in the present study[7]. The maze was elevated to a height of 25 cm. During 5 min test session the following parameters were noted: (a) number of entries the animal made in open and enclosed arms, (b) the total time spent in each arm and (c) choice of open/enclosed arm as the first arm entry. Animals were individually placed at the centre of the plus-maze facing towards an open arm at the beginning of the test. All the drugs were administered 30 min prior to the test, either alone or in combination. Each animal was used only once.

Elevated plus-maze: Measurement of TL: The method used to measure TL was essentially the same as described by Itoh *et al.*[5] The mice were placed individually at the end of one open arm facing away from the centre of the maze and the time the mouse took to move from open arm to either of the enclosed arms (TL) was recorded. On the 1st day the mouse was allowed to explore the plus-maze for 20s after the measurement of TL. The mice were returned to their home cages after the first trial. Twenty four hours later, the mice were placed on the elevated plus-maze individually as before and TL was recorded again. If the mouse did not enter the enclosed arm within 60s on the second trial, TL was assigned to 60s. TL measured on 1st and 2nd day served as parameters for acquisition and retrieval respectively. All the drugs were administered 30 min prior to the 1st trial.

Drugs: The drugs used in the study were obtained from the following sources: BR-16A (Himalaya Drug Co., Bombay, India), scopolamine hydrobromide (Merck and Co., Inc., Rahway, NJ, USA); aniracetam (F. Hoffman-La Roche, Basel, Switzerland) and FG 7142 (Schering, Berlin).

BR-16A was administered orally while the remaining drugs were given intraperitoneally in a constant volume of 1 ml/ 100 g of body weight.

Statistical analysis: One-way analysis of variance (ANOVA) was performed on % open arm entries, % time spent in open arms or total number of entries. Posthoc comparisons were made using Dunett's t-test. Probability levels of less than 5% were considered significant.

Results and Discussion

In elevated plus-maze mice show natural aversion to open and high spaces and, therefore, spend more time in the enclosed arms which forms the basis for its use in the measurement of anxiety[8]. The behavioural results of the present study showed that the naive mice spent a significantly lesser time in the open arms, and also entered them less frequently than the enclosed arms. The preference is likely to reflect an aversion towards the open arms caused by fear or anxiety. This aversion was, however, not consistently present as early as the first arm entry, since saline-treated mice showed a consistent tendency to enter an open arm first. It is, therefore, possible that the aversive quality of the open arms is not apparent until the mice enter them.

BR-16A (50-500mg/kg) reduced the percentage preference for the open arm as the first arm entry but failed to influence significantly the total number of entries in both the arms and the percentage of open arm entries. The lower doses (50, 100 mg/kg) failed to affect the percentage of time spent in open arms as compared to saline-treated control but the higher doses (250, 500 mg/kg) produced a significant decrease in the percentage of time spent in the open arms.

Chronic administration of BR-16A (100, 500 mg/ kg) for 7 and 14 days respectively reduced significantly the percentage of time spent in the open arms.

Table 1. Effect of acute administration of various doses of BR-16A on various parameters of anxiety on elevated plus-maze in mice

Group No.	Treatment mg/kg	n	% preference for open arm entry	% open arm entries (mean±SE)	% time spent in open arms (mean±SE)	Total No. of entries (mean±SE)
1	Saline	20	55	26.0 ± 3.0	28.0 ± 3.0	12.5 ± 0.92
2	BR-16A, 50	9	56	34.2±5.1	33.0 ± 4.2	12.2 ± 1.4
3	BR-16A, 100	8	50	32.3 ± 6.2	25.1 ± 3.2	12.8 ± 1.4
4	BR-16A, 250	9	33	26.4±5.2	19.3±3.1*	11.1±1.4
5	BR-16A, 500	15	12	24.8 ± 4.0	9.6 ± 3.0***	12.0 ± 1.5

**P*< 0.05, ****P*< 0.001 as compared to saline group. The data was analysed by one-way ANOVA followed by Dunett's t-test. ANOVA, F-ratio (12, 111) = 9.79, P< 0.05 for % open arm entries; F-ratio (12, 111) = 4.69, P< 0.05 for % time spent in open arms; F-ratio (12, 111) = 7.8, P<0.05 for total No. of entries.

Table 2. Effect of chronic (7, 14 days) administration of various doses of BR-16A on various parameters of anxiety on elevated plus-maze in mice.

Group No.	Treatment mg/kg	n	% preference for open arm entry	% open arm entries (meant ± SE)	% time spent in open arms (meant ± SE)	Total No. of entries (meant ± SE)
1	Saline	20	55	26.0 ± 3.0	28.0 ± 3.0	12.5 ± 0.92
2	BR-16A, 100 (7 days)	15	27	22.2±3.3	15.8±2.0*	13.8 ± 1.47
3	BR-16A, 100 (14 days)	8	12.5	19.4 ± 5.2	13.8±5.0*	11.8 ± 1.9
4	BR-16A, 500 (7 days)	14	28	19.0 ± 2.1	18.8 ± 5.0*	10.0 ± 1.37
5	BR-16A, 500 (14 days)	6	16.7	24.3 ± 5.2	12.4 ± 3.3*	13.8 ± 1.67

*P< 0.05 as compared to saline group. ANOVA, F-ratio (12, 111) = 9.79, P< 0.05 for % open arm entries; F-ratio (12, 111) = 4.69, P< 0.05 for % time spent in open arms; F-ratio (12, 111) = 7.8, P< 0.05 for total no. of entries.

There was no significant reduction in the percentage of open arm entries and the total number of entries in both the arms but the percentage preference for the open arm entry was significantly reduced as compared to saline-treated control.

Table 3. Effect of combined administration of BR-16A plus FG-7142 on various parameters of anxiety on elevated plus-maze in mice

Group No.	Treatment mg/kg	n	% preference for open arm entry	% open arm entries (meant SE)	% time spent in open arms (meant SE)	Total No. of entries (meant SE)
1	Saline	20	55	26.0±3.0	28.0 ± 3.0	12.5±0.92
2	FG 7142, 10	6	66	24.3±5.2	23.1 ±4.2*	9.0±0.63**
3	FG 7142, 20	5	40	11.2 ± 4.1	15.0 ± 5.1 **	7.8 ± 1.4*
4	FG 7142, 10 + BR-16A, 100	4	60	22.2 ± 3.3	9.0±4.3**	7.4±0.8***
5	FG 7142, 10 + BR-16A, 250	5	40	9.0 ± 2.0***	4.1 ± 3.2	4.0±1.08***
6	FG 7142, 10 + BR-16A, 500	5	20	4.0±0.8**	4.6±4.0*	3.4 ±0.4***

*P<0.05, **P<0.01, ***P<0.001 as compared to respective control values. ANOVA, F-ratio (12,111) = 9.79, P<0.05 for % open arm entries; F-ratio (12,111)= 4.69, P<0.05 for % time spent in open arms; F-ratio (12,111)= 7.8, P<0.05 for total no. of entries.

Table 4. Effect of the combination of BR-16A with scopolamine and aniracetam on the transfer latency (TL) as studied on elevated plus-maze in mice

Group No.	Treatment, mg/kg	n	Transfer latency (TL) in sec (mean ± SE)	
			1st day	2nd day
1	Saline	8	36.25 ± 9.50	28.87 ± 3.56
2	Scopolamine, 0.3	7	101.43 ± 10.89***	39.97 ± 7.04
3	Scopolamine, 0.3 + BR-16A, 50	8	58.25 ± 7.20*	37.25 ±4.82
4	Scopolamine, 0.3 + BR-16A, 100	8	29.50 ± 5.64***	25.50 ± 3.06
5	Aniracetam, 50	9	72.22 ± 11.15*	40.44 ±6.72
6	Aniracetam, 50 + Scopolamine, 0.3	6	39.2 ± 7.01 *	28.00 ± 7.70
7	Aniracetam, 50 + Scopolamine, 0.3+ BR-16A, 50	6	27.83 ± 3.20**	23.30 ± 3.33

**P<0.05, **P<0.01, ***P<0.001* as compared to respective control values. ANOVA, F-ratio (6,48)=15.45, *P<0.05.*

The selective decrease in the exploration of open-arms following acute as well as chronic administration of BR-16A suggests an anxiogenic action of the drug. Since BR-16A selectively affects the percentage of time spent in open arms, it appears that this parameter is more sensitive to drug effects than the number of entries.

FG 7142, a β-carboline and a central benzodiazepine inverse agonist[9], at 20 mg/kg dose showed a significant decrease in the percent preference, percentage of open arm entries and the time spent in open arms, thus demonstrating an anxiogenic response. At the lower dose (10 mg/kg), FG 7142 did not show such an effect. The combined administration of FG 7142 (10 mg/kg) and increasing doses of BR-16A (100-500 mg/kg) produced a further decrease in the exploration of the open arms. This lends credence to the proposal that BR-16A possesses anxiogenic action as revealed by the behaviour of mice on elevated plus-maze.

When elevated plus-maze was utilized for the evaluation of short-term memory, the time the mice took to go over to the enclosed arm (TL) on the 2nd day was shorter than that on the 1st day but the effect was not statistically significant probably due to large variations in the response. Scopolamine (0.3 mg/kg), an anticholinergic agent, injected 30 min prior to the 1st trial, produced a significant elevation of TL on the 1st day. However, the TL of the amnestic mice was shortened by the administration of BR-16A (50, 100 mg/kg).

The reversal effect of BR-16A on TL measured on 1st day was significantly enhanced by its combined administration with aniracetam (50 mg/kg) in scopolamine-treated mice. This study demonstrates that BR- 16A reverses scopolamine-induced deficit in acquisition[10], an effect enhanced by aniracetam. The lack of effect of any of these drugs on TL measured on 2nd day suggests the possible lack of any forceful motivation for learning.

In conclusion, the evaluation of behaviour of mice on elevated plus-maze suggests that BR-16A possesses an anxiogenic action and reveses acquisition deficit induced by cholinergic hypofunction. The anxiogenic action of BR-16A may also contribute to its facilitatory action on learning in mice, when evaluated using TL as a parameter on elevated plus-maze.

Acknowledgement

This work was supported by grants from Himalaya Drug Co., Bombay, India.

REFERENCES

1. Iyengar M A, *Study of crude drugs,* edited by Iyengar M A (Manipal Power Press, India) 1981.
2. Pellow S, Chopin P, File S E & Briley M, *J Neurosci Meth,* 14 (1985) 149.
3. Lister R G, *Psychophamacology,* 92 (1987) 180.
4. Fellow S & File S E, *Pharmacol Biochem Behav,* 24 (1986) 525.
5. Itoh J, Nabeshima T & Kameyama T, *Psychopharmacology,* 101 (1990) 27.
6. Verma A & Kulkarni S K, *Ind J Pharmacol* 23 (1990) 8 (Abstr).
7. Sharma A C & Kulkarni S K, *Drug Dev Res,* 22 (1991) 251.
8. Harro J, Kiivert R-A, Pbld M & Rago L, *Acta Comment Univ Tartuensis,* 839 (1988) 117.
9. Shanbhogue R, Hrishikeshavan H J, Devi K & Munonyedi S, *Prog Neuropsychopharmacol Biol Psychiat,* 14 (1990) 249.
10. Sharma A C & Kulkarni S K, *Meth Find Exp Clin Pharmacol,* 12 (1990) 175.

Paper Published In:
I.J.E.B. (Vol. 29, December 1991, pp. 1120-1123)

20

Effect of reserpine, chlorpromazine and meprobamate on stress induced metabolic alterations in urinary excretion of 3-Methoxy-4-Hydroxymandelic acid

S.K. KULKARNI, P.C. DANDIYA & K.P. KHUTETA
Department of Pharmacology & Physiology S.M.S. Medical College, Jaipur

Influence of tranquillizers, namely reserpine, chlorpromazine and meprobamate, on the urinary excretion of vanillylmandelic acid was determined in rabbits subjected to either heat or cold stress by keeping them at 40°±1°C or -2°±1°C for 1 hr respectively. Both the types of stress caused a significant increase in the urinary excretion of vanillyl mandelic acid. Preadministration of reserpine, chlorpromazine and meprobamate produced a varying degree of protection against stress induced changes.

It has been reported that physiological stress produces highly integrated metabolic activities in the organism[1-3]. A number of changes are known to take place in blood and other tissue constituents during stress besides the release of catecholamines and corticosteroids from the adrenals during stressful condition. Dandiya *et al.*[1,2] have reported that psychopharmacological agents, viz. reserpine, chlorpromazine and meprobamate, have successfully prevented some of the biochemical alterations produced by heat and cold stress. The present study was undertaken to study the effects of tranquillizers in conditions of physiological stress with special reference to the catecholamine metabolism. The influence of tranquillizing agents on the urinary excretion of 3-methoxy-4-hydroxymandelic acid (VMA), an end product of catecholamine metabolism, has been studied.

Urinary excretion of vanillyl mandelic acid (VMA) was determined by the method of Pisano *et al.*[4]. All estimations were done on healthy rabbits of either sex weighing between 1.3 and 1.6 kg at room temperature (26°±2°C). No food was given to the animals for 24 hr before the experiment. Urine was collected for 24 hr by keeping the animals separately in metabolic cages.

Reserpine, chlorpromazine and meprobamate were used in the study. The animals were subjected to either heat or cold stress by keeping them at an environmental temperature of 40°±1°C and -2°±1°C respectively for 1 hr. When drugs were administered, reserpine (0.3 mg/kg), chlorpromazine (3 mg/kg) and meprobamate (30 mg/kg), animals were subjected to stress 4 hr after reserpine; 1 hr after chlorpromazine and 45 min after meprobamate.

All the drugs were administered intraperitoneally.

Both types of stress caused a significant increase in the urinary excretion of VMA (Fig. 1). Premedication with different psychopharmacological agents produced varying effects. Reserpine itself produced a stress-like effect on VMA level. Pre- treatment with chlorpromazine and reserpine failed to offer protection against cold stress but meprobamate pretreatment produced a partial protection which was not significant. All the 3 drugs, given before heat stress, protected the animals from stress induced increase in the urinary excretion of VMA.

In the present study the urinary excretion of VMA was increased significantly on subjecting the animals to heat and cold stress. It is

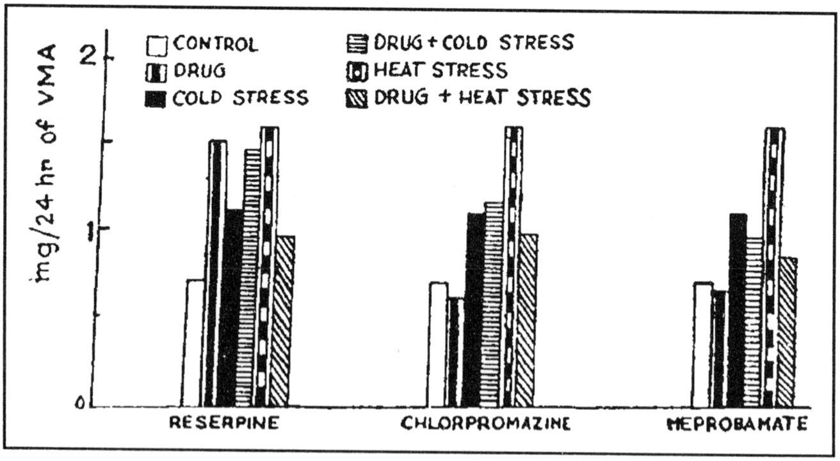

Fig. 1. Effect of psychopharmacological agents on vanillylmandelic acid (VMA) excretion

well known that different kinds of stress enhance the sympathetic activity directly by release of catecholamines and indirectly through the activation of the hypophyseal adrenocortical systems[5]. Further, McDonald and Weises[6] have shown that about 80-90% of endogenous catecholamines are converted to VMA under normal conditions.

Reserpine, when administered alone, caused a stress-like effect as the urinary excretion of VMA was significantly increased. Dandiya *et al.*[2] have also shown that reserpine produced some stress-like effect in animals. Present findings are consistent with the observations of McDonald and Weise[7] who have reported that acute reserpine administration caused an increased urinary excretion of VMA, both in normal and schizophrenic patients. On the other hand, chlorpromazine when given alone did not alter the urinary excretion of VMA. Similarly, meprobamate did not show remarkable effect when administered alone or before subjecting the animals to stress as this drug does not affect the overall turnover of catecholamines[7].

All the 3 drugs (reserpine, chlorpromazine and meprobamate) protected the animals from the heat stress-induced increase in the urinary excretion of VMA, but failed to offer significant protection in cold stress. In the earlier reports from our laboratory, Varma *et al.*[8] have also shown that these tranquillizers protected the animals from heat stress induced metabolic changes on the glutathione content of brain and blood and also on the brain neurohormonal changes.

The authors are thankful to Indian Council of Medical Research for providing liberal grants for this study. The authors are also thankful to pharmaceutical laboratories for supply of drugs, chlorpromazine hydrochloride, May & Baker Ltd, Dagenham, England; reserpine, Ciba of India Ltd, Bombay; meprobamate, John Wyeth Pharmaceuticals Ltd, Bombay.

REFERENCES

1. Dandiya, P. C., Verma, R. R., Khuteta, K. P. & Sogani, R. K., *Rajasthan Univ. Studies*, 1 (1966), 8.
2. Dandiya, P. C., Varma, R. R., Sogani, R. K. & Khuteta, K. P., *J. Pharm. Sci.*, 56 (1967), 300.
3. Menon, M. K. & Dandiya, P. C., *Europ. J. Pharmac.*, 8 (1969), 284.
4. Pisano, J. J., Court, J. R. & Abraham, D., *Clin. Chem. Acta*, 7 (1962), 285.
5. Mallov, S., *Am. J. Physiol.*, 204 (1963), 157.

6. McDonald, R. K. & Weise, V. K., *Proc. Soc. Exp. Biol. Med.*, 127 (1968), 748.
7. McDonald, R. K. & Weise, V. K., *J. Pharm. Exp. There.*, 136 (1962), 26.
8. Varma, R. R., Khuteta, K. P. & Dandiya, P. C., *Psychopharmacologia*, 12 (1968), 170.

Paper Published In:
I.J.E.B. (Vol. 11, No. 3. May 1973, pp. 229-230)

21

Basic mechanisms of pain and inflammation: Regulators and their inhibitors

S. K. KULKARNI AND VIJAY PAL SINGH
Pharmacology Division, University Institute of Pharmaceutical Sciences, Panjab University, Chandigarh 160 014, India

Introduction

The word pain is derived from the Latin word **poena**, meaning **punishment**. It is defined as an unpleasant sensory and emotional experience associated with actual or potential tissue damage, or described in terms of such damage. Pain, therefore, is a defense mechanism that helps to protect an organism by influencing it to withdraw from harmful stimuli. It is a complex sensory experience with many subjective components i.e. 1) discriminative, 2) learning and memory - associate pain with certain events, 3) unpleasantness or displeasure and 4) suffering, escape[1].

Commonly pain is categorized into somatic or visceral, based on where in the body the pain is felt. Somatic pain is caused by the activation of pain receptors either in the cutaneous (body surface) or deep tissues (musculoskeletal tissues). When it occurs in the musculoskeletal tissues, it is called deep somatic pain. Surface somatic pain is usually sharper and may have a burning or pricking quality whereas deep somatic pain is usually described as dull or aching but localized. Common examples of somatic pain include postsurgical pain from a surgical incision (cutaneous pain) and pain due to bone metastasis (deep tissue pain). In contrast, the visceral pain refers to the pain from internal areas of the body that are enclosed within a cavity. It is caused by activation of pain receptors resulting from infiltration, compression, extension, or stretching of the thoracic (chest), abdominal, or pelvic viscera. The pain associated with pancreatic cancer and metastases in the abdomen are well known examples of visceral pain. Characteristically, visceral pain is not well localized and is usually described as pressure-like, deep squeezing.

Clinically, pain has been classified into two major types, acute and chronic/persistent pain. Acute (fast) pain is felt within 0.1 sec after a painful stimuli (mechanical: pinch; thermal: heat or cold; chemical: acid or a bee sting; artificial: electric shock) is applied to the skin and disappears after the noxious stimuli has been removed. Whereas chronic (slow) pain is spontaneous in nature that begins after 1 sec and increases slowly. Chronic or persistent pain is subclassified into inflammatory and neuropathic pain. Inflammatory pain may last for hours, days, months, or years. Examples include scrapes, bruises, burns, minor infection, muscle joint pain, back pain, and tension headache. The second type of chronic pain i.e. neuropathic pain arises from injury to the peripheral or central nervous system. Examples of neuropathic pain include postherpetic neuralgia, extremity pain in diabetes, phantom limb pain, and sciatica. Neuropathic pain is often burning in quality and is sometimes paroxysmal, stabbing, buzzing and electric shock-like. The persons with neuropathic pain may also additionally experience allodynia (pain due to a stimulus which does not normally provoke pain), hyperalgesia (an increased response to a stimulus which is normally not painful), paraesthesia, dysesthesia, or hyperpathia (abnormal sensations, whether spontaneous or evoked). The nerve injury is associated with alteration in electrical properties, neurochemistry, and central connectivity of neurons. The result is the combination of axonal damage (axonopathy, axotomy) and damage to the axon's myelin sheath (dys- and demyelination). The nerve injury sites and the associated ganglions also develop ectopic hypersensitivity to thermal and chemical stimuli. These abnormalities can amplify signals leading to accumulation (wind up) and spreading of the sensation from the point of stimulation. Drugs that have proven efficacy in neuropathic pain include-anticonvulsants, tricyclic antidepressants, antiarrhythmics and local anesthetics. All of them posses membrane stabilizing property which is likely to be their mode of action while relieving the neuropathic pain[1,2].

Basic mechanisms - *Primary afferent nociceptors and pain pathways*

Although there are no pain fibers, there are anatomically and physiologically specialized peripheral sensory neurons called nociceptors, which respond to noxious stimuli. These are thin myelinated Aδ-fiber and unmyelinated C-fiber afferents that end as free, uncapsulated peripheral nerve endings in most of the tissues like muscles, joints, and viscera. Interestingly, the brain itself is not served by these sensory fibers and for this reason injury to brain tissue is painless. The myelinated Aδ-fiber afferents typically respond to light tactile stimuli and transmit sharp fast pain signals to spinal cord at the velocity of 6-30 m/sec. They also respond to noxious stimuli, but they do not increase their response when stimuli changes from moderate to strong. Conversely, slow chronic type of pain stimuli are transmitted by type C fibers at a velocity of 0.5 and 2 m/sec. Both A-δ and C-type fibers enter the spinal cord from dorsal roots and terminate on neurons in the dorsal horn. From these neurons originates the ascending pathways of pain[3] (Fig.1).

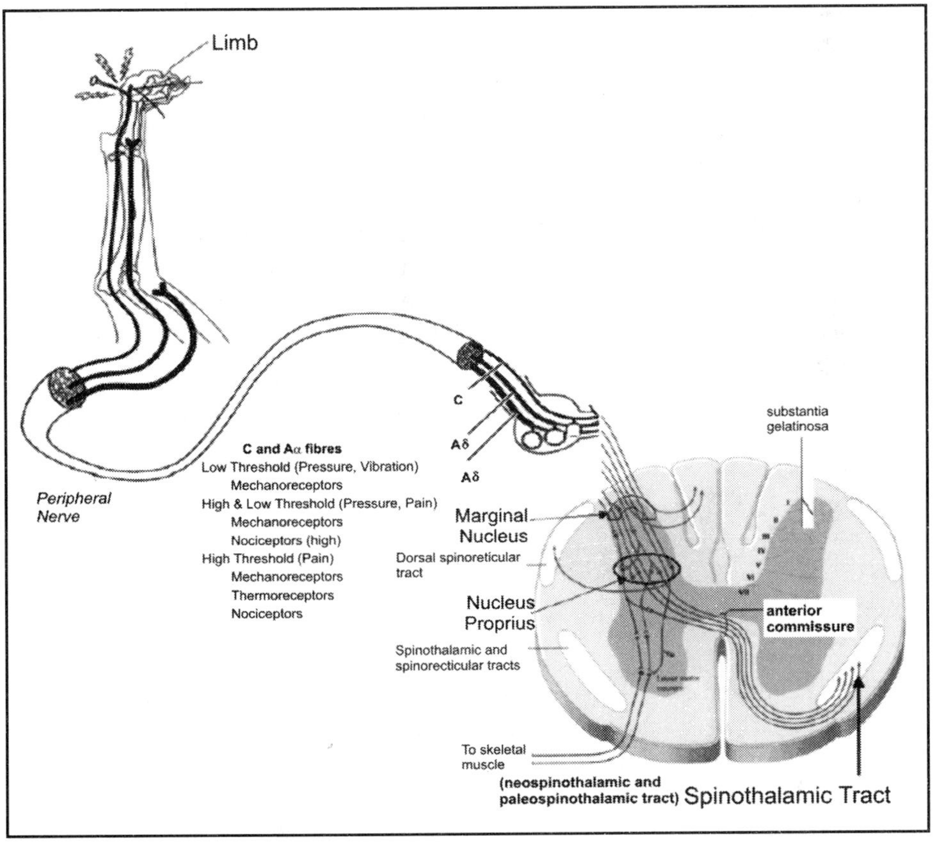

Fig. 1. Diagram illustrating termination of A-δ and C-fibers in dorsal horn of the spinal cord and generation of ascending pathways of pain[4].

Neospinothalamic tract (NSTT) for fast pain originates from the cells located in laminae I and the majority of fibers cross locally in the anterior commissure and ascend to contralateral quadrant. NSTT axons then terminate in ventroposterior thalamus nucleus, thalamus or intralaminar nuclei. *Paleospinothalmic pathway* transmits slow chronic pain. In this pathway, the peripheral fibers terminate almost entirely in laminae II and III of the dorsal horns, which together are called substantia gelatinosa. The fibers then pass through anterior commissure to the opposite side of the cord and finally to the brain. *Spinoreticular tract (*SRT*)* is located in the anterolateral quadrant of dorsal horn of spinal cord. Some of its axons terminate on cells involved in the clinical phenomenon of counter-irritation, whereby one reduces the severity of another. Other SRT cells make up the spinoreticulothalamic tract, which terminates in the medial thalamus. *Spinomesencephalic tract* terminates primarily in the superior colliculus and the periaqueductal grey. This tract activates neurons that are involved in the autonomic and somatomotor aspects of the defense reactions.

Another tract of ascending pain pathway is postsynaptic dorsal column pathway that includes ascending neurons from the lamina V and is particularly important for transmission of visceral pain. Apart from these systems, spino-parabrachial-amygdala system is normally involved in the fear and memory of pain, as well as in the behavioral and autonomic reactions to noxious events, such as vocalization, flight, freezing, pupil dilation, and cardiorespiratory responses[5-6]. Fig.2 represents summary of the neural and hormonal systems that mediate pain and pain inhibition.

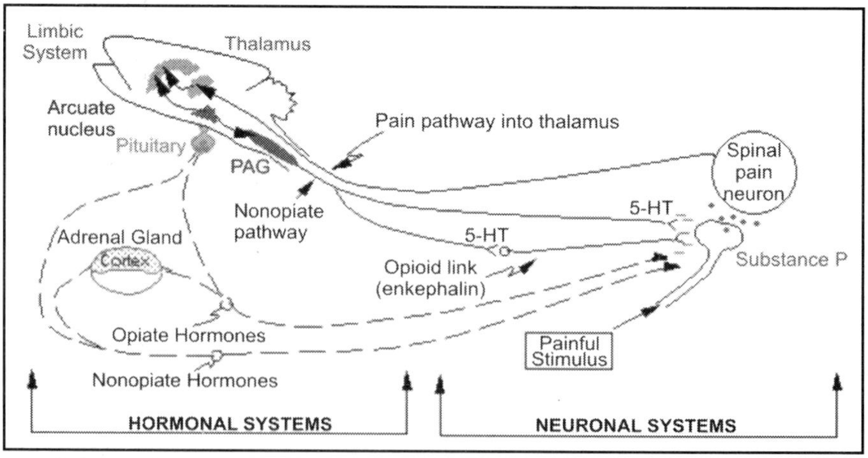

Fig. 2. Schematic summary of the neural and hormonal systems that mediate pain and pain inhibition, 5-HT: 5-hydroxytryptamine, PAG: Periaqueductal gray

Pain control mechanisms

Segmental mechanisms: Gate control theory

Melzack and Wall way back in, 1965, proposed a theory popularly known as **Gate Control Theory (GCT)** of pain[5]. The GCT postulated spinal 'gates' in the dorsal horn at each segmental level in the spinal cord, determining which of the competing impulses (pain, heat or touch) would be transmitted at any particular moment. Soon after the first publication, this theory was expanded to describe the neural system beyond the gate[7]. The expanded theory suggested different systems for the motivational, affective and cognitive aspects of pain experience. The neospinothalamic projection serves to process sensory discriminative information (location, intensity and duration). The information passing through the paleospinothalamic system activates the reticular and limbic areas, giving rise to the unpleasant affect and aversive (motivational) drive, which ultimately produces action. The higher centres in the brain (neocortical) influence the sensory-discriminative and the motivational-affective systems having evaluated the input in the light of past experience. This new model which retained the original GCT is represented in Fig.3.

Supraspinal mechanisms of pain control: brain stimulation produced analgesia

Powerful pain inhibitory mechanisms are also found in the brain. Electrical stimulation of midbrain area i.e., periaqueductal gray (PAG), produces analgesia in both humans and laboratory animals and also inhibit the firing of dorsal horn neurons that respond to noxious stimulation. Descending control is mediated via an excitatory connection from PAG to serotonin-containing neurons in the nucleus raphe magnus of the medulla. The serotonin axons from the nucleus raphe magnus inhibit the firing of the neurons in the laminae I and V of the dorsal horn[9]. Jain and Kulkarni, 1998[10], have shown that sumatriptan, a 5-HT_{1A} agonist, produced analgesia in acetic-acid induced writhing in mice which was antagonized by cholinomimetic drug phytostigmine and reversed by atropine. This suggested involvement of cholinergic mechanism in descending pathways of pain *(for details see Jain and Kulkarni, 1998)*. Besides, there are also parallel descending noradrenergic inhibitory controls which have been presumed as one of the major site of analgesic action of antidepressant drugs in neuropathic pain. This PAG-to-spinal circuit constitutes the brain's endogenous pain control system[11].

It is also evident that dopamine receptor mediated mechanisms play an important role in modulating pain. The use of dopamine

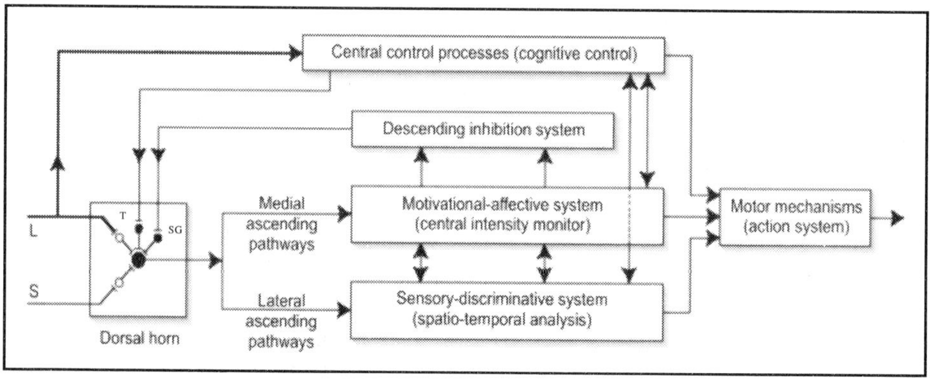

Fig. 3. Gate control theory of pain. The fibers project to the substantia gelatinosa (SG) and first central transmission (T) cells. The inhibitory effect exerted by the SG on the afferent fiber terminals is increased by activity in large (L) fibres and decreased by activity in small (S) fibres. The output of the transmission (T) cell in the dorsal horn projects to the sensory–discriminative system via the lateral ascending system and to the motivational–affective system via the medial ascending system. The central control 'trigger' composed of the dorsal column and the dorsolateral projection systems, is represented by a heavy line running from the large fibre system to the central control processes, which take place in the brain. These in turn project back to the dorsal horn as well as to the sensory–discriminative and motivational–affective systems. The brainstem inhibitory control system activated by impulses in the medial descending system provides descending control on the dorsal horn. Moreover, there is much interaction between the motivational–affective and the sensory–discriminative systems as indicated by the arrows. The net effect of all of these interacting systems is activation of the motor (action) system[8].

agonists suppresses the central pain in thalamic syndrome, herpes zoster or Parkinson's disease. A study by Ninan and Kulkarni, 1998[12], demonstrated that use of roxindole, a dopamine agonist blocked the nociception in tail-flick test in mice. In the same study, roxindole was demonstrated to possess significant analgesic effect in naloxone- or reserpine-induced hyperalgesia in mice which was antagonized by sulpiride or pindolol. These experiments therefore, suggested an interaction of dopaminergic with opioidergic and serotoninergic pathways in pain behavior in mice (*for details see Ninan and Kulkarni, 1998*). Similarly, Naidu et al., 2003[13], while studying the pharmacology of quercetin reinforced the role of dopaminergic, noradrenergic, and opioidergic pathways in nociception. Quercetin is a plant polyphenolic compound which is found abundantly in plants such as *Gingko biloba, Hypericium perforatum, Sambucus Canadensis,* etc. It is reported to possess a variety of beneficial effects including analgesic and anti-inflammatory activity. Here, mice treated with quercetin demonstrated a significant increase in tail-flick latency that was antagonized by naloxone, haloperidol (a D_1 and D_2 dopamine receptor antagonist), sulpiride (a D_2 receptor antagonist), yohimbine (a alpha-2 receptor antagonist) but not by SCH 23390 (a selective D_1 receptor antagonist). Further, quinpirole (a selective D_2 receptor agonist) but not SKF 38393 (a D_1 receptor agonist) enhanced the antinociceptive effect of quinpirole in mice. The authors therefore, highlighted the role of D_2-dopaminergic and α_2- adrenoreceptor receptors in pain response (*for details see Naidu, Singh, and Kulkarni, 2003*).

One of the recent studies has proposed the involvement of immunophilins in nociceptive responses of mice. Immunophilins are the receptor proteins for the major immunosuppressant drugs such as cyclosporine, tacrolimus and are highly expressed in the central nervous system. In this direction, Singh et al., 2003[14], observed that administration of immunosuppressants like tacrolimus (FK-506) to mice significantly increased the tail withdrawal latency to radiant source. An increase in nitric oxide levels in brain areas that execute pain response has been reported to induce hyperalgesia. Tacrolimus inhibited the production of nitric oxide, suggesting a possible role of nitric oxide as second messenger during immunophilin activation (*Singh, Kumar, Naidu, and Kulkarni, 2003*).

Overall there are three primary sites, the periphery, the spinal cord, and the brain areas, at which modification of pain transmission can occur. The following text will focus on the responsiveness of nociceptors to mediators released at the site of injury.

Mediators of pain and inflammation

Tissue injury or application of a noxious stimuli results in pain, which is probably the most common symptom causing people to seek medical attention. It is well established that primary afferent nociceptors (A-δ and C fibers) transmits the painful information from periphery to spinal and supraspinal centers for integration and response. During a noxious challenge the conductance of nociceptors is increased by direct action of inflammatory mediators on nociceptors[15]. Several mediators have been implicated as acting directly on the primary afferent nociceptors to sensitize them and produce pain (Fig.4).

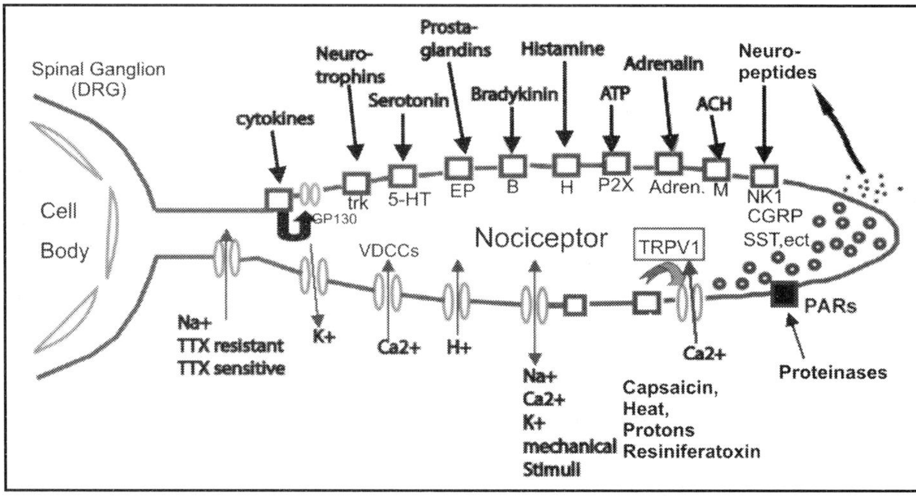

Fig. 4. Various mediators involved in sensitizing the nociceptor following injury or noxious stimuli[17]. CGRP: Calcitonin gene related protein, TTX: tetradotoxin

Amongst these the most well understood mediators of pain and inflammatory episodes are prostaglandins (PGs) which directly act on the peripheral terminals of A-δ and C fibers and lower their threshold to noxious stimuli[16-19]. PGs are generated by action of cyclooxygenase (COX) on arachidonic acid (AA). The mammalian COX pathway is represented in (Fig. 5).

Cyclooxygenase enzyme, prostanoids, and non-steroidal anti-inflammatory drugs

In early 1990s, the enzyme COX was demonstrated to exist in two isoforms, COX-1 and COX-2[20,21]. The 3 - dimensional structure of these two COX isoenzymes is strikingly similar to each other (Fig.6).

Recently, a third isoform COX-3 has been discovered. However, its expression is skeptic in humans at the present[22-24]. The similarities and differences in expression, structure and tissue distribution of these isoforms are summarized in table 1.

COX-1 is constitutively expressed as housekeeping enzyme in nearly all tissues, and mediated physiological responses (e.g. cytoprotection of the stomach, platelet aggregation and renal function). On the other hand, COX-2, expressed by inflammatory cells (e.g. macrophages, monocytes, synoviocytes) has been considered as inducible isoform. This isoform is primarily responsible for the synthesis

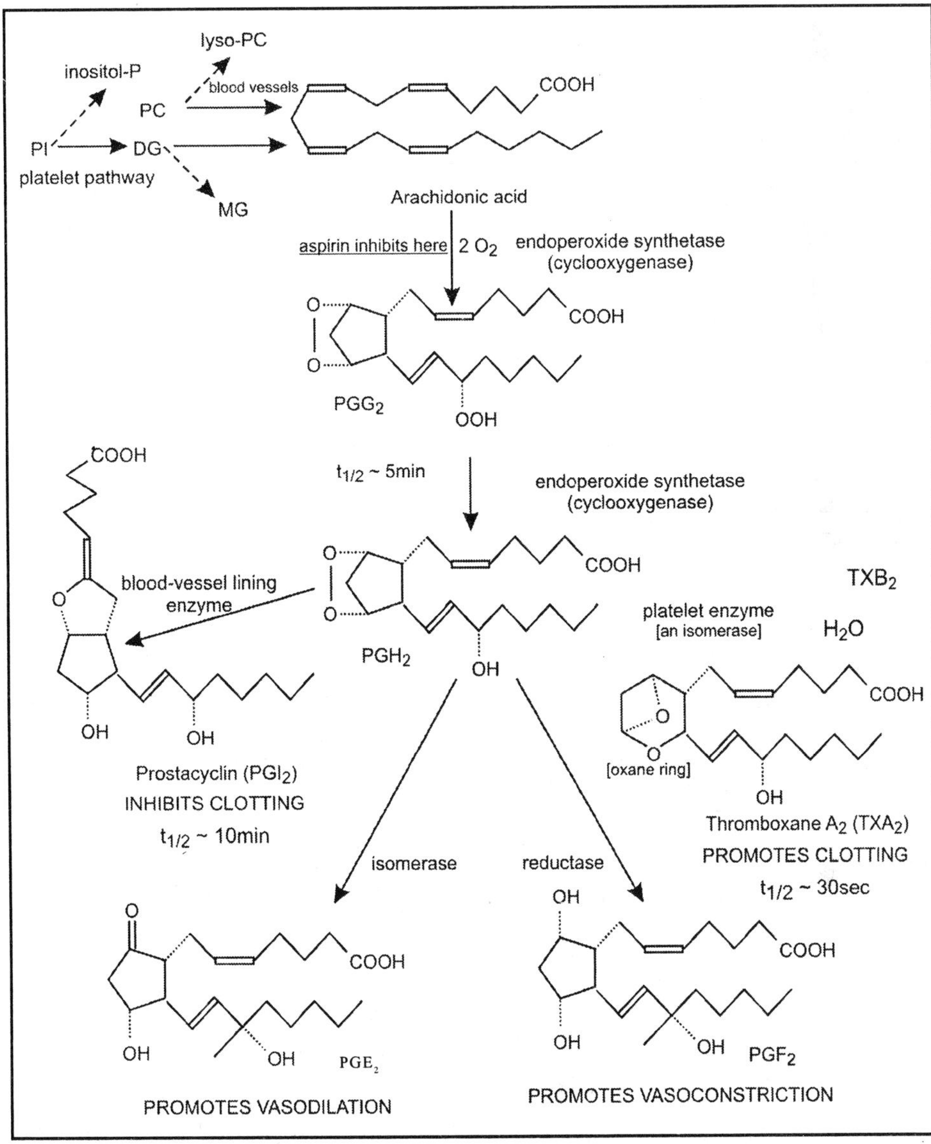

Fig. 5. The cyclooxygenase and lipoxygenase pathways of arachidonic acid metabolism. (a) The cyclooxygenase (COX) pathway results in the formation of prostaglandin G_2 (PGG_2) from arachidonic acid by a cyclooxygenase reaction. In a subsequent peroxidase reaction, PGG_2 undergoes reduction to prostaglandin H_2 (PGH_2). Both of these reactions are catalyzed by COX (PGH synthase). PGH_2 serves as a substrate for cell-specific isomerases and synthases, producing prostanoids such as prostacyclin (PGI_2), thromboxane A_2 (TXA_2), $PGF_{2\alpha}$, PGE_2, and PGD_2.

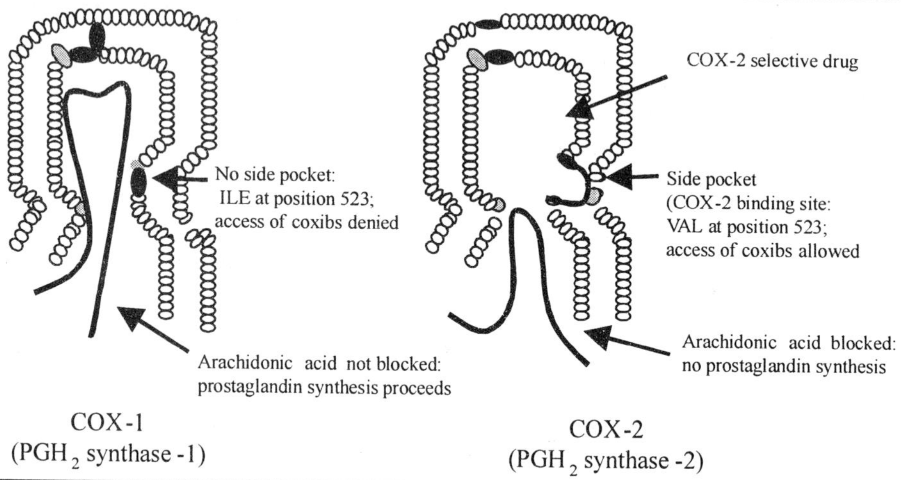

Fig. 6. Structure of the COX-1 and COX-2 isoenzymes. Picture shows active site similarities and differences. ILE = isoleucine; VAL = valine

of PGs that are involved in pathological processes such as acute and chronic inflammatory conditions[25]. A study by Padi and Kulkarni, 2005[26], have shown an extended role of COX-2. The authors evaluated the effect of ketoroloc, a non-selective anti-inflammatory drug (NSAID), and parecoxib (a prodrug of valdecoxib), a selective COX-2 inhibitor against the lipopolysaccharide (LPS) challenge in formalin treated mice paw. Here, intravenous administration of ketorolac or parecoxib significantly inhibited the nocifensive response (licking and biting behaviour) in late-phase but did not affect the early-phase after formalin challenge in mice. These findings therefore, provided a behavioural evidence for the delayed expression of COX-2 in LPS-induced hyperalgesia in mice (*for details see Padi and Kulkarni, 2005*).

Prostanoids are the major cyclooxygenase products. The term prostanoid includes prostaglandins, prostacyclin, thromboxanes, and related substances. Prostaglandins are mainly found in free form but several combined structures (amides and esters) are also described. Prostaglandins (PGs) were discovered in the seminal plasma around 1930. Ulf Von Euler in 1935 demonstrated their physiological properties and lipid nature. His contribution was recognized with the Nobel Prize in 1970. Their chemical structure was revealed by Bergstrom in 1962 who isolated the first prostaglandin. His student, Samuelsson, isolated and determined the structure of several of most significant prostaglandins while Sir John Vane not only discovered prostacyclin

Table 1. Similarities and differences in expression, structure and tissue distribution of COX isoforms

	COX-1	COX-2	COX-3
Physiology	• Constitutive form of COX • "Housekeeping enzyme" producing prostaglandins that help to regulate normal kidney, gastrointestinal functions and vascular homeostasis	• Inducible form of COX • "Inflammatory response enzyme" induced during inflammation and produce prostaglandins that are involved in inflammation • behaves as immediate early gene and controls mitogenesis and cell growth	• COX-3 is a splice variant of COX-1which when glycosylated displays COX-1 activity • inducible isoenzyme expressed in later resolving stages of inflammation
Localization	• Present in platelets, endothelial cells, stomach, kidney, smooth muscle, and most of the other tisuues • lumen of endoplasmic reticulum	• Present in brain-cortical and limbic neurons • recent studies have identified its constitutive expression in kidney, gastrointestinal tract • endoplasmic reticulum and nuclear envelope	• Expression in humans is skeptic (found in canine brains)
Amino acids	• 599 amino acid • additional 17 amino acid sequence at N - terminal • N-terminal sequence begins with ADPGA	• 604 amino acid • additional 18 amino acid sequence at c-terminal • N-terminal begins with ANPCC	• COX-3 gene has an insertion of 30 - 44 amino acids in the signal sequence of COX-1
Molecular weight	• 67000 d	• 72000 d	• 72000 d
Acetylation by aspirin	• Acetylation at ser 530 causing complete inhibition	• Acetylation at ser 523 modifies the enzyme to produce 15R -HETE - 15R hydroxyeicosatetraenoic acid and lipoxins	preferential acetylation by acetaminophen (others with low anti-inflammatory effect)
Regulation of expression	• Gene is 22 Kb in length with 11 exons • gene located on chromosome 9 • mRNA transcript is 2.8 to 3.0 kd • promoter region of gene has poor inducibility • post transcriptional addition of 3 high mannose oligosaccharides • not inhibited by glucocorticoids	• Gene is 22 Kb in length with 11 exons • gene located on chromosome 1 • mRNA transcript is 4.0 to 4.5 kd • promoter region contains may transcriptional factors which can be upregulated by pro-inflammatory cytokines • post transcriptional addition of 4 high mannose oligosaccharides • Inhibited by glucocorticoids	• 5.2 kb mRNA in fram deletion spanning exons 5-8
Active site	• Smaller active site due to presence of isoleucine amino acid at position 523	• Larger active site due to presence of valine amino acid at position 523	• Not reported
Substrate	• OnlyC20 carboxylic acids	• Both C18 and C20 carboxylic acids	• Only C20 carboxylic acids

but also demonstrated that aspirin acted by inhibiting COX enzyme. All the three were recipients of the Nobel Prize for physiology and medicine in 1982.

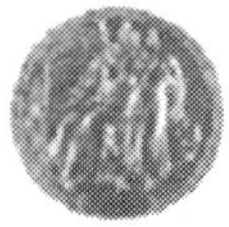

The Nobel Prize in Physiology or Medicine 1982

"for their discoveries concerning prostaglandins and related biologically active substances"

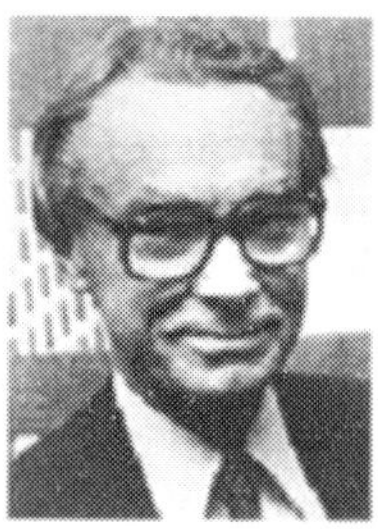

Sune K. Bergstrom
1/3 of the prize
Sweden
Karolinska Institutet Stockholm, Sweden
b. 1916
d. 2004

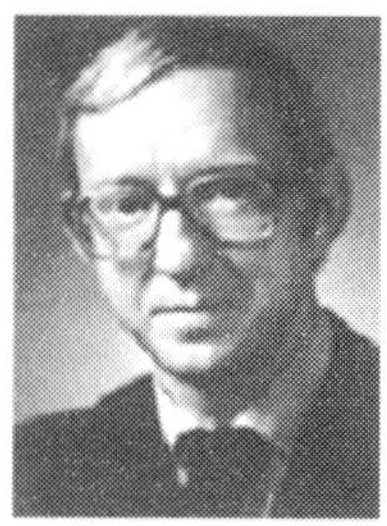

Bengt I. Samuelsson
1/3 of the prize
Sweden
Karolinska Institutet Stockholm, Sweden
b. 1934

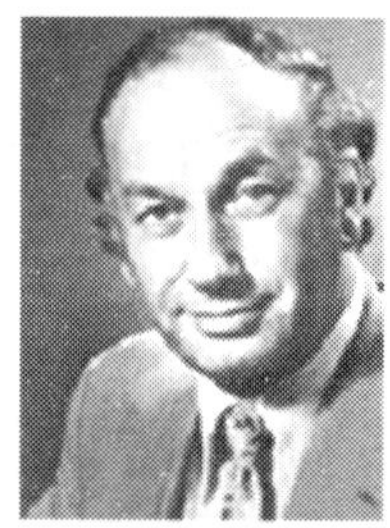

John R. Vane
1/3 of the prize
United Kingdom
The Wellcome Research Laboratories Beckenham, United Kingdom
b. 1927
d. 2004

Around 14 natural prostaglandins are known and their number is continually growing. The major prostanoids include prostaglandin D_2 (PGD_2), prostaglandin E_2 (PGE_2) and prostaglandin E_1 (PGE_1), prostaglandin $F_{2\alpha}$ ($PGF_{2\alpha}$), prostaglandin H_2 (PGH_2), prostaglandin I_2 (PGI_2), thromboxane A_2 (TXA_2). Besides, prostaglandins of the A and B series, thromboxane B_2 (TXB_2) (stable but biologically inactive) is other bioactive prostanoid which has a very short half-life in the tissues (some minutes). Other biologically active prostanoids derivatives include F2-isoprostanes (F2-IsoP or iso-prostaglandins), phytoprostanes F1, punaglandins and isofurans, prostamides, and glyceryl prostaglandins[27].

Almost thirty years ago, the mechanism of action of aspirin-like drugs or non-steroidal anti-inflammatory drugs (NSAIDs) was proposed as their ability to inhibit prostaglandin biosynthesis. NSAIDs bind to the active site of COX enzyme which catalyses the transformation of arachidonic acid to PGs by reaction with two molecule of oxygen. They do not affect peroxidase activity that reduces 15S-hydroperoxide PGG_2 to 15S-alcohol PGH_2. Since then a number of NSAIDs have been developed and marketed for the treatment of pain and inflammation. Broadly NSAIDs are classified as COX-1 or COX-2 selective based on their selectivity to COX isoforms. They have been further subclassified on the basis of relative selectivity. Table 2 summarizes the classification of NSAIDs[28].

Table 2. Classification of NSAIDs

COX-1 selective		
Highly selective COX-1	**Relatively selective COX-1**	**Equally selective (COX-1 = COX-2)**
Flurbioprofen	Fenoprofen	Aspirin
Ketoprofen	Piroxicam	Ibuprofen
		Indomethacin
		Keterolac
		Naproxen
		Tenoxicam
		Tolmetin

COX-2 selective		
Preferential selective	**Highly selective**	
	First generation	**Second generation**
Etodoloc	Celecoxib	Valdecoxib
Meloxicam	Rofecoxib	Etoricoxib
Nabumetone		Lumaricoxib
Nimesulide		Parecoxib*

*Parecoxib is an injectable pro-drug of valdecoxib

The classical NSAIDs like aspirin, indomethacin, ibuprofen, and naproxen have no enzyme selectivity and inhibit both COX-1 and COX-2 with similar potency. According to the COX hypothesis these drugs exert anti-inflammatory action by blocking COX-2 activity and, at the same time, produce unwanted side effects, mainly gastrointestinal (GI) and renal toxicity, due to the inhibition of COX-1 activity[25,29-37]. Consequently, the hypothesis that specific inhibition of COX-2 might have therapeutic advantages over the classical NSAIDs was proposed and the specific inhibitors of COX-2 isoenzyme were developed as safer and newer NSAIDs. The new generation of selective COX-2 inhibitors came to be commonly known as "coxibs". However, the experimental and clinical studies have indicated that the tolerability of coxibs is similar to the classical mixed-type NSAIDs[38]. The pharmacological studies employing COX-2 knock-out mice have shown a constitutive expression of COX-2 in several organs where it synergizes the COX-1 in maintaining homeostasis in kidney, platelets, gastrointestinal tract[39,40]. The Vioxx Gastrointestinal Outcomes Research (VIGOR) study and Adenomatous Poly Prevention on Vioxx (APPROVe) trial have shown that selective COX-2 inhibitors cause significant ulceration at about half the rate of conventional NSAIDs[41] and exhibit significant renal and cardiovascular toxicity. As a result, the liberal use of coxibs have received a major set back of withdrawal of rofecoxib from market. Subsequently, USFDA has recommended a warning label to be inserted for all NSAIDs, including coxibs[42]. Recent studies have now confirmed that COX-2 derived PGs, particularly PGI_2, is a potent inhibitor of platelet aggregation and prevents adhesion of leukocytes, and accumulation of cholesterol in vascular cells. Therefore, the use of COX-2 inhibitors, which do not inhibit platelet COX-1, might (at least in theory) unfavorably alter the thromboxane-prostacyclin balance by inhibiting COX-2-dependent synthesis of vasoprotective PGI_2 in endothelial cells and predispose to cardiovascular toxicity.

Although, a prompt change in the labeling of these drugs has been implemented, the unresolved cardiovascular risk and multiple COX protein pose a particular challenge for discovery of safer NSAIDs with high isoform specificity and selectivity. It is note worthy to consider the observations of Sharma et al., 2005[43], who reported the analgesic and anti-inflammatory effect of aspartame in acetic acid-induced writhing in mice and carrageenan-induced paw oedema in rats, respectively. The authors have argued the therapeutic effect of aspartame like sweeteners due to their ability to inhibit prostaglandin synthesis suggesting that such alternatives can be effective in pain and inflammation management. However, their gastrotolerability and cardiotoxic potential is yet to be explored (*for details see Sharma, Jain, Kulkarni, 2005*).

Other alternatives to NSAIDs for the management of pain have been mentioned in the studies by Kumar et al., 2000[44], and Patil et al., 2004[45]. Cumulatively, these studies have evaluated the efficacy of phosphodiesterase (PDE) enzyme inhibitors in experimental paradigms of nociception in rodents. PDE enzymes occur widely in the mammalian tissues in at least eleven isoforms. Amongst these PDE-IV and V are responsible for degradation of cyclic nucleotides. PDE-IV and PDE V hydrolyses cyclic adenosine monophosphate (cAMP) and cyclic guanosine monophosphate (cGMP), respectively, to corresponding inactive monophosphates. Therefore, inhibition of hydrolyzing enzymes in either of the case leads to increase in the levels of respective cyclic nucleotides which are reported to produce analgesia and suppress inflammation at cellular level. Kumar et al., 2000[44], observed that rolipram, a PDE IV inhibitor or theophylline, a non-specific PDE inhibitor dose dependently produced analgesic and anti-inflammatory effect in acetic acid-induced writhing in mice and carrageenan-induced paw oedema in rat, respectively. In the same study, combination of nimesulide (a preferential COX-2 inhibitor) and rolipram but not with other PDE inhibitors was found to have enhanced effect as compared to their effect *per se* (*for detail see Kumar, Jain, Kulkarni, 2000*). Similarly, Patil et al., 2004[45], demonstrated that systemic or local administration of sildenafil, a PDE V inhibitor, produced antinociception in acetic acid-induced abdominal constrictions in mice and reversed carrageenan-induced mechanical hyperalgesia in rat hind paw. The local antinociceptive effect of sildenafil was enhanced by acetylcholine or neotigmine and effectively blocked by L-NAME (a non-selective nitric oxide synthase inhibitor) or methylene blue (a guanylate cyclase inhibitor). Likewise, the effect of combination too was sensitive to same drugs suggesting that sildenafil mediated antinociception presumably involves cGMP-nitric oxide pathway and interaction with cholinergic pathway (*for details see Patil, Jain, Singh, and Kulkarni 2004*).

Besides, recent evidences indicate that metabolites of arachidonic acid other than COX-pathway are putatively involved in producing and maintaining inflammation. For example, most NSAIDs inhibit COX activity without decreasing generation of lipoxygenase (LOX)-produced leukotrienes (LTs). This newer concept of 5-lipoxygenase in pathological conditions with prospects of its inhibition is being considered by numerous researchers, including our own research group.

5-Lipoxygenase and leukotrienes

Arachidonic acid is also a substrate for another group of enzymes called lipoxygenases (LOXs). Of all the LOX isoforms (5-LOX, 12-LOX, 15-LOX), 5-LOX is the key enzyme of the leukotriene (LT) pathway that catalyzes the initial two steps of LT biosynthesis (Fig.7.).

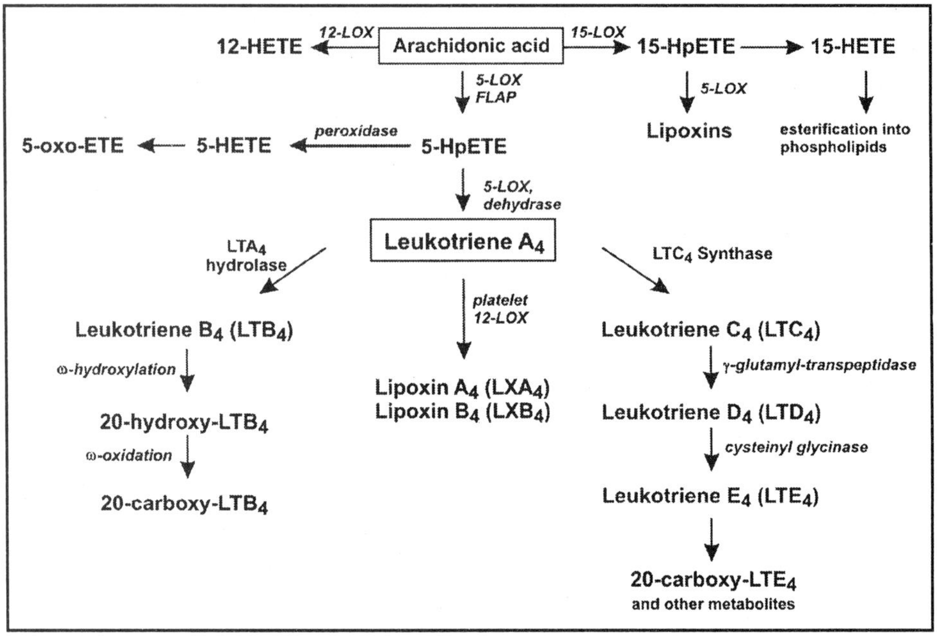

Fig. 7. The free arachidonic acid is oxidized by 12-, 15-, or 5-lipoxygenase (12- 15-, or 5- LOX) to 12-, 15- or 5- hydroperoxy derivative (hydroperoxyeicosatrienoic acid; 12-, 15- or 5-HpETE), respectively. 15-HpETE is subsequently reduced by glutathione peroxidase to create a more stable hydroxy acid (HETE). Simultaneously, 5-HpETE formed by 5-LOX in the presence of FLAP (5-lipoxygenase activating factor) undergoes subsequent dehydration to form short-lived epoxide leukotriene A_4. This unstable compound is the precursor of the biologically active of leukotrienes B_4 (LTB_4), C_4 (LTC_4), D_4 (LTD_4) and E_4 (LTE_4). These last three products, known as cysteinyl leukotrienes (CysLTs) make up the biologic mixture previously defined as "slow-reacting substance" (SRS) of anaphylaxis.

Among the leukotrienes LTB_4, and cysteinyl leukotrienes (LTC_4, LTD_4, LTE_4,) are the potent mediators of inflammation. LTB_4 has a chemotactic effect on neutrophils, and as such help to bring the necessary cells to the inflamed tissue. LTB_4 has been implicated in the pathogenesis of certain inflammatory diseases (rheumatoid arthritis, and ulcerative colitis) as it stimulates the production and release of proinflammatory cytokines from macrophages, lymphocytes or synovial membrane[46-48]. Recently, Haribabu et al., 2000[49], have demonstrated that deletion of LTB_4 receptor in mice leads to a reduction in vascular and cellular components of inflammation, suggesting that inhibition of LTB_4 activity could be an effective drug target for inflammatory conditions. A more recent study has confirmed these findings to note that LTs are important mediators in chronic inflammation and joint destruction in rheumatoid arthritis (RA)[50]. Further, Zouboulis et al., 2003[51], reported a potential involvement of LTB_4 in the development of acne where it induces proliferation, differentiation and apoptosis of sebaceous glands of skin. Similarly Singh et al., 2005[52], reported that LTs are responsible for inflammatory cascade in damaged rat colon. Zileuton, a 5-LOX inhibitor was investigated for its effect in dextran sodium sulphate induced inflammation in rat distal colon. Zileuton treatment significantly prevented the development of inflammation in rat colon and inhibited neutrophil recruitment and caused an increase in prostaglandins (which, may be protective) at the site of inflammation (*for details see Singh, Patil, and Kulkarni, 2004*).

Cysteinyl leukotrienes (CysLTs), formerly known as slow reacting substance related to anaphylaxis, have long been known to be involved in the pathogenesis of bronchial asthma[53]. However, their proinflammatory effects in other conditions have recently been considered. They are released during inflammation, rheumatoid arthritis and hypersensitivity reactions leading to oedema and smooth muscle contraction[54]. The experimental trials have demonstrated that CysLTs may also participate in idiopathic and stimuli (e.g. NSAIDs)-evoked gastric inflammation. CysLTs induce vasoconstriction and reduce blood flow in the gastric mucosa leading to ulceration[55]. In addition, 5-LOX expression in neurons has been reported to significantly promote neurodegeneration. Activation of 5-LOX favors oxidative stress and lipid peroxidation which increases the brain vulnerability to neurodegeneration[56,57]. Furthermore, the pharmacological evidence supports the pathological role of LTs in atherosclerosis, unstable angina or cardiac infarction. The increased production of LT results in adhesion of polymorphonuclear cells to the vascular endothelium which leads to vascular permeability and endothelial dysfunction[58,59]. Besides pro-inflammatory role, the LOX interaction products act as anti-inflammatory signals. These products, commonly known as lipoxins (LXs), are generated during cell-cell interactions by one of at least three biosynthetic routes. These pathways are 1) 15- and 5-LOX, 2) 12- and 5-LOX mediated metabolism of arachidonic acid, and 3) aspirin-triggered biosynthesis of lipoxins (Fig.16) which may work independently or in concert[60] (Fig.8).

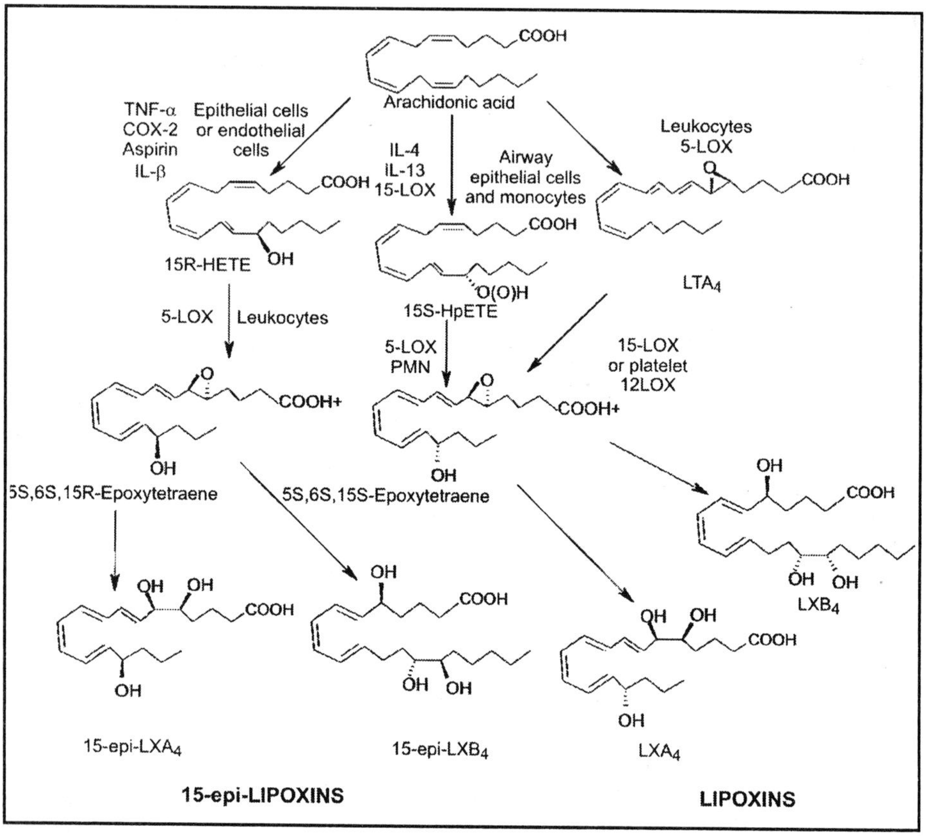

Fig. 8. Lipoxin (LX) and aspirin - triggered 15-epi-lipoxin biosynthesis. Illustration of the three main transcellular routes to generate lipoxins and 15-epi-lipoxins in mammalian tissues. Each of these is an independent route initiated by site selective addition of molecular oxygen to arachidonic acid in the donor cell type of origin. LOX- lipoxygenase; LT - leukotriene; PMN - polymorphoneutrophils; 15*S*-HpETE - 15*S*-hydroxyperoxyeicosatetraenoic acid; 15*R*-HETE - 15*R*-hydroxyeicosatetraenoic acid; COX-2 - cyclooxygenase-2; IL-1β - interleukin 1β; TNF-α - tumor necrosis factor –alpha[60].

Lipoxins display counter regulatory roles and exert putative anti-inflammatory or immunomodulatory actions that are likely to have a physiological role during homeostasis and illness as well[61].

A thorough understanding of COX and LOX pathways therefore, suggest that both PGs and LTs play a complementary role in a variety of inflammatory diseases. As a consequence, new dual inhibitors of COX and 5-LOX are now being studied as new potential drugs to treat inflammation with curtailed side effects.

Dual inhibitors of COX and 5-LOX - Background and pharmacological rationale

An interesting paper published in 1996 by Nickerson-Nutter and Medvedeff observed that combination of LT synthesis inhibitor and naproxen, a non-selective COX inhibitor, produced a significant reduction in the collagen-induced arthritis in mouse. No compound alone produced any inhibition of arthritis[62]. This observation was the beginning of a new era in the therapeutic approach i.e. use of inhibitors of COX and 5-LOX in the management of inflammatory disorders.

Both conventional NSAIDs and the selective COX-2 inhibitors primarily exert their effect by reducing the production of PGs that are induced during an inflammatory event. In recent years it has been clarified that, along with PGs, other key lipid mediators; LTs and LXs complimentarily participate in the development and persistence of inflammatory processes. Since LTs are non-responsive to the effect of NSAIDs, it is suggested that the simultaneous dual inhibition of COX and 5-LOX pathways might have synergistic effects and achieve optimal wider spectrum of anti-inflammatory effect[63]. Bishnoi et al., 2006[64], studied the analgesic effect of combining NSAIDs with acetyl 11 - keto - beta bosewellic acid (AKBA), a 5-LOX inhibitor in mice. The combinations of AKBA with naproxen, nimesulide or rofecoxib produced more pronounced analgesia in acetic acid-induced writhing and tail-flick test in mice (Table 3a and b) indicating that dual inhibition approach might provide better management of pain with reduced dose of either of the drugs. Further, the combination is also expected to be more gastrotolearble *(for details see Bishnoi, Patil, and Kulkarni, 2005).*

Recent studies have demonstrated that in the presence of COX (COX-1/-2 alone or combined) inhibition, LTs (LTB_4 and CysLTs) generated via shunt pathway induce chemotaxis and local vasoconstriction that enhances the local blood flow to gastric mucosa[65]. A recent study by Singh et al., 2005[66], has reported the relevance of 5-LOX and COX interactions in modulating gastric ulceration to NSAIDs. This experimental work evaluated the effect of licofelone, a dual inhibitor of COX and 5-LOX on early and late events associated with indomethacin-induced gastric damage in rats and mice. Licofelone did not exacerbate the gastric damage caused by indomethacin while it significantly reduced the LTB_4 levels.

Licofelone also prevented indomethacin-induced increased vascularity in mice stomach. Besides, and more importantly, licofelone reversed the adherence of neutrophils in mesenteric venules (intravital microscopy) caused by indomethacin (Fig 9 and 10). Further, licofelone per se treatment spared the rat stomach and did not increase LTB_4 levels or vascularity of the stomach (Fig.9 and Table 4). These

Table 3a. Effect of COX and 5-LOX inhibitiors and their combinations at different doses in acetic acid-induced writhing in mice. (n = 6)

Treatment (mg/kg)	Number of wriths (mean ± S.E.M.)	% inhibition
Control	61.0 ± 1.6	
Naproxen (5)	41.33 ± 2.5 [a]	32.2
Naproxen (10)	35.0 ± 2.1 [a]	42.6
Nimesulide (1)	36.0 ± 4.3 [a]	40.9
Nimesulide (2)	32.4 ± 5.1 [a]	46.9
Rofecoxib (1)	43.3 ± 1.2 [a]	29.0
Rofecoxib (2)	38.6 ± 1.2 [a]	36.7
AKBA (50)	41.33 ± 1.8 [a]	32.2
AKBA (100)	36.0 ± 4.3 [a]	40.9
Naproxen (5) + AKBA (100)	30.2 ± 1.2 [ac]	50.5
Nimesulide (1) + AKBA (100)	22.6 ± 2.5 [abd]	62.9
Rofecoxib (1) + AKBA (100)	30.6 ± 1.9 [ae]	49.8

[a]$P < 0.05$ as compared to control values, [b] as compared to AKBA (100 mg/kg), [c] as compared to naproxen (5 mg/kg), [d] as compared to nimesulide (1 mg/kg),[e] as compared to rofecoxib (1 mg/kg). AKBA: acetyl 11 - keto - beta bosewellic acid. *(For Details see Bishnoi, Patil, and Kulkarni, 2005)*

Table 3b. Effect of COX and 5-LOX inhibitors and their combinations at different doses on tail-flick latency in tail-flick test in mice. Values are mean ± S.E.M. (n=6)

Treatment (mg/kg)	% MPE (30 min)	% MPE (60 min)	% MPE (120 min)
Control	15.2 ± 2.2	10.4 ± 4.1	3.8 ± 3.3
Naproxen (5)	24.4 ± 1.5	36.4 ± 3.2	30.6 ± 2.2
Naproxen (10)	48.4 ± 5.6 [a]	86.4 ± 6.9 [a]	48.4 ± 3.9 [a]
Nimesulide (1)	32.4 ± 3.5 [a]	54.3 ± 4.5 [a]	38.2 ± 4.5
Nimesulide (2)	62.6 ± 3.5 [a]	136.4 ± 5.4 [a]	58.3 ± 9.6 [a]
Rofecoxib (1)	28.6 ± 1.6 [a]	42.5 ± 5.3 [a]	39.6 ± 4.5
Rofecoxib (2)	56.4 ± 9.3 [a]	98.2 ± 8.2 [a]	60.0 ± 6.6 [a]
AKBA (50)	29.3 ± 2.5 [a]	46.8 ± 5.6 [a]	9.17 ± 3.3
AKBA (100)	58.3 ± 6.5 [a]	97.3 ± 4.9 [a]	29.9 ± 3.5 [a]
Naproxen (5) + AKBA (100)	36.2 ± 1.25 [ac]	106.4± 6.9 [ac]	72.2 ± 6.4 [abc]
Nimesulide (1) + AKBA (100)	64.5 ± 5.2 [ad]	156.3 ± 9.3 [ad]	84.5 ± 9.9 [abd]
Rofecoxib (1) + AKBA (100)	48.2 ± 3.5 [ae]	110.2 ± 8.2 [ae]	82.5 ± 7.2 [abe]

[a]$P < 0.05$ as compared to control values, [b] as compared to AKBA (100 mg/kg), [c] as compared to naproxen (5 mg/kg), [d] as compared to nimesulide (1 mg/kg),[e] as compared to rofecoxib (1mg/kg). AKBA: acetyl 11 - keto - beta bosewellic acid. % MPE refers to percent maximal possible effect. *(For Details see Bishnoi, Patil, and Kulkarni, 2005)*

observations suggested that the dual inhibitors of 5-LOX and COX-1/ -2 might be less irritant on the stomach relative to COX inhibitors *(for details see Singh, Patil, and Kulkarni, 2005).*

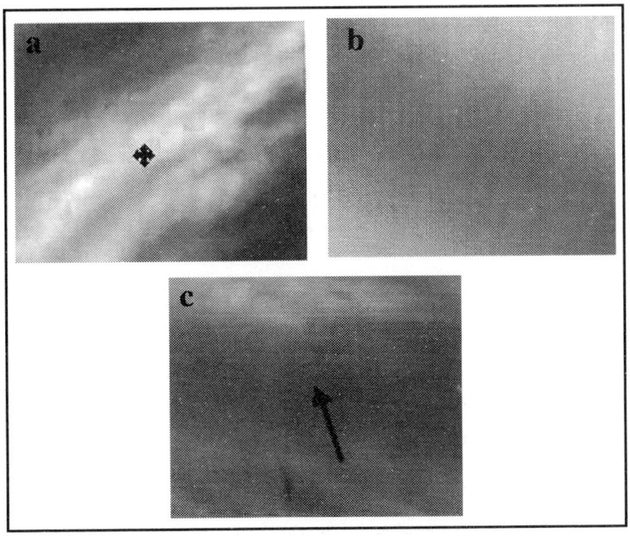

Fig. 9. Representative intravital microscopic photographs of mesenteric venules of rats treated with **(a)** indomethacin (100 mg/kg, po), **(b)** licofelone (100 mg/kg, po), **(c)** licofelone (30 mg/kg, po) + indomethacin (100 mg/kg, po). Arrow (() indicates clear blood flow through mesenteric venule, (ȷ) indicates accumulated neutrophils seen as white debris (For details see Singh, Patil, and Kulkarni, 2005).

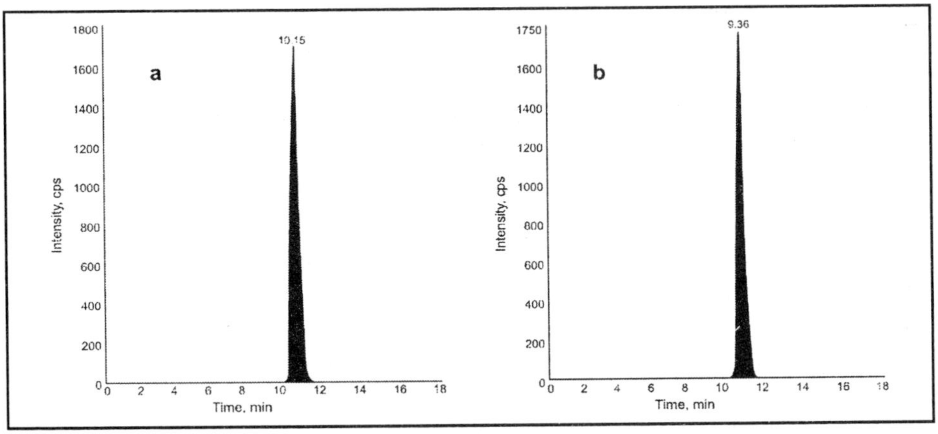

Fig. 10. LCMS/MS chromatogram of (a) leukotriene B_4 (Retention time 10.15 min, Mass selection 337.5 to 249.5) (b) leukotriene internal standard (Retention time 9.36 min, Mass selection 411.1 to 380.1. *(For details see Singh, Patil, and Kulkarni, 2005).*

Table 4. Leukotriene B_4 (LTB_4) levels of stomach of rats treated with indomethacin, licofelone or indomethacin + licofelone (n = 5-6 rats per group)

Treatment (mg/kg)	LTB_4 levels (ng/g of stomach ± S.E.M.)
Vehicle	25.9 ± 3.0
Indomethacin (100)	40.2 ± 2.1*
Licofelone (30)	23.2 ± 4.1
Licofelone (30) + Indomethacin (100)	28.0 ± 4.2^a

*$P < 0.019$ as compared to vehicle control, $^aP < 0.05$ as compared to indomethacin [F=4.21, (3,25)] (For details see Singh, Patil, and Kulkarni, 2005).

Thus, the dual inhibitors of COX and 5-LOX may have two theoretical advantages of stronger anti-inflammatory and a protective effect on GI mucosa. In addition to this, COX and 5-LOX dual inhibition does not block the 12- or 15-LOX pathways, which contribute to the formation of anti-inflammatory LXs[63].

Apart from these two advantages the dual inhibition approach of inhibiting COX-1/-2 and 5-LOX might also provide additional cardioprotection. Platelets and leukocytes on endothelial cells constitute an early mechanism of vascular inflammatory damage and consequent vessel occlusion. Pro-aggregatory thromboxane A_2 (TXA_2) synthesised by COX-1 in platelet, vasodilator PGI_2 by COX-2 in leukocytes and platelets with LTs synthesized by 5-LOX in neutrophils or by cell-cell interaction contribute to coronary vasoconstriction. Once activated, platelet-leukocyte aggregation within the injured regions of vasculature induces chemokine synthesis and respiratory burst of neutrophils. Under such circumstances, selective inhibition of either COX-1 or -2 or 5-LOX might not be effective in downregulating the vascular inflammation and thrombosis. It is therefore, suggested that inhibition of 5-LOX enzyme together with COX-1/-2 would result into (i) inhibition of COX-1 to prevent platelet TXA_2 formation, (ii) inhibition of COX-2 to downregulate leukocyte activation and widespread vascular inflammation, and (iii) inhibition of 5-LOX to further, and specifically, reduce leukocyte inflammatory and thrombogenic potential, and to counteract the gastric damage associated with the inhibition of COX-1[67]. The advancement in understanding the role and targeting these enzyme systems therefore, suggest a promising pharmacological approach in post-COX-2 era to reduce the cardiovascular events (pro-thrombotic risk) of selective COX-2 inhibition without gastric side effects of non-specific inhibition of COX.

Not only this, a few observations have highlighted a possibility that dual inhibitors of 5-LOX/COX might also be free from the acute renal toxicity[68], a side effect shared by available NSAIDs. If this is the case, development of dual inhibitors of 5-LOX and COX will offer an additional advantage over existing NSAID therapy, a proposition awaiting clinical evidence.

Several distinct inhibitors of COX and 5-LOX have been synthesized. The chemical structures of few such compounds are given below (Fig.11).

The oldest one was benoxaprofen, which was withdrawn from use in 1982 because of hepatotoxic and photosensitizing potential.

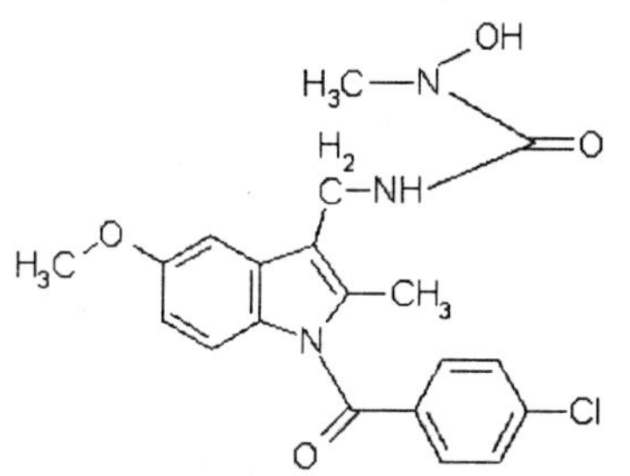

Indomethacin Derivative

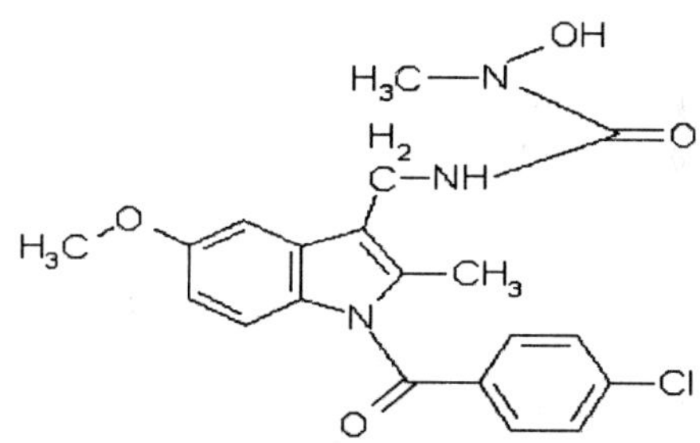

Fenamate Derivatives

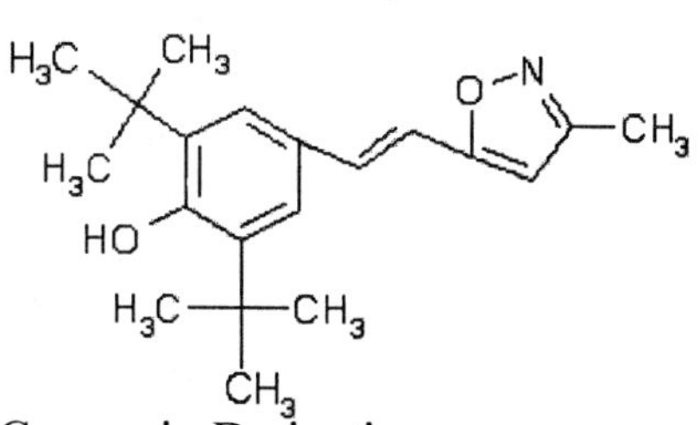

Curcumin Derivatives

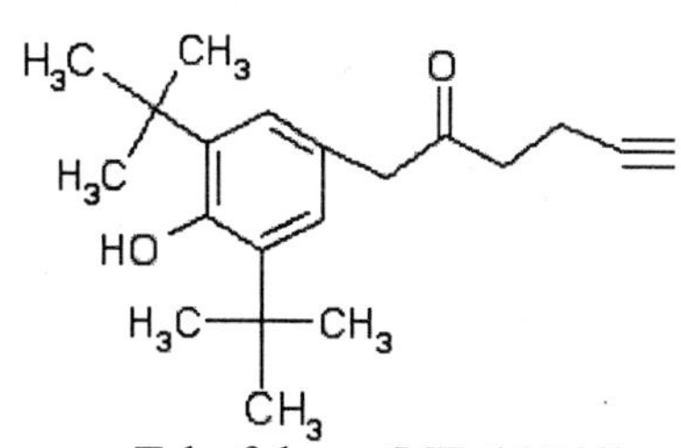

Tebufelone (NE-11740)

Di-tert-butylphenones

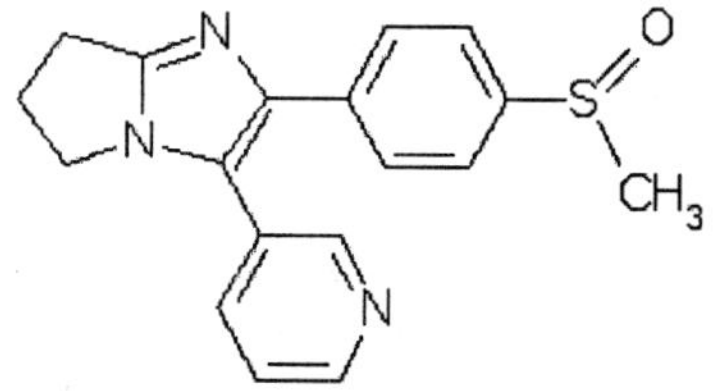

SK&F 105809

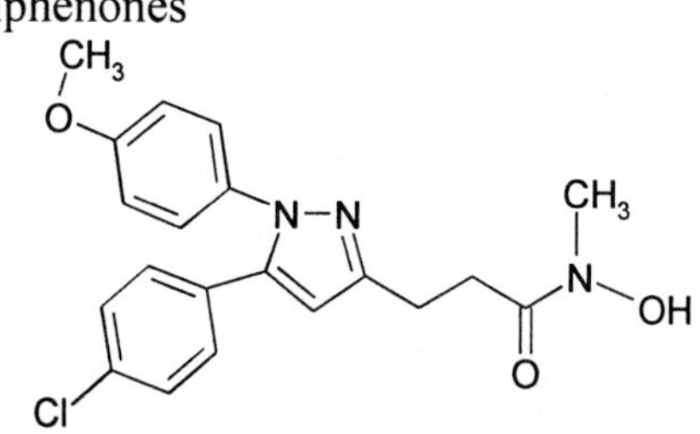

Tepoxalin

Fig. 11. Contd...

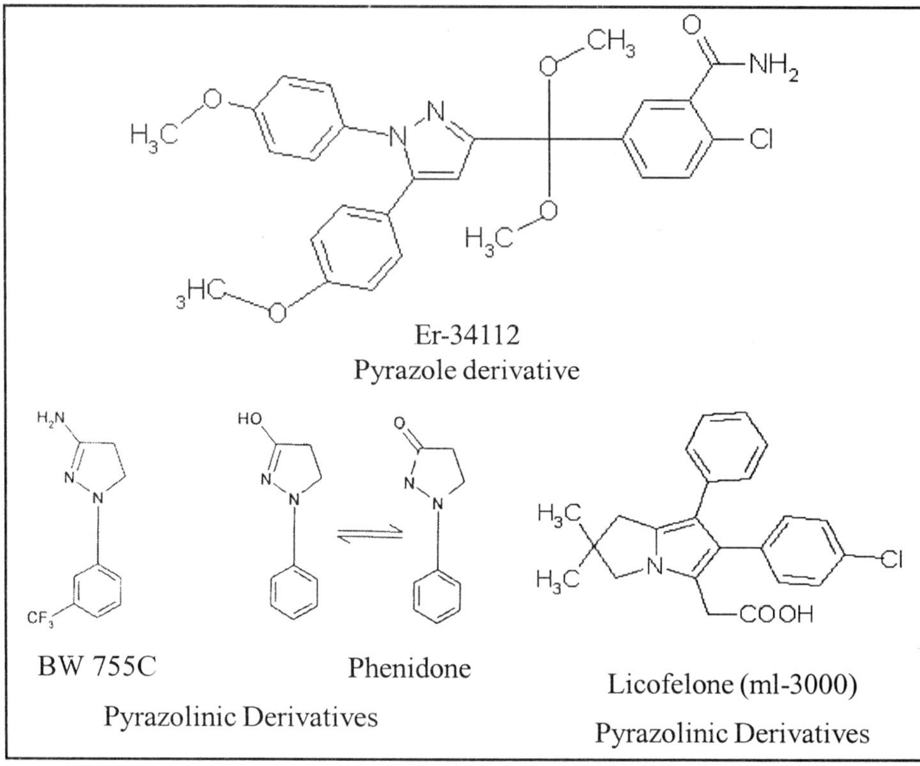

Fig. 11. Structures of dual inhibitors of COX and 5-LOX

Others (tepoaxalin and tebufelone) displayed broad inhibition of redox enzymes and liver toxicity.

Presently darbufelone and licofelone (ML 3000) are in phase-III clinical trials. They are devoid of redox potential and act as substrate competitors. Table 5 summarizes the *in vitro* and *in vivo* activities of some potential dual inhibitors developed

Licofelone, ([2,2-dimethyl-6-(4-chloropheny-7-phenyl-2,3-dihydro-1H-pyrrazoline-5-yl] acetic acid), is the most promising of the dual inhibitor of COX and 5-LOX enzymes. Originally discovered by Merckle GmbH and developed by EuroAllaince (a consortium of Alfa Wassermann SpA, Lacer SA and Merckle), it is presently under clinical evaluation (Phase III) for the treatment of osteoarthritis (OA)[69].

The major pharmacodynamic studies of licofelone including those carried out by our own research group are summarized in table 6.

Table 5. Dual inhibitors of COX and 5-LOX with their IC_{50} values and *in vivo* activity[67]

Compound	*In vitro* IC_{50} (μM)			*In vivo* activity
	COX-1	COX-2	5-LOX	
Tepoxalin (Zubrin™)	0.80 (Both COX-1/-2)		0.15	Adjuvant induced arthritis in rats (ED_{50} = 3 mg/kg)
Tebufelone	1.50	0.02	20-22	Anti-inflammatory; antipyretic in humans (50mg vs. 600mg aspirin)
di-7-tert-butyl-2,3-dihydro-3,3-dimethylbenzofuran (DHDMBF)	0.06	0.02	6.0	Anti-inflammatory

Compound	*In vitro* IC_{50} (μM)			*In vivo* activity
	COX-1	COX-2	5-LOX	
BF389		0.84	3.65	Adjuvant arthritis in rat paw oedema (1.2 mg/kg for oedema inhibition and 1.7 mg/kg for bone damage inhibition)
RJW63556	>10.0	1.81	1.02	Adjuvant arthritis in rat paw oedema (3mg/kg)
PGV20229	7.00	0.22	8.00	Adjuvant arthritis in rat paw oedema (6.6mg/kg)
C-1986	0.80 (Both COX-1/-2)		2.8	Carrageenan-induced foot paw oedema
Licofelone (ML 3000)	0.16-0.2 (Both COX-1/-2)		0.1-0.23	Licofelone (10mg/kg) significantly decreased the secondary lesion in rat adjuvant- arthritis
				Licofelone (10 mg/kg, po) was more effective than aspirin (50 mg/kg, po) in phenylquinone-induced writhing in mice
				Licofelone (10mg/kg) showed a significant analgesic effect over 3h in Brewer's yeast-induced hyperthermia in rats
				Licofelone co-administered to aspirin-treated rats did not exacerbate acute gastric injury and also did not alter the gastric adaptation to aspirin. Licofelone (10 to 100 mg/kg, po) did not produce any acute damage
				Licofelone (10, 30, 100mg/kg, po) demonstrated significant antithrombotic effect, comparable to aspirin

Table 6. Summary of pharmacodynamic activity of licofelone

Licofelone (ML 3000)		
Effect studied	**Experimental model**	**Result**
Anti-inflammatory	Carrageenan-induced rat paw oedema	ED_{50} = 19.1 mg/kg, po (onset 2h, short duration) (Singh, Patil and Kulkarni, 2005a[70])
	Bradykinin-induced rat paw oedema	ED_{50} = 13.0 mg/kg, po (onset 1h, long duration) (Singh, Patil and Kulkarni, 2005a[70])
	Archidonic acid-induced rat paw oedema	ED_{50} = 16.8 mg/kg, po (onset 1h, long duration) (Singh, Patil and Kulkarni, 2005a[70])
	Freund's adjuvant-induced acute inflammation	ED_{50} = 18.2 mg/kg po (Singh, Patil and Kulkarni unpublished observation)
	Freund's adjuvant-induced established inflammation	ED_{50} = 17.5 mg/kg, po (Singh, Patil and Kulkarni unpublished observation)
	Rat adjuvant- arthritis	Licofelone (10mg/kg) significantly decreased the secondary lesion[71]
Analgesic	Acetic acid-induced writhing	ED_{50} 31.33 mg/kg, po (Singh, Patil and Kulkarni unpublished observation)
	phenylquinone-induced writhing in mice.	Licofelone 10 mg/kg, po was more effective than aspirin 50 mg/kg, po[71]
Anti-hyperalgesic effect	Carrageenan-induced rat hind paw mechanical hyperalgesia	ED_{50} = 47.6 mg/kg, po (onset 1h, long duration) (Singh, Patil and Kulkarni, 2005a[70])
	Bradykinin-induced rat hind paw mechanical hyperalgesia	ED_{50} = 78.6 mg/kg, po (onset 2h, medium duration) (Singh, Patil and Kulkarni, 2005a[70])
	Arachidonic-induced rat hind paw mechanical hyperalgesia	ED_{50} = 92.2 mg/kg, po (onset 1h, medium dur ation) (Singh, Patil and Kulkarni, 2005a[70])
	Freund's adjuvant-induced acute hyperalgesia	4.6 mg/kg, po (Singh, Patil and Kulkarni unpublished observation)
	Freund's adjuvant-induced established inflammation	12.0 mg/kg, po (Singh, Patil and Kulkarni unpublished observation)
	Incision pain in rats	2.92 mg/kg, po (onset 3h, long duration) (Singh, Patil and Kulkarni, 2005b[72])
Anti-allodynic effect	Incision pain in rats	36.77 mg/kg, po (onset 1h, long duration) (Singh, Patil and Kulkarni, 2005b[72])
Antipyretic	Brewer's yeast-induced hyperthermia in rats	licofelone (10mg/kg) showed a significant analgesic effect over 3h[71]
Anti-thrombic	laser-induced thrombus in rats	licofelone (10, 30, 100 mg/kg, po) demonstrated significant anti-thrombotic effect, comparable to aspirin[73]

An unpublished study by Singh, Patil and Kulkarni, demonstrated the ability of licofelone, to ameliorate the intracerebroventricular N-methyl D-aspartate (NMDA)-induced cellular damage in mice. Authors observed that licofelone when administered pre - (1 day) or post - (3 days) NMDA, significantly attenuated the brain oedema and cellular damage. It also inhibited NMDA-induced malondialdehyde (MDA) and nitrite generation in mouse whole brain and the neuroprotection was still evident when licofelone treatment was initiated 8 hr after NMDA administration, but not when administered 20 h later. The study therefore, suggested that dual inhibitors of COX and 5-LOX, like licofelone can prevent *in-vivo* NMDA excitotoxicity with long therapeutic window. A brief summary of the clinical trials conducted on Licofelone is summarized in Table 7.

Table 7. Summary of clinical trial results on licofelone

Effect studied	Model used	Result
Safety and tolerability	Phase I trials in healthy volunteers (n=121) with normal gastric mucosa and duodenal mucosa	After 4 weeks, the gastric mucosa was completely normal in 93% of volunteers given licofelone (200mg, bid), 89% given licofelone (400mg, bid), 90% given placebo and 37% naproxen (500mg, bid)[76,77]
Efficacy and safety	Phase II trials in osteoarthritis (OA) patients (n=107)	Doses of 100, 200, and 400 mg, bid of licofelone for 4 weeks demonstrated a significant, superior effect compared to placebo, similar effect to diclofenac (50mg, bid). Licofelone was well tolerated[76,78,79]
Efficacy and safety	Phase II trails in OA patients (n=148)	Efficacy was similar to patients given licofelone (200mg, bid) or naproxen (500 mg, bid) for 12 weeks. Only 14% of licofelone-treated patients reported GI side effects compared with 26% of those treated with naproxen[80,81].
Safety and efficacy	Phase II trails in patients (n=710) with OA of knee	Doses of 100, and 200 mg, bid of licofelone for 4 weeks demonstrated similar efficacy to naproxen (500mg, bid) for 4 weeks. The general tolerability of and GI tolerability of licofelone were better than naproxen[82].
Comparing licofelone with celecoxib	OA patients (n=608)	Licofelone (200mg, bid) was as effective as celecoxib 200mg once daily. Low adverse event rate was reported with licofelone (31.9%) than the celecoxib group (36.4%). No comparison of relative GI toxicity was conducted[83,84]
Comparing licofelone with celecoxib	OA patients (n=608)	Licofelone (200mg, bid) was as effective as celecoxib 200mg once daily. Low adverse event rate was reported with licofelone (31.9%) than the celecoxib group (36.4%). No comparison of relative GI toxicity was conducted[83,84]
GI safety of licofelone with aspirin comedication	Two multicentric, randomized, double blind, and endoscopy trials (licofelone n=35, naproxen n=41); (licofelone n=95, naproxen n=106)	The superior GI tolerability of licofelone compared to naproxen was confirmed in both the studies. In the first study the GI ulcer index for licofelone or naproxen was 2.9 and 26.8%, respectively, and 2.1 and 20.8%, respectively in second study[84,85].

The experimental data therefore, suggested that dual inhibitors of COX and 5-LOX are at least as effective as NSAIDs with advantage of remarkable gastrointestinal safety. Besides, these drugs are expected to be devoid of cardiovascular complications, a recently reported adverse effect with coxibs. Therefore, in view of the literature discussed above, it appears that simultaneous inhibition of COX and 5-LOX pathways could offer opportunities to treat painful and inflammatory conditions with more efficient and better tolerated drugs. Also this class of compounds will certainly be of great interest for the treatment of other pathologies such as neurodegeneration, carcinogenesis and angiogenesis.

REFERENCES

1. Basbaum A & Bushell C, Pain: Basic mechanisms. In: Pain 2005- an updated review. Justins Dm (Ed.). IASP Press: Seattle; 2005. p 3-9.
2. Guyton AC, Hall JE (Eds.). Somatic sensations: II, Pain, headache, and thermal sensations. In Textbook of medical physiology. 10th ed. Harcourt Publishers International Company: Singapore; 2001. p. 552.
3. Greenspan JD, Noc and the peripheral nervous system's role in pain, *J Hand Ther* 10 (1997) 78.
4. vanat.cvm.umn.edu/NeuroLectPDFs/LectNociceptionI.pdf. [Cited 2002].
5. Melzack R & Wall PD, Pain mechanisms: a new theory. *Science* 34 (1965) 102.
6. Light AR, The initial processing of pain and its descending control : spinal and trigeminal systems. Reichmann H (Ed.). 12th Vol. S. Karger AG, Basel. 1992.
7. Melzack R & Wall PD, The challenge of pain. New York, NY: Penguin Press; 1984.
8. www.fleshandbones.com/readingroom. Introduction to the pain management.
9. Robinson AJ, Central nervous system pathways for pain transmission and pain control; issues relevant to practicing clinician. *J Hand Ther* 10 (1997) 64.
10. Jain NK & Kulkarni SK, Antinociceptive effect of sumatriptan in mice. *Ind J Exp Biol* 36 (1998) 973.
11. Siddall PJ & Cousins MJ, Neurobiology of pain. *Int Anethesiol Clin* 35 (1997) 1.
12. Ninan I & Kulkarni SK, Involvement of dopamine D2 and 5-HT1A receptors in roxindole-induced antinociception. *Ind J Exp Biol* 37 (1998) 234.

13. Naidu PS, Singh A & Kulkarni SK, (D2 -dopamine and $\alpha2$ - adrenoreceptor - mediated analgesic response of quercetin. *Ind J Exp Biol* 41 (2003) 1400.

14. Singh A, Kumar G, Naidu PS & Kulkarni SK, Antinociceptive effect of FK506 in mice. *Ind J Exp Biol* 41 (2003) 1405.

15. Levine JD & Taiwo YO, Hyperalgesic pain: a review. *Anesth Prog* 37 (1990) 133.

16. Taiwo YO, Bjerknes LK, Goetzl EJ & Levine JD, Mediation of primary afferent peripheral hyperalgesia by the cAMP second messenger system. *Neuroscience* 32 (1989) 577.

17. Taiwo YO, Goetzl EJ & Levine JD, Hyperalgesia onset latency suggest hierarchy of action. *Brain Res* 423 (1987) 333.

18. Southall MD & Vasko MR, Prostaglandin E(2)-mediated sensitization of rat sensory neurons is not altered by nerve growth factor. *Neurosci Lett* 32 (1989) 577.

19. Aley KO & Levine JD, Contribution of 5- and 12-lipoxygenase products to mechanical hyperalgesia induced PGE_2 and epinephrine in the rat. *Exp Brain Res* 148 (2003) 482.

20. Fu JY, Masferrer JL, Seibert K, Raz A & Needleman P, The induction and suppression of prostaglandin H2 synthase (cyclooxygenase) in human monocytes. *J Biol Chem* 265 (1990) 16737.

21. Chandrasekharan NV, Dai H, Roos KL, Evanson NK, Tomsik J, Elton TS & Simmons DL, COX-3, a cyclooxygenase-1 variant inhibited by acetaminophen and other analgesic/antipyretic drugs: cloning, structure, and expression. *Proc Natl Acad Sci USA* 99 (2002) 13926.

22. Xie W, Chipman JG, Robertson DL, Erikson RL & Simmons DL, Expression of a mitogen-responsive gene encoding prostaglandin synthase is regulated by mRNA splicing. *Proc Natl Acad Sci USA* 88 (1991) 2692.

23. Kis B, Snipes JA & Busija DW, Acetaminophen and the cyclooxygenase-3 puzzle: sorting out facts, fictions, and uncertainties. *J Pharmacol Exp Ther* 315 (2005) 1.

24. Burdan F, Chalas A & Szumilo J, Cyclooxygenase and prostanoids-biological implications. *Postepy Hig Med Dosw* 60 (2006) 129.

25. Vane JR, Bakhle YS & Botting RM, Cyclooxygenases 1 and 2. *Ann Rev Pharmacol Toxicol* 38 (1998) 97.

26. Padi SV & Kulkarni SK, Role of cyclooxygenase-2 in lipopolysaccharide-induced hyperalgesia in fomalin test. *Ind J Exp Biol* 43 (2005) 53.

27. http://www.cyberlipid.org/prost1/pros0001.htm. Prostanoids and related compounds. [Cited: 2006, May 1].

28. Kulkarni SK, Jain NK & Singh A, Cyclooxygenase isoenzymes and newer therapeutic potential for cyclooxygenase inhibitors. *Methods Find Exp Clin Pharmacol* 22 (2000) 291

29. Wu KK, Inducible cyclooxygenase and nitric oxide synthase. *Adv Pharmacol* 33 (1995) 179.

30. Smith WJ, Garavito RM & DeWitt DL, Prostaglandin endoperoxidase H synthases (cyclooxygenases)-1 and -2. *J Biol Chem* 271 (1996) 33157.

31. Smith WL & Langenbach R, Why there are two cyclooxygenases isoenzymes. *J Clin Invest* 107 (2001) 1491.

32. Siebert K, Zhang Y, Leathy K, Hauiser S, Masferrer J & Isakson P, Distribution of COX-1 and COX-2 in normal and inflamed tissues. *Adv Exp Med Biol* 400A (1997) 167.

33. DuBois RN, Abramson SB, Crofford L, Gupta RA, Simon LS, Van De Putte LBA & Lipsky PE, Cyclooxygenase in biology and disease. *FASEB J* 12 (1998) 1063.

34. Mitchell JA & Warner TD, Cyclooxygenase-2: pharmacology, physiology, biochemistry and relevance to NSAID therapy. *Br J Pharmacol* 128 (1999) 1121.

35. Smith WL, DeWitt DL & Gravito RM, Cyclooxygenases: structural, cellular and molecular biology. *Annu Rev Biochem* 69 (2000) 145.

36. FitzGerald GA & Patrono C, The coxibs, selective inhibitors of cyclooxygenase-2. *N Engl J Med* 345 (2001) 433.

37. Warner TD 7 Mitchell JA, Cyclooxygenases: new forms, new inhibitors, and lessons from the clinic. *FASEB J* 18 (2004) 790.

38. Celloti F & Laufer S, Anti-inflammatory drugs: New multitarget compounds to face an old problem. The dual inhibition concept. *Pharmacological Res* 43 (2001) 429.

39. Langenbach R, Loftin C, Lee C & Tiano H, Cycloocygenase knockout mice. Models for elucidating isoform-specific functions. *Biochem Pharmacol* 58 (1999) 1237.

40. Lipsky PE, Brooks P, Crofford LJ, DuBois R, Graham D, Simon LS, van de Putte LB & Abramson SB, Unresolved issues in the role of cyclooxygenase-2 in normal physiologic processes and disease. *Arch Intern Med* 160 (2000) 913.

41. Bombardier C, Laine L, Reicin A, Shapiro D, Burgos-Vargas R, Davis B, Day R, Ferraz MB, Hawkey CJ, Hochberg MC, Kvien TK & Schnitzer TJ, VIGOR Study Group. Comparison of upper gastrointestinal toxicity of rofecoxib and naproxen in patients with rheumatoid arthritis. VIGOR Study Group. *N Engl J Med* 343 (2000)1520.

42. http://www.fda.gov/cder. USFDA (home page on internet). Center for Drug Evaluation and Research. [Cited: 2004, Nov 18].

43. Sharma S, Jain NK & Kulkarni SK, Possible analgesic and anti-inflammatory interactions of aspartame with opiods and NSAIDs. *Ind J Exp Biol* 43 (2005) 498.

44. Kumar A, Jain NK & Kulkarni SK, Analgesic and anti-inflammatory effects of phosphodiesterase inhibitors. *Ind J Exp Biol* 38 (2000) 26.

45. Patil CS, Jain NK, Singh VP & Kulkarni SK, Cholinergic-NO-cGMP mediation of sildenafil-induced antinociception. *Ind J Exp Biol* 42 (2004) 361.

46. Rainsford KD, Ying C & Smith F, Effects of 5-lipoxygenase inhibitors on interleukin production by human synovial tissues in organ culture: comparison with interleukin-1 synthesis inhibitor. *J Pharm Pharmacol* 48 (1996) 46.

47. Lewis RA, Austen KF & Soberman RJ, Leukotrienes and other products of the 5-lipoxygenase pathway. Biochemistry and relation to pathobiology in human diseases. *N Engl J Med* 192 (2000) 439.

48. He W, Pelletier JP, Martel-Pelletier J, Laufer S & Di Battista JA, The synthesis of interleukin-1 beta, tumor necrosis factor-á and interstitial collagenase (MMP-1) is eicosanoid dependent in human OA synovial membrane implants: interactions with anti-inflammtory cytokines. *J Rheumatol* 29 (2002) 546.

49. Haribabu B, Verghese MW, Steeber DA, Sellars DD, Bock CB & Snyderman R, Targeted disruption of the leukotriene B(4) receptor in mice reveals its role in inflammation and platelet-activating factor-induced anaphylaxis. *J Exp Med* 192 (2000) 433.

50. Alten R, Gromnica-Ihle E, Pohl C, Emmerich J, Steffgen J, Roscher R, Sigmund R, Schmolke B & Steinmann G, Inhibition of leukotriene B4-induced CD11B/CD18 (Mac-1) expression by BIIL 284, a new long acting LTB_4 receptor antagonist, in patients with rheumatoid arthritis. *Ann Rheum Dis* 63 (2004) 170.

51. Zouboulis CC, Nestoris S, Adler YD, Orth M, Orfanos CE & Picardo, M, A new concept for acne therapy: a pilot study with zileuton, an oral 5-lipoxygenase inhibitor. *Arch Dermatol* 139 (2003) 668.

52. Singh VP, Patil CS & Kulkarni SK, Effect of 5-lipoxygenase inhibition on events associated with inflammatory bowel disease in rats. *Ind J Exp Biol* 42 (2004) 667.

53. Penrose JF, Austan KF & Lam BK, Leukotriens: biosynthetic pathways, release and receptor mediated actions with relevance to disease states. In: Inflammation basic principles and clinical correlates. Gallin JL, Snyderman R (Eds). Lippicort Williams and Wilkins; Phildalpheia: 1999. p 361-372.

54. Sala A & Folco G, Neutrophils, endothelial cells, and cysteinyl leukotrienes, a new approach to neutrophil-dependent inflammation? *Biochem Biophys Res Commun* 283 (2001) 1003.

55. Fiorucci S, Distrutti E, de De Lima OM, Romano M, Mencarelli A, Barbanti M, Palazzini E, Morelli A & Wallace JL, Relative contribution of acetylated cyclo-oxygenase (COX)-2 and 5-lipoxygenase (LOX) in regulating gastric mucosal integrity and adaptation to aspirin. *FASEB J* 17 (2003) 1171.

56. Manev H, Uz T, Sugaya K & Qu T, Putative role of neuronal 5-lipoxygenase in an aging brain. *FASEB J* 14 (2000) 1464.

57. Kim GW & Chan PH, Oxidative stress and neuronal DNA fragmentation mediate age-dependent vulnerability to the mitochondrial toxin, 3-nitropropionic acid, in the mouse striatum. *Neurobiol Dis* 8 (2001) 114.

58. Lee CC, Appleyard RF, Byrne JG & Cohn LH, Leukotrienes D_4 and E_4 are produced in myocardium impair coronary flow and ventricular function after two hours of global ischemia in rat heart. *Cardiovas Res* 27 (1993) 770.

59. Sala A, Rossoni G, Buccellati C, Berti F, Folco G & Maclouf J, Formation of sulphidopeptide-leukotrienes by cell-cell interaction causes coronary vasoconstriction in isolated, cell-perfused heart of rabbit. *Br J Pharmacol* 110 (1993) 1206.

60. Fierro IM & Serhan CN, Mechanisms in anti-inflammation and resolution: the role of lipoxins and aspirin-triggered lipoxins. *Braz J Med Biol Res* 34 (2001) 555.

61. Weylandt KH & Kang JX, Rethinking lipid mediators. *Lancet* 366 (2005) 618.

62. Nickerson-Nutter CL & Medvedeff ED, The effect of leukotriene synthesis inhibitors in models of acute and chronic inflammation. *Arthritis Rheum* 39 (1996) 515.

63. Pelletier JM, Lajeunesse D, Reboul P & Pelletier JP, Therapeutic role of dual inhibitors of 5-LOX and COX, selective and non-selective non-steroidal anti-inflammatory drugs. *Ann Rehum Dis* 62 (2003) 501.

64. Bishnoi M, Patil CS & Kulkarni SK, Potentiation of antinociceptive effect of NSAIDs by specific lipoxygenase inhibitor, acetyl 11-keto-beta boswellic acid. *Ind J Exp Biol* 44 (2005)128.

65. Wallace JL, Keennan CM & Granger DN, Gastric ulceration induced by Nonsteroidal anti-inflammatory drugs is a neutrophil-dependent process. *Am J Physiol* 259 (1990) G462.

66. Singh VP, Patil CS & Kulkarni SK, Effect of licofelone against NSAIDs-induced gastrointestinal ulceration and inflammation. *Ind J Exp Biol* 43 (2005) 247.

67. Gaetano G de, Donati MD & Cerletti, C, Prevention of thrombosis and vascular inflammation: benefits and limitations of selective or combined COX-1, COX-2 and 5-LOX inhibitors. *Trends Pharmacol Sci* 24 (2003) 245.

68. Algate DR, Augustin J, Atterson PR, Beard DJ, Jobling CM, Laufer S, Munt PL & Tries S, General pharmacology of [2,2-dimethyl-6-(4-chlorophenyl)-7-phenyl-2,3- dihydro-1H-pyrrolizine-5-yl]-acetic acid in experimental animals. *Arzneimittelforschung* 45 (1995) 159.

69. Ding C & Cicuttini F, Licofelone Merckle. *Drugs* 6 (2003) 803.

70. Singh, VP, Patil CS, & Kulkarni SK, Anti-inflammatory effect of licofelone against various inflammatory challenges. *Fundam Clin Exp Pharmacol* 20 (2005a) 65.

71. Tries, S & Laufer, S, The pharmacological profile of ML 3000: A new pyrrolizine derivative inhibiting the enzymes cyclooxygenase and 5-lipoxygenase. *Inflammopharmacology* 9 (2001) 113.

72. Singh VP, Patil CS, Kulkarni SK, Effect of licofelone against mechanical hyperalgesia and cold allodynia in the rat model of incisional pain. *Pharmacol Rep*. 57 (2005b) 380.

73. Tries S, Laufer S, Radziwon P, Breddin HK, Antithrombotic and platelet function inhibiting effects of ML3000, a new antiinflammatory drug with COX/5-LOX inhibitory activity. *Inflamm Res* 51 (2002) 129.

74. Jovanovic, DV, Fernandes JC, Martel-Pelletier J, Jolicoeur FC, Reboul P, Laufer S, Tries S & Pelletier JP, *In vivo* dual inhibition of cyclooxygenase and lipoxygenase by ML3000 reduces the progression of experimental osteoarthritis: suppression of collagenase 1 and interleukin-1beta synthesis. *Arthritis Rheum* 44 (2001) 2320.

75. Lajeunesse, D, Pelletier JM, Fernandes JC, Laufe S, Pelletier JP, Treatment with licofelone prevents abnormal subchondreal bone cell metabolism in experimental dog arthritis. *Ann Rheum Dis* 63 (2004) 73.

76. Alfa Wassermann SpA, ML 3000, the parent drug of new category of anti-inflammatory agents, double acting anti-inflammatory drugs (DAAD), shows outstanding gastroduodenal tolerability in clinical studies. Alfa Wassermann SpA Press Release 1999; June 16.

77. Forest laboratories Inc, Forest laboratories announces positive results with ML 3000 in early clinical trials. Forest laboratories Inc. Press Release 2000, March 29.

78. Alfa Wassermann SpA, Positive ML 3000 clinical trial results announced by EuroAlliance at OARSI meeting in Barcelona. Alfa Wassermann SpA Press Release 2000; October.

79. Albrecht W, Bias P, Lammerich A, Carre C & Clerch, L, Pharmacokinetics, safety, and tolerability of licofelone (ML3000) 200 mg bid given with food

in young and elderly healthy volunteers. *Ann Eur Congr Rheumatol* 12-15 (2002a) AB0293.

80. Albrecht W, Bias P& Lammerich A, Investigation of the single-dose pharmacokinetics of warfarin during repeated administration of licofelone (ML 3000) 200 mg bid to healthy volunteers *Ann Eur Congr Rheumatol* 12-15 (2002b) AB0295.

81. Reginster J, Bias P & Buchner A, First clinical results of licofelone (ML3000), an inhibitor of COX-1, COX-2, and 5-LOX, for the treatment of osteoarthritis. *Ann Rheum Dis* 61 suppl (2002) 116.

82. Blanco FJ, Buchner A& Bias P, Licofelone, an inhibitor of COX-1, COX-2, and 5-LOX, is as effective as naproxen and shows improved safety during 12 weeks treatment in patients with osteoarthritis of the knee. *Ann Rheum Dis* 62 suppl (2003) 261.

83. Skelly MM & Hawkey CJ, Potential alternatives to COX-2 inhibitors. New molecules may overtake the COX-2 inhibitors debate. *Br Med J* 324 (2002) 1289.

84. Langman MJS, Adverse effects of conventional non-steroidal anti-inflammatory drugs on the upper gastrointestinal tract. *Fundam Clin Pharmacol* 17 (2003) 393.

85. Bias P, Buchner A, Klesser B & Laufer S, The gastrotolearbility of the LOX/ COX inhibitor, licofelone is similar to placebo and superior to naproxen therapy in healthy volunteers. *Am J Gastroenterol* 99 (2004) 611.

22

Potentiation of antinociceptive effect of NSAIDs by a specific lipooxygenase inhibitor, acetyl-11-keto-beta boswellic acid

MAHENDRA BISHNOI, CHANDRASHEKAR S. PATIL, ANIL KUMAR AND S.K. KULKARNI
Pharmacology Division, University Institute of Pharmaceutical Sciences, Panjab University, Chandigarh 160 014, India

The present study was aimed to assess the combined effects of cyclooxygenase and 5-lipoxygenase (COX/5-LOX) inhibitors in different animal models of nociception. Naproxen, nimesulide and rofecoxib are well-established antinociceptive agents acting *via* COX inhibition. AKBA (acetyl-11-keto-beta-boswellic acid) is a 5-LOX inhibitor. AKBA (50-200 mg/kg) produced a dose dependent and significant antinociceptive effect in different animal models of nociception. Based on the earlier reports from our laboratory, subeffective doses of all the three COX Inhibitors were selected and they were administered (naproxen, 5 mg/kg; nimesulide, 1 mg/kg; and rofecoxib, 1 mg/kg) with AKBA (100 mg/kg). This produced a more significant antinociceptive effect as compared to *per se* effect observed in all the three models of nociception. However, the effect of combination of nimesulide with AKBA was more pronounced as compared to naproxen and rofecoxib and their combination with AKBA. The present finding provided an evidence for the potentiation of antinociceptive effect of NSAIDs with AKBA. Such a combination may help to reduce the therapeutic doses of conventional NSAIDs and also reduce side effects (gastric, cardiac and renal) that are popularly associated with the NSAIDs.

Keywords: Antinociception, Boswellic acid, Nociception, NSAID

Oxidized arachidonic acid derivatives, collectively termed as eicosanoids (prostaglandins and leukotrienes) have important modulatory role in inflammation, blood clotting, control of vascular tone, renal functions, reproductive functions as well as pain[1]. Role of prostaglandins (PGs) in pain is long and extensively studied. PGs act directly on the peripheral terminals of the nociceptors through G protein coupled receptors to modulate (*via* cAMP/PKA second messenger) the tetrodotoxin resistant sodium channel and to produce pain. Besides this, leukotrienes, especially LTB_4, result into increase in vascular permeability and chemotaxis of polymorphonuclear leukocytes as well as release of chemicals from leukocytes, which produce the sensitization of nociceptors[2,3]. The lipoxygenase products of arachidonic acid metabolism have also been implicated directly in activating the capsaicin sensitive vanilloid receptors. 5-lipooxygenase products are also involved in hyperalgesia[4,5].

Acetyl-11-keto-beta-boswellic acid (AKBA) is one of the four major pentacyclic triterpenic acids present in the acidic extract of the *Boswellia serrata* gum resin, which is used for a variety of inflammatory disorders, such as rheumatoid arthritis, osteoarthritis, and cervical spondylitis[6]. AKBA is a novel and highly specific inhibitor of 5-lipooxygenase, the key enzyme in leukotriene biosynthesis. AKBA inhibits 5-LOX either directly interacting with the enzyme itself or interacting with 5-lipooxygenase activating proteins (FLAP)[6,7].

Based on the possible role of the leukotrienes in the sensitization and provocation of nociceptors and the already established role of cyclooxygenase metabolites, we studied the effect of different COX inhibitors (naproxen, nimesulide and rofecoxib) and LOX inhibitor, acetyl-11-keto-beta-boswellic acid (AKBA), and their combination. The study was undertaken to determine whether the combined inhibition showed better analgesic activity than single inhibition in different models of pain.

Materials and Methods

Animals: Laca mice (20-30 g) of either sex, bred in central animal house of Panjab University, Chandigarh maintained at 12 hr light and dark cycle were used in the study. Animals were housed under standard laboratory conditions, with free access to food and water. All experiments were carried out between 0900 and 1700 hrs and the experimental protocol was approved by IAEC of the university.

Drug, dose, route: The drugs, nimesulide (1 and 2 mg/kg), naproxen (5 and 10 mg/kg), rofecoxib (1 and 2 mg/kg) and test substance AKBA (50 and 100 mg/kg) were prepared in 0.5% carboxy methylcellulose (CMC) and administered orally (po) half an hour before subjecting to nociceptive stimulus in the different models of nociception. They were administered simultaneously whenever a combination was attempted.

All the substances were obtained from M/s Panacea Biotec, Ltd., Lalru, India.

Assessment of anti-nociceptive activity

The anti-nociceptive activity of the given drugs and their combination was assessed using different models of nociception as follows:

Acetic acid-induced writhing (abdominal contractions): Abdominal contractions were induced by 1% acetic acid solution (0.1 ml/10 g, ip) in mice. The number of abdominal wriths was scored over 20 min after the injection of acetic acid[8].

Tail flick test: The antinociceptive effect was also determined by using the tail flick test. The response was recorded at 30, 60 and 120 min after drug administration[8].

Tail-immersion test: The distal end (2 cm) of the mouse-tail was marked and this part of the tail was immersed in a water bath containing warm water at 55°C. Withdrawal of the tail from the water was taken as the endpoint. The reaction time was determined before and at various time intervals (30,60,120 min) after different treatments. A cut off time of 10 sec was observed to avoid injury to the tail[8]. Results were expressed in % maximum possible effect (% MPE)

$$\%MPE = \frac{(\text{Post treatment latency} - \text{pre treatment latency}) \times 100}{\text{Pre treatment latency}}$$

Statistical analysis: The data was expressed as mean±SEM and was analyzed using Students t-test. $P<0.05$ was considered as significant.

Results

Acetic acid induced-writhing (abdominal contractions)–Animals from the control group showed 61±1.58 abdominal writhes during an observation period of 20 min after acetic acid injection. All the 4 test drugs studied nimesulide (1, 2 mg/kg), naproxen (5,10 mg/kg), rofecoxib (1, 2 mg/kg) and AKBA (50,100 mg/kg) showed significant and dose-dependent decrease in the number of abdominal constrictions as compared to the control group. Nimesulide (2 mg/kg, po) showed the maximum effect. When the sub-effective dose of COX inhibitors (nimesulide, 1 mg/kg; naproxen, 5 mg/kg; rofecoxib, 1 mg/kg) was combined with 5-LOX inhibitor AKBA (100 mg/kg) the analgesic effect of all the three drugs was potentiated significantly as compared to control as well as their *per se* effect. Effect of combination of nimesulide with AKBA was more prominent than other two COX inhibitors (Table1).

Table 1. Effect of COX and 5-LOX inhibitors and their combination at different doses on acetic acid induced writhing in mice (Values are mean±SEM of 6 animals)

Drug treatment (mg/kg)	Number of wriths	% Inhibition
Control	61.0±1.58	
Naproxen,		
5	41.33±2.48 [a]	32.24
10	35±2.15 [a]	42.62
Nimesulide,		
1	36.0±4.31 [a]	40.98
2	32.4±5.11 [a]	46.88
Rofecoxib,		
1	43.3±1.24 [a]	29.01
2	38.6±1.24 [a]	36.72
AKBA,		
50	41.33±1.80 [a]	32.24
100	36±4.31 [a]	40.98
Naproxen, 5 + AKBA, 100	30.2±1.24 [ac]	50.49
Nimesulide, 1+ AKBA, 100	22.6±2.49 [abd]	62.95
Rofecoxib, 1 + AKBA, 100	30.6±1.85 [ae]	49.83

[a]$P< 0.05$ as compared to control values, [b]as compared to AKBA (100 mg/kg) values, [c]as compared to naproxen (5mg/kg) values, [d]as compared to nimesulide (1 mg/kg) values, [e]as compared to rofecoxib (1 mg/kg) values. Drugs were administered orally.

Tail- flick test: All the 4 test drugs, nimesulide (1, 2 mg/kg), naproxen (5, 10 mg/kg), rofecoxib (1, 2 mg/kg) and AKBA (50, 100 mg/kg) showed significant and dose-dependent increase in % MPE as compared to control. The effect was maximum at 60 min in all the 4 drugs and after that the effect started decreasing and at 120 min it was minimum. Combination of AKBA with naproxen or rofecoxib appeared to potentiate the effect of these NSAIDs at 30 and 60 min, though the maximum effect was lesser than that observed for AKBA alone. However, the observation at 120 min revealed a clear potentiation in terms of duration of action as well as efficacy when compared to their individual effects.

Combination of AKBA with nimesulide clearly exhibited a potentiation at all periods of observation when compared to their individual effects. Effect of combination of nimesulide with AKBA was more prominent than other two COX inhibitors (Table 2).

Table 2. Effect of COX and 5-LOX inhibitors and their combination at different doses on tail-flick test in mice (Values are mean±SEM of 6 animals)

Drug treatment (mg/kg)	%MPE 30min	%MPE 60min	%MPE 120min
Control	15.23±2.20	10.47±4.15	3.80±3.32
Naproxen,			
5	24.42±1.51	36.42±3.20	30.64±2.24
10	48.46±5.61 [a]	86.42±6.98 [a]	48.34±3.98 [a]
Nimesulide,			
1	32.42±3.54	54.36±4.45	38.20±4.51
2	62.59±3.52 [a]	136.42±5.4 [a]	58.34±9.62 [a]
Rofecoxib,			
1	28.62±1.65	42.48±5362	39.64±4.50
2	56.42±9.35 [a]	98.24±8.21 [a]	60.04±6.65 [a]
AKBA,			
50	29.35±2.54	46.78±5.63	9.17±3.33
100	58.37±6.58 [a]	97.28±4.89 [a]	29.86±3.56 [a]
Naproxen, 5 + AKBA, 100	36.24±1.25 [ac]	106.42±6.98 [ae]	72.25±6.42 [abc]
Nimesulide, 1+ AKBA, 100	64.5±5.21 [ad]	156.32±9.32 [abd]	84.56±9.98 [abd]
Rofecoxib, 1 + AKBA, 100	48.2±3.25 [ae]	110.26±8.25 [ae]	82.49±7.21 [abe]

[a]$P< 0.05$ as compared to control values, [b]as compared to AKBA (100 mg/kg) values, [c]as compared to naproxen (5mg/kg) values, [d]as compared to nimesulide (1 mg/kg) values, [e]as compared to rofecoxib (1 mg/kg) values. Drugs were administered orally.

Tail immersion test: All the 4 test drugs (nimesulide, 1 and 2 mg/kg; naproxen 5 and 10 mg/kg; rofecoxib, 1 and 2 mg/kg; and AKBA 50, 100 mg/kg) showed significant and dose-dependent increase in %

MPE as compared to the control. The effect was maximum at 60 min in all the drug treated groups and the effect started decreasing thereafter. Nimesulide (2 mg/kg, po) showed the maximum effect. When sub-effective dose of COX inhibitors (nimesulide, 1 mg/kg; naproxen, 5 mg/kg; and rofecoxib, 1 mg/kg) were combined with 5-LOX inhibitor AKBA (100 mg/kg) the analgesic effect of all the three drugs was potentiated significantly as compared to control as well as their *per se* effect at 60 min. Although the effect was potentiated at 30 and 120 min, it was not significant. The effect of combination was also not increased significantly as compared to AKBA *per se*. The effect of the combination of nimesulide with AKBA was more prominent than the other two COX inhibitors (Table 3).

Table 3. Effect of COX and 5-LOX inhibitors and their combination at different doses on tail-withdrawal latency in tail-immersion test in mice (Values are mean±SEM of 6 animals)

Drug treatment (mg/kg)	%MPE 30min	%MPE 60min	%MPE 120min
Control	4±2.21	8.33±1.2	33.1±8.54
Naproxen,			
5	24.58±2.21	68.32±3.54	40.21±3.65
10	31.12±1.56 [a]	92.20±7.52 [a]	52.64±5.54 [a]
Nimesulide,			
1	28.95±1.54	88.90±6.39	38.52±3.69
2	58.25±4.54 [a]	162.70±8.54 [a]	70.45±6.58 [a]
Rofecoxib,			
1	32.41±3.24	72.61±6.35	68.5±5.24
2	42.60±4.58 [a]	132.52±9.87 [a]	103.2±10.4 [a]
AKBA,			
50	22.14±3.65	50.71±5.56	22.44±1.24
100	38.88±6.88 [a]	115.5±10.21 [a]	46.11±5.65 [a]
Naproxen, 5 + AKBA, 100	32.25±3.65 [ac]	116.32±9.25 [ac]	62.10±3.69 [abc]
Nimesulide, 1+ AKBA, 100	40.42±5.16 [ad]	146.92±8.97 [abd]	62.58±5.64 [abd]
Rofecoxib, 1 + AKBA, 100	38.2±3.98 [a]	124.5±9.94 [ae]	60.0±6.04 [ab]

[a]*P*< 0.05 as compared to control values, [b]as compared to AKBA (100 mg/kg) values, [c]as compared to naproxen (5mg/kg) values, [d]as compared to nimesulide (1 mg/kg) values, [e]as compared to rofecoxib (1 mg/kg) values. Drugs were administered orally.

Discussion

Evidences clearly indicate that prostanoids, especially PGE_2 are involved in the hyperalgesia and act synergistically with other mediators to produce inflammatory pain. They also sensitize the receptors on the afferent nerve endings and produce synergistic effect to the actions of bradykinin and histamine[1].

There are also evidences supporting the role of leukotrienes in acute pain. LTB_4 and HETE are potent chemo-tactic factors for the polymorphs, which in turn lower the firing threshold of the pain fibers and thus stimulate the nociceptor directly[3]. Capsaicin receptors (VR-1) that are cloned recently are reported to be activated by noxious heat and acid suggesting their role in thermal and chemical pain[9]. Several reports had confirmed that the metabolic products of the lipoxygenase enzyme are the able candidates for the endogenous activation of capsaicin receptors[10].

Besides this, the inhibition of epinephrine induced hyperalgesia (which act directly on primary afferent nociceptors) by different selective and non-selective 5 and 12 lipoxygenase inhibitors also supports the suggestion that lipooxygenase products might be involved in the nociceptive sensitization[11]. 5-lipoxygenase products of arachidonic acid metabolism also act as the second messenger, downstream to protein kinase A and protein kinase C and modulate the action of these kinases in primary afferent nociceptors to mediate their sensitization to mechanical and chemical noxious stimuli. 5 and 12 lipooxygenase products act synergistically with PGE_2 to produce the mechanical hyperalgesia[12,13].

Acetyl-11-keto-beta-boswellic acid (AKBA) is one of the four major pentacyclic triterpenic acids present in the acidic extract of *Boswellia serrata* gum resin[14]. Earlier studies indicate that the primary mode of action involves the inhibition of the 5-lipoxygenase, the key enzyme responsible in the formation of inflammatory compounds, leukotrienes[15]. The mechanism of inhibition is poorly understood as it might inhibit 5-LOX either directly interacting with the enzyme itself or interacting with 5-lipooxygenase activating proteins (FLAP) [6]. Other studies report that AKBA is devoid of any significant side effect and toxicity[7].

Hence, the role of prostaglandin and leukotrienes were supposed to act synergistically to produce mechanical and chemically induced inflammatory pain. Therefore, the combination of their inhibitors might have pronounced effect than their individual effect. Results obtained from different experimental proofs suggest that dual inhibitors of COX and 5-LOX isoenzymes are more pronounced analgesic agents than individual COX inhibitors, whether selective and nonselective[16].

In the present study, there was dose-dependent increase in the analgesic activity of all the given drugs, nimesulide, 1, 2 mg/kg; naproxen, 5, 10 mg/kg; rofecoxib, 1, 2 mg/kg; and AKBA, 50,100 mg/kg in all the three nociceptive models. Effect of all the drugs was maximum after 60 min of noxious stimuli, which started to decline thereafter. Results of above experiments provided evidence that metabolites of COX isoenzymes as well as metabolites of the other pathway of the arachidonic acid metabolism namely, LOX pathway had a role in the acute pain. Further, combination of sub-maximal dose of COX inhibitors nimesulide (1 mg/kg), naproxen (5 mg/kg), rofecoxib (1 mg/kg) with 5-LOX inhibitor AKBA (100 mg/kg) not only synergistically increased the analgesic effect of submaximal doses of COX inhibitors, but also increased the duration of their action. The analgesic activity and the duration of action of combination were equivalent or even better than individual maximal dose treatment of different COX inhibitors. The study also indicated that the combination of AKBA (5-LOX inhibitor) with nimesulide (selective COX-2 inhibitor) produced a more pronounced effect than its combination with naproxen (nonselective COX inhibitor) or rofecoxib (selective COX-2 inhibitor).

In conclusion, the present finding provided evidence that combination of a safe 5-LOX inhibitor like AKBA might reduce the therapeutic doses of conventional NSAIDs and also spared the different side effects (gastric, renal, cardiac), which are associated with the conventional NSAIDs therapy. It will be more advantageous to identify molecules that inhibit both the pathways of AA metabolism namely COX and LOX for better antinociceptive effect.

Acknowledgement

Authors are grateful to the Panacea Biotech, Lalru, Punjab, India for providing drug samples for this work.

REFERENCES

1. Reichling D B & Levine J D, The primary afferent nociceptor as the pattern generator, *Pain*, 6 (1999) S 103.

2. Piomelli D, The ligand that comes from within, *Trends Pharmacol Sci*, 22 (2001) 17.
3. Boden S E, Schweizer S, Dufer M, Drews G & Safayhi H, Stimulation of leukotrienes synthesis in intact polymorph nuclear cells by 5-lipoxygenase inhibitor 3-oxo-tirucallic acid, *J Neurosci*, 60 (2002) 267.
4. Aley K O & Messing R O, Mochly-Rosen D & Levine J D, Chronic hypersensitivity for inflammatory nociceptor sensitization mediated by the epsilon isozyme of protein kinase C, *J Neurosci*, 20 (2000) 4680.
5. Cunha F Q, Teixeira M M & Ferriera S H, Pharmacological modulation of secondary mediator systems-cyclic AMP and cyclic GMP on inflammatory hyperalgesia, *Br J Pharmacol*, 127 (1999) 671.
6. Safayhi H, Sailor E R & Ammon H P T, 5-lipooxygenase inhibition by Acetyl- 11-keto-beta- boswellic acid (AKBA) by a novel mechanism, *Phytomedicine* 3(1996) 71.
7. Singh G B, Singh S & Bani S, Anti-inflammatory actions of boswellic acids, *Phytomedicine*, 3 (1996) 81.
8. Jain N K, Singh A & Kulkarni S K, Analgesic, antiinflammatory and ulcerogenic activity of zinc naproxen complex in mice and rats, *Pharm Pharmacol Commun*, 5 (1999) 599.
9. Hwang S W, Cho H, Kwak S Y & Oh U, Direct activation of capsaicin receptors by products of lipooxygenases: Endogenous capsaicin like substances, *Proc Natl Acad Sci USA*, 97 (2000) 6155.
10. Craib S J, Ellington H C, Pertwee R Q & Ross R A, A possible role of lipooxygenase in the activation of vanilloid receptors by anandamide in the guinea pig bronchous, *Br J Pharmacol*, 134 (2001) 30.
11. Khasar S G, Mccarter G & Levine J D. Epinephrine produces a beta-adrenergic receptor mediated mechanical hyperalgesia and *in vitro* sensitization of rat nociceptors, *J Neurophysiol*, 81 (1999) 1104.
12. Aley K O, Martin A, Mcmohan T, Mok J & Levine J D, Nociceptor sensitization by extracellular signal regulated kinases, *J Neurosci*, 21 (2001) 6933.
13. Aley K O & Levine J D, Contribution of 5 and 12 lipooxygenase products to mechanical hyperalgesia induced by prostaglandin E_2 and epinephrine in the rats, *Exp Brain Res*, 148 (2003) 482.
14. Ammon H P T, Safayhi H & Mack T, Mechanism of antiinflammatory actions of curcumin and boswellic acids, J *Ethnopharmacol*, 38 (1993) 113.
15. Singh G B & Atal C K, Pharmacology of an extract of salai guggal, *Boswellia serrata, a* new non-steroidal anti inflammatory agent, *Agents Action*, 18 (1986) 407.

16. Rioja I, Terencio C, Ubeda A, Molina P & Alcaraz M J, A pyrroloquinazoline derivative with anti-inflammatory and analgesic activity by dual inhibition of cyclooxygenase-2 and 5-lipoxygenase, *Euro J Pharmacol,* 434 (2002) 177.

—•—

Paper Published In:
I.J.E.B. (Vol. 44, February 2006, pp.128-132)

23

Role of cyclooxygenase-2 in lipopolysaccharide-induced hyperalgesia in formalin test

SATYANARAYANA S.V. PADI AND S.K. KULKARNI
Pharmacology Division, University Institute of Pharmaceutical Sciences,
Panjab University, Chandigarh 160014, India

Lipopolysaccharide (LPS)-induced hyperalgesia and the role of cyclooxygenase (COX) isoforms in acute and chronic nociceptive assays have been well established. However, the role of COX isoforms in LPS-induced hyperalgesia in the formalin test is not clear. Thus, the present study was undertaken to characterize the time course of formalin-induced nociceptive response in LPS-pretreated mice and to investigate possible effects of COX inhibitors to address the potential role of COX isoforms in LPS-induced hyperalgesia in the formalin test. All the animals showed typical biphasic response to formalin challenge. At 0 hr (immediately) and 4 hr after LPS pretreatment, animals did not show any alteration in formalin-induced tonic pain. However, 12 and 16 hr after LPS pretreatment, there was a significant increase in the late phase of formalin-induced nocifensive response as compared to control mice. Treatment with intravenously administered ketorolac (a nonselective COX inhibitor) significantly and dose-dependently inhibited the late phase of formalin-induced nociceptive behaviour in saline and LPS-pretreated mice. In contrast, parecoxib (prodrug of valdecoxib, a selective COX-2 inhibitor) or dexamethasone (COX-2 transcription inhibitor), when administered intravenously or intraperitoneally, respectively, did not show antinociceptive effect in the formalin test in saline-pretreated mice. However, both the agents significantly and dose-dependently decreased the late phase nociceptive behaviour of the formalin test in LPS-pretreated mice to the level of the animals that received saline pretreatment. These results suggest that induction of COX-2 by proinflammatory mediators and subsequent release of prostaglandins could be responsible for LPS enhancement of formalin-induced nocifensive behaviour and supports an important role of COX-2 in LPS-induced hyperalgesia in the formalin test.

Keywords: Cyclooxygenase isoforms, Formalin test, Hyperalgesia, Lipopolysaccharide.

Peripheral tissue injury or inflammation causes exaggerated pain behaviour that includes hyperalgesia, an increased responsiveness to noxious stimuli. Prostaglandins (PGs) specifically in the spinal cord, have long been thought to play a key role in inflammatory process, sensitisation of nociceptors, generation of pain and nociceptive processing[1,2]. Nonsteroidal anti-inflammatory drugs (NSAIDs) act by inhibiting cyclooxygenase (COX), which is the rate limiting enzyme, that catalyses conversion of arachidonic acid to generate PGs. There are two isoforms of COX, namely COX-1 and COX-2. COX-1 is constitutively expressed in most cells for housekeeping functions, while COX-2 is present in low levels in physiological conditions, but is rapidly induced by cytokines, growth factors and inflammatory stimuli[2,3]. Recently, COX-3 has been identified but its physiological and pathological roles are yet to be characterized[4].

Lipopolysaccharide (LPS), also known as endotoxin, a major constituent of the outer membrane of the cell wall of gram-negative bacteria, is reported to produce number of pathophysiological changes in the organism[5,6]. It is also known to release proinflammatory cytokines such as interleukin-1 (IL-1), IL-6, and tumour necrosis factor-alpha (TNF-α) by activated monocytes and macrophages[5-7]. In addition to proinflammatory cytokines, the subsequent release of nitric oxide (NO) and prostaglandins (PGs) has been found to induce long-lasting hyperalgesia after central, systemic and local administration of LPS[8-11]. Recently, many studies have been performed using various classes of pharmacological agents including COX inhibitors to characterize and delineate possible underlying mechanisms involved in LPS-induced hyperalgesia in various nociceptive assays[10,12-15].

It is generally agreed that the formalin test reproduces various aspects of acute inflammatory pain analogous to human postoperative pain. Further, the pain intensity in this nociceptive assay is a reproducible and quantifiable behavioural response and has been used for the evaluation of the analgesic activity of various pharmacological agents[16,17]. The diluted formalin when injected into hind paw of mice and rats shows characteristic biphasic licking and biting behaviours to continuous (tonic) noxious stimuli and this complex nociceptive patterns last for approximately 60 min. The first or acute phase lasts for about 5 min which is followed by a longer-lasting, more persistent phase (about 40 min) that is characterized by shaking or licking and biting behaviours of the paw[17]. It is generally agreed that the first phase results at least in part from direct activation of primary afferent fibres, both low-threshold mechanoreceptive and nociceptive types, whereas the second phase reflects a facilitated state of central sensitisation driven by the persistent primary afferent inputs and this ongoing activity releases excitatory amino acids and neuropeptides that are necessary for the development of the second phase[1,18].

The role of COX isoforms and the effects both peripherally and centrally administered COX inhibitors in formalin-induced nocifensive behaviour have been well established[1,19,20]. Despite extensive studies reported on LPS-induced hyperalgesia, the role of COX isoforms in LPS-induced hyperalgesia in the formalin test is not known. Thus, the present study has been carried out to examine time course and characteristics of LPS-induced hyperalgesia in the formalin test and to investigate the effects of COX inhibitors to address the role of COX isoforms on LPS enhanced formalin-induced nocifensive behaviour in animals.

Materials and Methods

Materials: Parecoxib sodium (Panacea Biotec Ltd., India) and ketorolac tromethamine (Ketanov® 15 mg/ml) intravenous injection (Ranbaxy Ltd., India), dexamethasone (Unichem Labs, India), lipopolysaccharide from *Salmonella typhimurium* (Sigma, USA), and formalin (37% formaldehyde) (SD Fine Chemicals, India) were used in this study. Parecoxib sodium, 2% formalin and lipopolysaccharide were freshly prepared by dissolving in normal saline to suitable concentration. All the drugs were administered in a dose volume of 1 ml/100 g body weight of mice.

Experimental animals: Albino Swiss mice (20-25 g) of either sex (bred in Central Animal House of Panacea Biotec Ltd., Punjab) were housed under standard conditions of light and dark cycle with food and water *ad libitum*. The protocol was approved by the Institutional Animal Ethics Committee of Panjab University, Chandigarh and carried out in accordance with the guidelines of the Indian National Science Academy. Newly acquired mice were acclimatised-to laboratory conditions 2 hr before being used in the experiment. Each animal was used for a single treatment and sacrificed by euthanasia after experimentation. Each group consisted of six animals.

Fommalin-induced tonic pain: The mouse paw formalin test was carried out according to a previous report[21]. Briefly, mice were injected with 20 ml of 2% formalin solution in normal saline subcutaneously into the plantar surface of the left paw with a 26-guage needle fitted to a microsyringe. Pain response was quantified by counting the time spent in licking and biting of the injected paw for 5 min periods from 0-45 min. Two phases of spontaneous licking was observed after formalin injection. The interval from 0-10 min was defined as early phase and the interval 10-45 min as late phase, respectively.

Experimental design: LPS dissolved in normal saline and injected 50 mg/0.1 ml/mouse was administered intraperitoneally at different time intervals. Control animals received normal saline 0.1 ml/mouse. The LPS pretreated and control animals were subjected to formalin-induced tonic pain at 0 hr (immediately), 4, 12, or 16 hr after LPS administration. Ketorolac (nonselective COX inhibitor) or parecoxib (selective COX-2 inhibitor) (1, 5 or 10 mg/kg) was administered intravenously 30 min before assessing formalin-induced tonic pain in saline or LPS-pretreated mice. A single injection of dexamethasone (0.5 mg/kg) was administered intraperitoneally 2 hr before saline or LPS pretreatment to mice and another injection of dexamethasone (0.5 mg/kg, ip) was administered 2 hr before formalin challenge. Saline pretreated and LPS pretreated control animals also received equivalent volume of normal saline intravenously 30 min before formalin challenge. In all these animals, formalin-induced nociceptive responses were observed 12 hr after saline or LPS pretreatment.

Statistical analysis: All the values were expressed as mean ±SE. The mean sum of licking and biting behaviour between two groups was analysed by unpaired Student's t-test. The mean sum of licking and biting behaviour in both early and late phases of the formalin test was analysed by one-way analysis of variance with Dunnett's t-test for multiple comparisons between different groups. A value of $P < 0.05$ was considered as statistically significant.

Results

Effect of lipopolysaccharide pre-treatment on the formalin-induced nociception in mice: All the mice subcutaneously challenged with formalin into hind paw showed characteristic biphasic response with an early and a late phase (Fig. 1). A preliminary study was performed to assess any gross difference in formalin-induced nociceptive behaviours of the LPS-injected mice compared to saline injected mice immediately after the treatment (0 hr). No significant difference between time course of formalin-induced nociceptive response was observed in various control groups of animals tested at various time intervals after saline injection i.e., at 0, 4, 12, and 16 hr, respectively indicating consistency and reproducibility of the measurements among groups (Fig. 1). LPS pretreatment at 0 hr (immediately) and for 4 hr did not show any significant difference in the sum of licking and biting behaviour responses in both early (Fig. 2A) and late phases (Fig. 2B) of the formalin challenge as compared to control mice that received saline pretreatment. In contrast, LPS pretreatment for 12 and 16 hr markedly increased the mean licking and biting responses during the time course of the formalin test resulting in a state of tonic hyperalgesia (Fig. 1B). A significant enhancement of formalin-induced nociceptive response as compared to saline pretreatment group was observed during the late phase (10-45 min) but not in the early phase (0-10 min) in mice with LPS pretreatment for 12 hr or more (Fig. 2). Therefore, in the subsequent experiments, formalin-induced nocifensive behaviour in saline or drug treated animals was observed 12 hr after LPS pretreatment.

Effect of cyclooxygenase inhibitors in lipopolysaccharide enhanced formalin-induced nociception in mice: Intravenous administration of ketorolac (1, 5, or 10 mg/kg) significantly and dose dependently decreased formalin-induced nociceptive behaviour as compared to saline treatment in control or LPS-pretreated mice (Fig. 3B). However, it did not alter nociceptive response in early phase of the formalin test in saline or LPS-pretreated mice (Fig. 3A). Both, parecoxib (1, 5 or 10 mg/kg, iv) and dexamethasone (0.5 mg/kg, ip) showed nociceptive responses similar to saline-treated mice following formalin injection (Figs 4 and 5). On the contrary, parecoxib significantly and dose-dependently reduced the enhanced number of licking and biting behaviour in late phase of the formalin test in LPS-pretreated mice to the level of the animals that received only saline, however it had no effect on early phase of the formalin test (Fig. 4). Pretreatment with dexamethasone before LPS pretreatment significantly inhibited the enhancement of late phase, but not early phase formalin-induced nocifensive behaviour (Fig. 5).

Discussion

In the present study, systemic administration of LPS enhanced formalin-induced licking and biting behaviours in the late phase, which

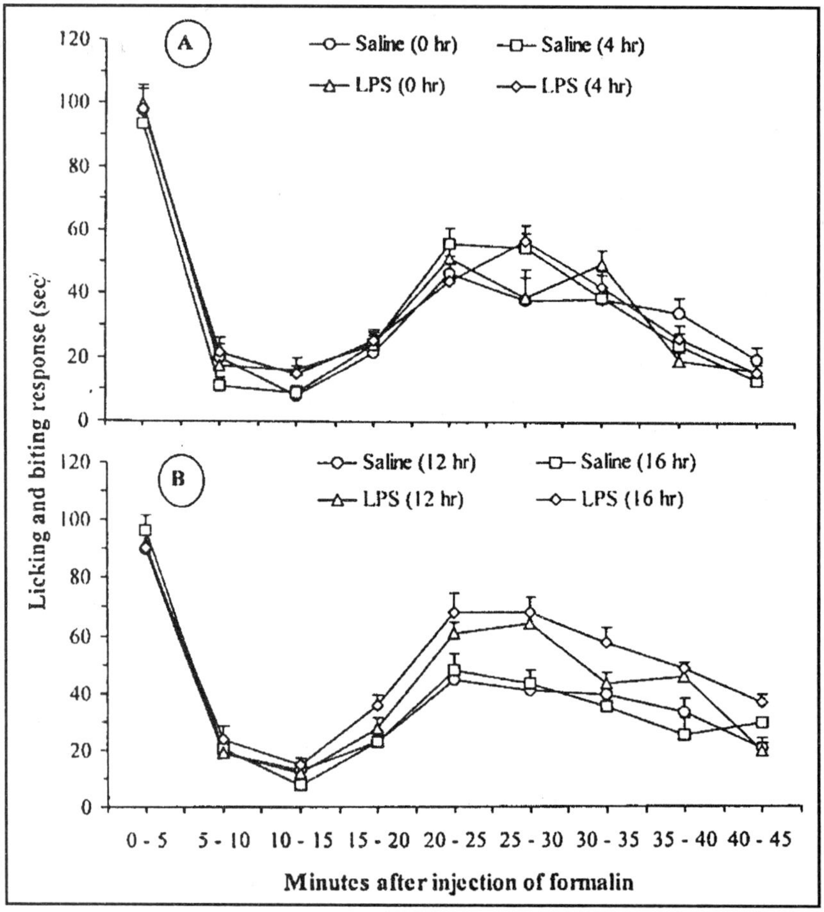

Fig. 1. Time course of formalin response in mice pretreated with lipopolysaccharide (LPS) or saline (A) 0 and 4 hr and (B) 12 and 16 hr before the nociceptive test. Points represent the mean ±S.E. of formalin-induced licking and biting responses in seconds during 5 min intervals observed for 45 min.

is indicative of hyperalgesic response. The important aspect in this study is the time course of hyperalgesia that was most evident and consistent in all the LPS-pretreated animals. Although there was no significant difference in the tonic pain behaviour at 0 hr and after 4 hr, but there was a marked and significant potentiation of nociceptive response at 12 and 16 hr after LPS pretreatment in mice challenged with formalin resulting in a state of hyperalgesia. Although dose-dependent LPS potentiation of formalin-induced tonic pain was not studied, the same concentration of LPS was employed which was previously reported to cause hyperalgesia in mice[13,22]. Indeed, the late phase represents facilitated state of central sensitisation, however, marked enhancement of nociceptive response was observed in late phase following LPS pretreatment suggesting that increased release of nociceptive mediators and/or release of certain mediators other than those normally involved in formalin nociceptive responses are specifically induced by LPS pretreatment.

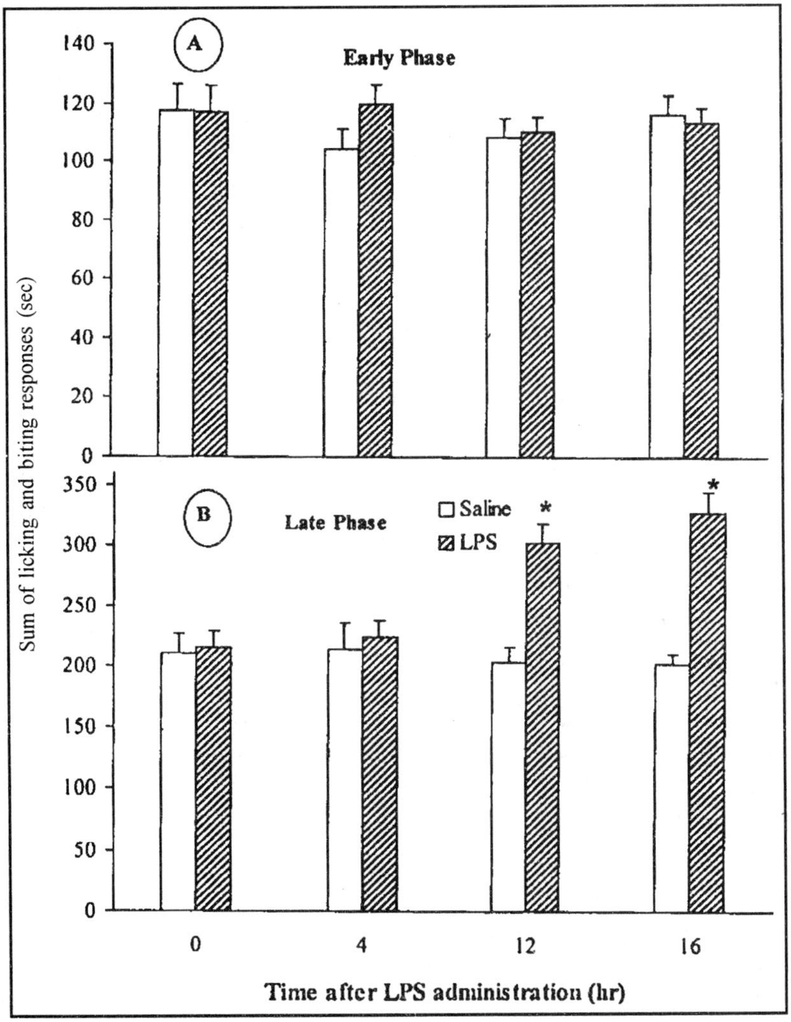

Fig. 2. Duration of nociceptive behaviour during (A) early phase (0 - 10 min) and (B) late phase (10-45 min) of the formalin test in mice pretreated with lipopolysaccharide (LPS) or saline 0, 4, 12, and 16 hr before formalin challenge. The data represent the mean ± S.E. of sum of formalin-induced licking and biting responses in seconds during the early and late phase. * P < 0.05 as compared to corresponding saline pretreated group (t-test).

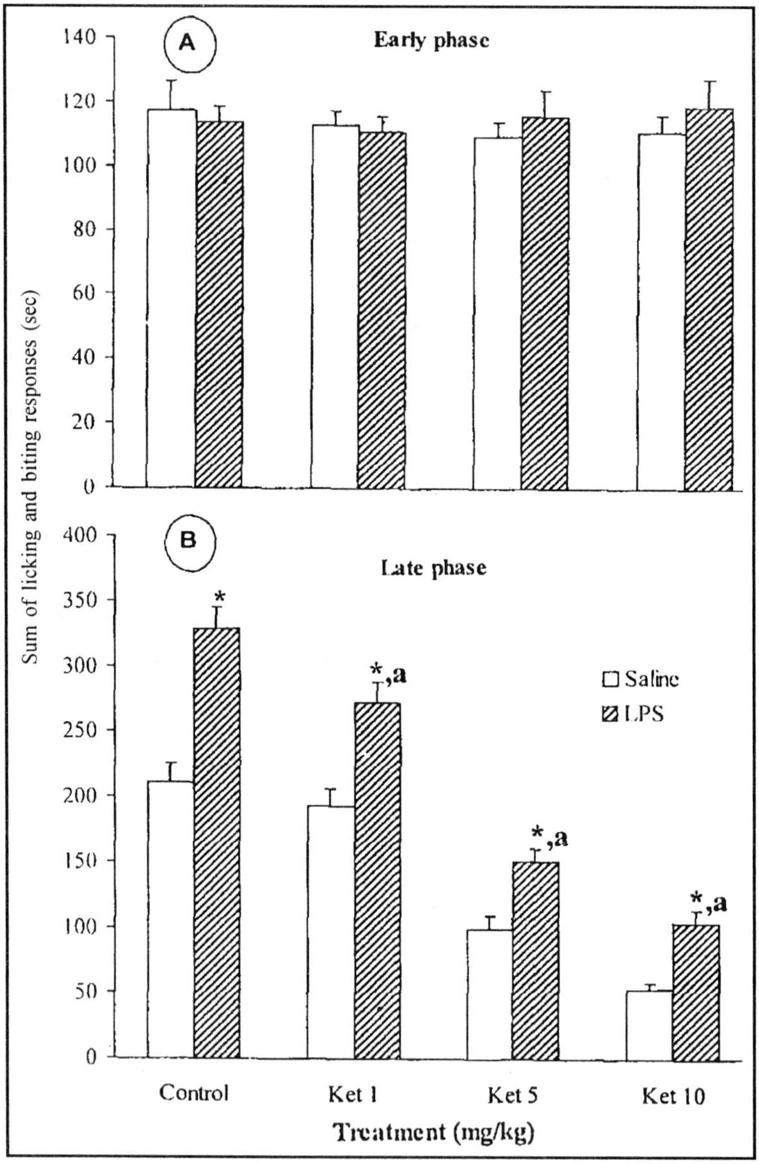

Fig. 3. Effect of ketorolac (Ket) on nociceptive behaviour during (A) early phase (0-10 min) and (B) late phase (10-45 min) of the formalin test in mice pretreated with saline or lipopolysaccharide (LPS) 12 hr before formalin challenge. Ketorolac was intravenously administered 30 min before nociceptive assay. The data represent the mean ± S.E. of sum of formalin-induced licking and biting responses in seconds during the early and late phase.* $P < 0.05$ as compared to corresponding saline pretreated group (t-test). [a] P < as compared to LPS-pretreated control animals (one way ANOVA followed by Dunnett's test).

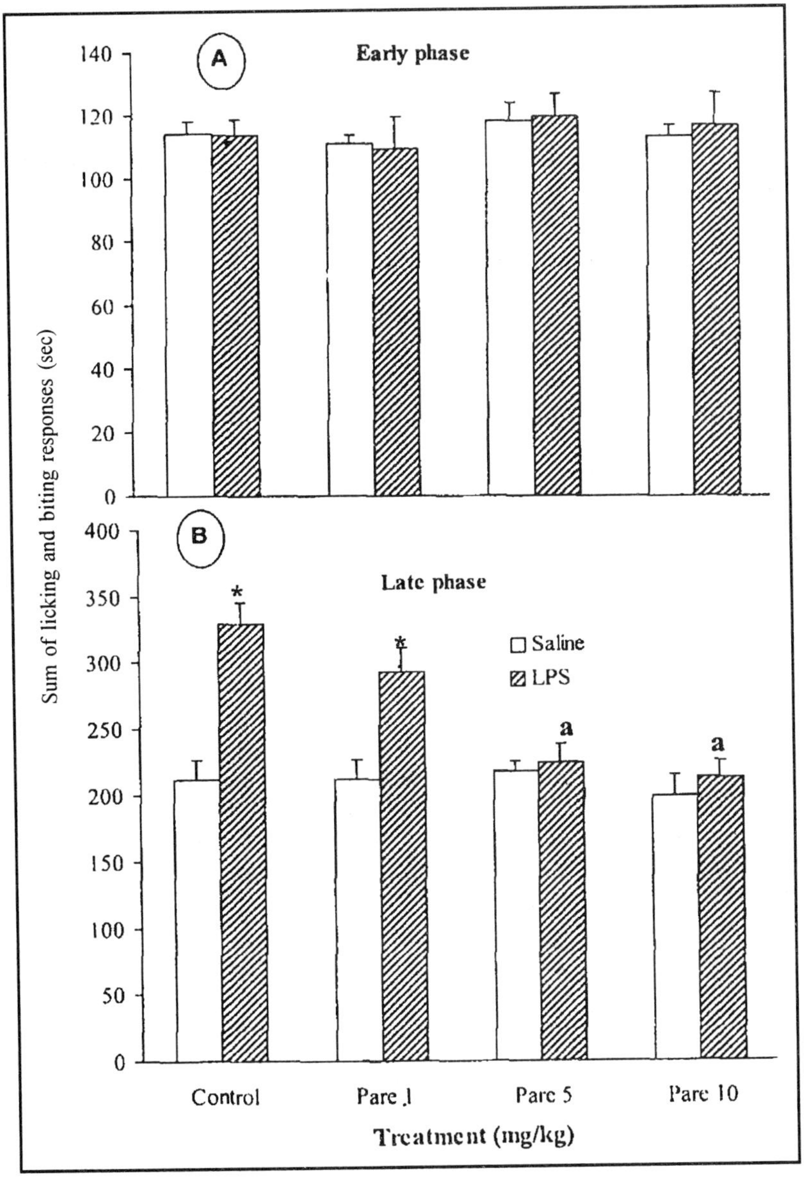

Fig. 4. Effect of parecoxib (Pare) on nociceptive behaviour during (A) early phase (0-10 min) and (B) late phase (10-45 min) of the formalin test in mice pretreated with saline or lipopolysaccharide (LPS) 12 hr before formalin challenge. Parecoxib was intravenously administered 30 min before nociceptive assay. The data represent the mean ±S.E. of sum of formalin-induced licking and biting responses in seconds during the early and late phase. * $P < 0.05$ as compared to corresponding saline pretreated group (t-test). [a] P < as compared to LPS-pretreated control animals (one way ANOVA followed by Dunnett's test).

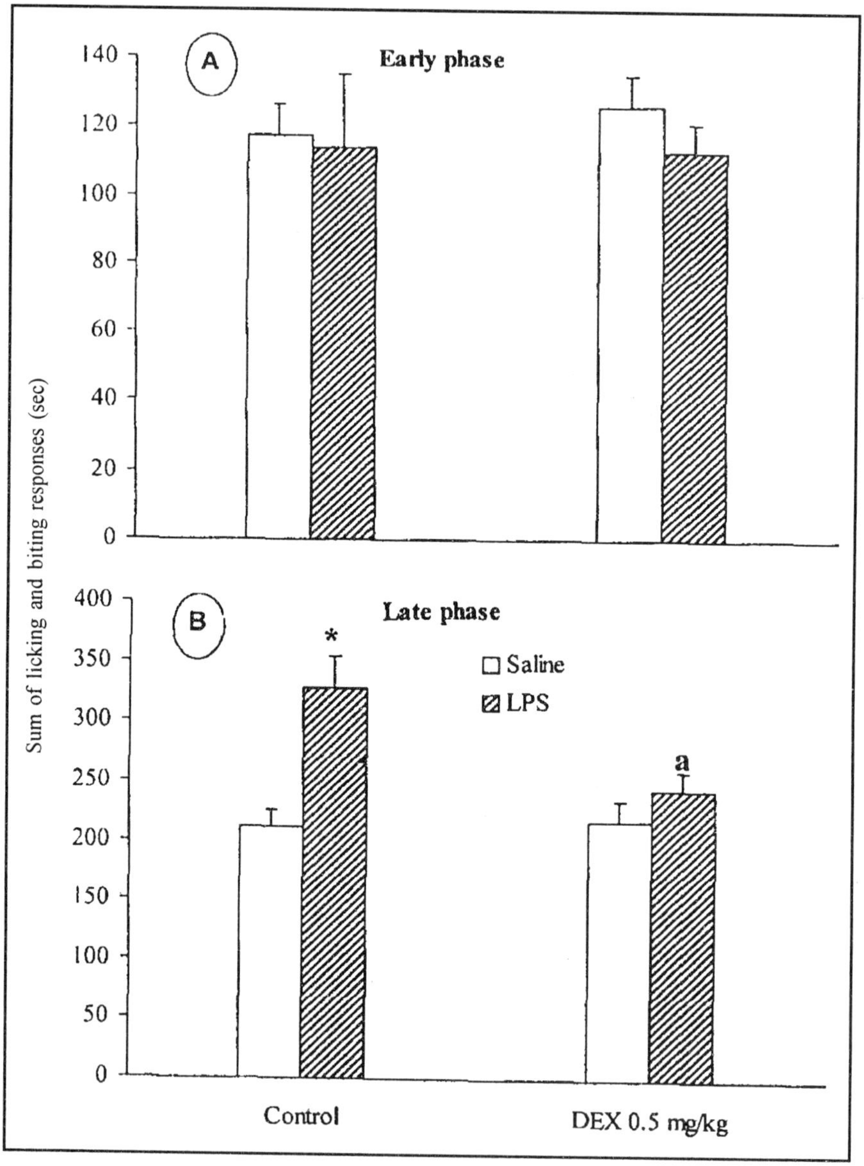

Fig. 5. Effect of dexamethasone (Dex) on nociceptive behaviour during (A) early phase (0-10 min) and (B) the late phase (10-45 min) of the formalin test in mice pretreated with saline or lipopolysaccharide (LPS) 12 hr before formalin challenge. Dexamethasone was intraperitoneally administered 2 hr before LPS pretreatment. The data represent the mean ± S.E. of sum of formalin-induced licking and biting responses in seconds during the early and late phase. * $P < 0.05$ as compared to corresponding saline pretreated group (t-test). [a]$p < 0.05$ as compared to LPS pretreated control animals (one way ANOVA followed by Dunnett's test).

Systemic administration of ketorolac, a nonselective COX inhibitor, but not parecoxib (a prodrug of valdecoxib, a selective COX-2 inhibitor) or dexamethasone (COX-2 transcription inhibitor) showed antinociceptive effect in the formalin test in saline-pretreated mice. Selective COX-1 and nonselective COX inhibitors, but not selective COX-2 inhibitors reduced formalin-induced nociceptive responses[1,19,20].

Consistent with previous reports, the results of the present study well support the role of COX-1 derived PGs for facilitation of nociceptive processing that occurs in inflammatory late phase of the formalin test. Importantly, ketorolac markedly decreased the late phase nociceptive behaviour of the formalin test in LPS-pretreated mice. Further, both parecoxib and dexamethasone also reduced LPS-induced hyperalgesia. However, both these agents reduced only the enhancement of nociceptive behaviour by LPS to the level of the animals that receive only saline treatment. These results implicate that PGs derived from COX-1 but not by COX-2 play a role in this acute nociceptive test in normal animals whereas PGs derived specifically from COX-2 may be involved in LPS potentiation of formalin-induced nociceptive responses.

In the recent past, a number of studies attempted to unravel the mechanisms underlying in LPS-induced hyperalgesia[10-13,15]. LPS, when administered intraperitoneally does not cross blood-brain barrier, however, it stimulates the expression and release of various immunological factors, cytokines such as IL-1, IL-6, and TNF-α by activated monocytes and macrophages and proinflammatory mediators in the periphery and in the central nervous system. In addition, these cytokines increase the expression of iNOS, and COX-2, and also induce the expression and release of various proinflammatory mediators including PGs and neuropeptides[10,11,14,23,24]. It is well known that LPS regulates COX isozymes expression differentially with downregulation of COX-1 and upregulation of COX-2 (refs. 25, 26). Previous studies have shown that the dramatic increase in levels of COX-2 isoform in response to proinflammatory cytokines in synovial joints, macrophages, monocytes, and spinal cord[14,27,28]. Further, various circulating factors increase the expression of COX-2 in the neuronal and nonneuronal elements besides macrophages and fibroblasts within 2 hr and subsides by 4 - 24 hr following LPS administration, but similar changes were also observed after peripheral tissue injury and inflammation[14,29-31]. In the spinal cord, LPS activates the signalling pathways such as nuclear factor kappaB (NF-kβ), AP-1,

CREB, mitogen activating protein kinase (MAPK) cascade leading to transcriptional activation of COX-2 expression in astrocytes, microglia, endothelial cells, and leptomeningeal cells[14,32].

Increased expression of COX-2 that catalyses arachidonic acid into PGH_2 and PGE synthase that produces PGE_2 from PGH_2 in skin, dorsal root ganglia, white and gray matter of spinal cord or synoviocytes was observed 4 - 24 hr after IL-1β or systemic LPS pretreatment, respectively[28,33]. The results of the present study are coherent to time course of increased expression of COX-2 where time-dependent hyperalgesia was observed 12-16 hr after LPS pretreatment. Importantly, the increased expression of COX-2 increases basal and evoked PGs release. These PGs sensitise peripheral nerve endings and facilitate central nociceptive processing in spinal cord resulting in exaggerated pain behaviour (hyperalgesia). These data indicate that the elevated COX-2 could be a major contributor to hypersensitivity after LPS administration.

In the present study, the effect of selective inhibition of COX-2 prior to LPS pre-treatment was not evaluated because marked hyperalgesia was observed 12 hr after LPS administration. Moreover, formalin-induced biting and licking for 60 min would not be sufficient for activation of COX-2 mRNA and generation of COX-2. In addition, COX-1 is present constitutively and readily releases PGs in response to tissue injury and noxious stimuli whereas COX-2 is inducible and not present constitutively in the periphery and in spinal cord where sensitisation of nociceptors and nociceptive processing occurs, respectively[2,3]. Indeed, selective COX-2 inhibitors have no role in the activation of COX-2 mRNA and generation of new enzyme. It is likely that COX-2 may not be associated with spinal prostanoid synthesis acutely or with facilitated nociception, which occurs within limited time frame of acute analgesic tests.

Although, COX-2 expression was not measured, the administration of dexamethasone, an inhibitor of COX-2 expression prior to LPS injection significantly prevented hyperalgesia in the present study. Further, clear inhibition of COX-2 expression by dexamethasone has been demonstrated in both *in vitro* and *in vivo*[10,28,34,35]. In various studies, enhancement of the late phase of formalin nociceptive responses have also been reported in rats that were already in a state of neuropathy-induced hyperalgesia due to spinal nerve ligation and diabetes[36-38]. It has also been reported that hyperalgesia in these neuropathy models is dependent on COX-2 and enhanced release of PGs in spinal cord[31,39,40]. Further, selective inhibition of COX-2 produced significant antihyperalgesic effect against chronic pain in experimental animals in which there is a marked increase in COX-2 mRNA and PGs in spinal cord[29,30]. Similarly, selective inhibition of COX-2 reversed cytokine and LPS-induced hyperalgesia in various peripheral and central nociceptive assays[8,10,13-15]. Taken together, the results provide support to the concept that the PGs released by COX-2 involve in central nociceptive processing that results in hyperalgesic behaviour in LPS-pretreated animals.

In conclusion, the above results indicate that LPS potentiated formalin-induced nociceptive response with marked hyperalgesia produced in the late phase. Further, LPS-mediated induction of COX-2 contributes to the development of inflammatory pain hypersensitivity in the formalin test.

Acknowledgement

Grant support to SSVP by M/s Panacea Biotec Ltd., Lalru, Punjab, India is appreciated.

REFERENCES

1. Malmberg A B & Yaksh T L, Antinociceptive actions of spinal non-steroidal anti-inflammatory agents on the formalin test in the rat, *J Pharmacol Exp Ther*, 263 (1992) 136.
2. Willingale H L, Gardiner N J, McLymont N, Giblet S & Grubb B D, Prostanoids synthesized by cyclooxygenase isoforms in the rat spinal cord and their contribution to the development of neuronal hyperexcitability, *Br J Pharmacol*, 122 (1997) 1593.
3. Kulkarni S K, Jain N K & Singh A, Cyclooxygenase isoenzymes and newer therapeutic potential for selective COX-2 inhibition, *Methods Find Exp Clin Pharmacol*, 22 (2000) 291.
4. Chandrasekharan N V, Dai H, Tarepu Roos K L, Evanson N K, Tomsik J, Elton T S & Simmons D L, COX-3, a cyclooxygenase-1 variant inhibited by acetaminophen and other analgesic/antipyretic drugs: Cloning, structure and expression, *Proc Natl Acad Sci USA*, 99 (2002) 13926.
5. Bluthe R M, Lestage J, Rees G, Bristow A & Dantzer R, Dual effect of central injection of recombinant rat interleukin-4 on lipopolysaccharide induced sickness behaviour in rats, *Neuropsychopharmacology*, 26 (2002) 86.
6. Kent R S, Bluthe R M, Kelly K W & Dantzer R, Sickness behaviour as a new target for drug development, *Trends Pharamcol Sci*, 13 (1992) 24.

7. Watkins L R, Wiertelak E P, Goehler L E, Smith K P, Martin D & Maier S F, Characterization of cytokine-induced hyperalgesia, *Brain Res*, 654 (1994) 15.
8. Jain N K, Patil C S, Kulkarni S K & Singh A, Modulatory role of nitric oxide and cyclooxygenase pathway in LPS-mediated hyperalgesia, *Inflammopharmacology*, 9 (2002) 373.
9. Hamilton L C & Warner T D, Interactions between inducible isoforms of nitric oxide synthase and cyclooxygenase *in vivo:* Investigations using the selective inhibitors, 1400W and celecoxib, *Br J Pharmacol*, 125 (1998) 335.
10. Matsumoto H, Naraba H, Ueno A, Fujiyoshi T, Murakami M, Kudo I & Oh-ishi S, Induction of cyclooxygenase-2 causes an enhancement of writhing response in mice, *Eur J Pharmacol*, 352 (1998) 47.
11. Safieh-Garabedian B, Kanaan S A, Haddad J J, Jaoude P A, Jabur S J & Saade N E, Involvement of interleukin-1β, nerve growth factor and prostaglandin E_2 endotoxin-induced localised inflammatory hyperalgesia, *Br J Pharmacol*, 121 (1997) 1619.
12. Anjaneyulu M & Chopra K, Reversal of lipopolysaccharide-induced thermal and behavioural hyperalgesia by quercetin, *Drug Dev Res*, 58 (2003) 248.
13. Jain N K, Patil C S, Kulkarni S K & Singh A, Rofecoxib reversal of lipopolysaccharide-mediated central and peripheral hyperalgesia, *Brain Pharmacol*, 1 (2001) 73.
14. Samad T A, Moore K A, Sapirstein A, Billet S, Allchome A, Poole S, Bonventre J V & Woolf C J, Interleukin-1-beta-mediated induction of COX-2 in the CNS contributes to inflammatory pain hypersensitivity, *Nature*, 410 (2001) 471.
15. Satyanarayana P S V, Jain N K, Singh S & Kulkarni S K, Effect of selective inhibition of cyclooxygenase-2 on lipopolysaccharide-induced hyperalgesia, *Inflammopharmacology*, 12 (2004) 57.
16. Abbott F V & Franklin K B J, Noncompetitive antagonism of morphine analgesia by diazepam in the formalin test, *Pharmacol Biochem Behav*, 24 (1986) 319.
17. Murray C W, Porreca F & Cowan A, Methodological refinement of the mouse paw formalin test, *J Pharmacol Meth*, 20 (1988) 175.
18. Abbadie C, Taylor K T, Peterson M A & Basbaum A I, Differential contribution of the two phases of the formalin test to the pattern of *c-fos* expression in the rat spinal cord: Studies with remifentanil and lidocaine, *Pain*, 69 (1997) 101.
19. Dirig D M, Konin G P, Isakson P C & Yaksh T L, Effect of spinal cyclooxygenase inhibitors in rat using the formalin test and *in vitro* prostaglandin E_2, *Eur J Pharmacol*, 331 (1997) 155.

20. Padi S S V, Jain N K, Singh S & Kulkarni S K, Pharmacological profile of parecoxib: A novel, potent injectable selective COX-2 inhibitor, *Eur J Pharmacol,* 491 (2004) 69.

21. Minami T, Nakano H, Kobayashi T, Sugimoto Y, Ushikubi F, Ichikawa A, Narumiya S & Ito S, Characterisation of EP receptor subtypes responsible for prostaglandin E_2-induced pain response by use of EP_1 and EP_3 receptor knockout mice, *Br J Pharmacol,* 133 (2001) 438.

22. Kanaan S A, Saade N E, Hadda J J, Abdelnoor A M, Atweh S F, Jabbur S J & Safeih-Grarbedian B, Endotoxin-induced local inflammation and hyperalgesia in rats and mice: A new model for inflammatory pain, *Pain,* 66 (1996) 373.

23. Eriksson C, Nobel S, Winblad B & Schultzberg M, Expression of interleukin-1a and b, and interleukin-1 receptor antagonist mRNA in the rat central nervous system after peripheral administration of lipopolysaccharides, *Cytokine,* 12 (2000) 423.

24. O'Neill L A & Lewis G P, Interleukin-1 potentiates bradykinin and TNF-alpha-induced PGE_2 release, *Eur J Pharmacol,* 166 (1989) 131.

25. Liu S F, Newton R, Evans T W & Barnes P J, Differential regulation of cyclooxygenase-1 and cyclooxygenase-2 gene by lipopolysaccharide treatment *in vivo* in the rat, *Clin Sci,* 90 (1996) 301.

26. Matsumoto H, Naraba H, Murakami M, Kudo I, Yamaki K, Ueno A & Ohshi S, Concordant induction of cyclooxygenase-2 leads to preferred production of prostaglandin E_2 to thromboxane and prostaglandin D_2, *Biochem Biophys Res Commun,* 230 (1997) 110.

27. Marziniak M & Sommer C, Upregulation of cyloxygenase-2 is dependent on tumor necrosis receptor factor 1 and 2 after chronic constriction injury, *J Neurol,* 247(III), (2000) 125.

28. Stichtenoth D O, Thoren S, Bian H, Peters-Golden M, Jakobsson P- H & Crofford L J, Microsomal prostaglandin E synthase is regulated by proinflammatory cytokines and glucocorticoids in primary rheumatoid synovial cells, *J Immmunol,* 42 (2001) 469.

29. Beiche F, Scheuerer S, Brune K, Geisslinger G & Goppelt-Struebe M, Up-regulation of cyclooxygenase-2 mRNA in the rat spinal cord following peripheral inflammation, *FEBS Lett,* 390 (1996) 165.

30. Ebersberger A, Grubb B D, Wilingale H L, Gardiner N J, Nebe J & Schaible H G, The intraspinal release of prostaglandin E_2 in a model of acute arthritis is accompanied by an up-regulation of cyclooxygenase-2 in the spinal cord, *Neuroscience,* 93 (1999) 775.

31. Ma W & Eisenach J C, Cyclooxygenase-2 in the infiltrating inflammatory cells in injured nerve is universally upregulated following various types of peripheral nerve injury, *Neuroscience,* 121 (2003) 691.

32. Hwang D, Jang B C, Yu G & Biudreau M, Expression of mitogen-inducible cyclooxygenase induced by lipopolysaccharide: mediation through by both mitogen-activated protein kinases and NF-kappaB signalling pathways in macrophages, *Biochem Pharmacol,* 54 (1997) 87.

33. Schuligoi R, Ulcar R, Peskar B A & Amann R, Effect of endotoxin treatment on the expression of cyclooxygenase-2 and prostaglandin synthase in spinal cord, dorsal root ganglia, and skin of rats, *Neuroscience,* 116 (2003) 1043.

34. Hempel S L, Monick M M & Hunninghake G W, Lipopolysaccharide induces prostaglandin synthase-2 protein and mRNA in human alveolar macrophages and blood monocytes, *J Clin Invet,* 93 (1994) 391.

35. Zhang Y, Shaffer A, Portanova J, Seibert K & Isakson P C, Inhibition of cyclooxygenase-2 rapidly reverses inflammatory hyperalgesia and prostaglandin E_2 production, J *Pharmacol Exp Ther,* 283 (1997) 1069.

36. Calcutt N A, Jorge M C, Yaksh T L & Chaplan S R, Tactile allodynia and formalin hyperalgesia in Streptozocin-diabetic rats: effects of insulin, aldose reductase inhibition and lidocaine, *Pain,* 68 (1996) 293.

37. Courteix C, Eschalier A & Lavarenne J, Streptozocin-induced diabetic rats: behavioural evidence for a model of chronic pain, *Pain,* 53 (1993) 81.

38. LaBuda CJ, Donahue R & Fuchs PN, Enhanced formalin nociceptive responses following L5 nerve ligation in the rat reveals neuropathy-induced inflammatory hyperalgesia, *Pain,* 94 (2001) 59.

39. Ma W & Eisenach J C Morphological and pharmacological evidence for the role of peripheral prostaglandins in the pathogenesis of neuropathic pain, *Eur J Neurosci,* 15 (2002) 1037.

40. Pop-Busui R, Marinescu V, Van Huysen C V, Li F, Sullivan K, Greene D A, Larkin D & Stevens M J, Dissection of metabolic, vascular, nerve conduction interrelationships in experimental diabetic neuropathy by cyclooxygenase inhibition and acetyl-l-carnitine administration, *Diabetes,* 51 (2002) 2619.

Paper Published In:
I.J.E.B. (Vol. 43, January 2005, pp.53-60)

24

Effect of licofelone against NSAIDs-induced gastrointestinal ulceration and inflammation

VIJAY PAL SINGH, CHANDRASHEKHAR S PATIL AND S.K. KULKARNI

Pharmacology Division, University Institute of Pharmaceutical Sciences, Panjab University, Chandigarh 160 014, India

The present study was aimed to evaluate the effect of licofelone, a dual inhibitor of cyclooxygenase1/2-5-lipoxygenase against indomethacin-induced gastric damage in rats and mice in order to assess the role of leukotrienes if any, in nonsteroidal anti-inflammatory drugs (NSAIDs)-induced gastrointestinal inflammation. Acute pretreatment with licofelone reversed the indomethacin-induced gastric ulceration, neutrophil adhesion in mesentery venules, neutrophil count in blood, lipid peroxides and vascularity in the stomachs of mice and rats. Further, chronic pretreatment of licofelone also prevented indomethacin-induced gastric morphological changes and cellular infiltration in mesentery venules. Moreover, acute administration of indomethacin elevated leukotriene B_4 levels in gastric mucosa, which was reversed by pretreatment with licofelone. The results suggest that licofelone offered gastroprotection against NSAIDs-induced gastropathy through its effect on leukotrienes and by inhibiting extravasation of neutrophils.

Keywords: Gastric ulceration, NSAIDs, Licofelone, LTB_4,LOX, Neutrophils

Gastrointestinal (GI) damage induced by nonsteroidal anti-inflammatory drugs (NSAIDs) is one of the most frequent associated adverse effects. These changes are presumably due to inhibition of cyclooxygenase (COX), the enzyme responsible for conversion of arachidonic acid (AA) to prostaglandins (PGs) that are needed to maintain the integrity of gastric mucosa[1]. However, the postulate that COX inhibition by NSAIDs diverts AA metabolism to 5-lipoxygenase (5-LOX) pathway, suggests the possible role of leukotrienes (LTs) in vascular changes and mucosal damage associated with the use of NSAIDs[2]. Thus, dual inhibitors of COX/LOX pathway, which would be gastrofriendly whilst retaining anti-inflammatoy effect, were developed.

However, role of LTs in NSAIDs-induced gastropathy is debatable. Both, supporting and opposing reports on the effect of 5-LOX inhibitor and leukotriene receptor antagonists against NSAIDs-induced gastric damage are available[3-7]. LTs cause chemotaxis, degranulation of neutrophils, increase vascular permeability and affect vascular tone[8]. Neutrophils have been implicated as mediators of the epithelial cell and microvascular dysfunction associated with several models of gastrointestinal mucosal injury including that induced by NSAIDs. The circulating activated neutrophils appeared to be important in the development of gastric erosions, and changes in vascular integrity following NSAIDs treatment[9]. Indeed, depletion of blood neutrophils or inhibition of their adherence is reported to prevent NSAID-gastropathy[10]. Also, the role of neutrophil derived oxygen free radicals in NSAIDs-induced disruption of gastric membrane integrity is documented[11].

Licofelone (ML3000), a dual inhibitor of COX/5LOX, has been reported to possess a potent antiinflammatory effect and a favorable gastrotolearbility properties[12,13]. The present study has been aimed to evaluate effect of licofelone, dual COX/LOX inhibitor against the events and on the effectors associated with NSAIDs-induced gastric damage in rats and mice.

Materials and Methods

Animals: Swiss mice (22-25 g), Wistar rats (180-200 g) (Central Animal House, Panacea Biotec Ltd., Lalru) of either sex were used. They were housed in plastic cages at room temperature (25±0.5°C) and 12:12 hr L:D cycle. Animals were given food and water ad libitum. Experiments were carried out between 0900 and 1500 hr. The experimental protocols were approved by the Institutional Animal Ethics Committee.

Drugs and regimen: Licofelone, indomethacin, and naproxen (Panacea Biotec Ltd., New Delhi, India), were obtained in house. All drugs were suspended in Tween 80 and administered orally in the dose volume of 10 ml/kg. Schematic drawings representing the drug regimen in early and late events of indomethacin-induced gastroinflammation is given in Fig 1a and b. The dose selection was based on earlier studies[9,12].

Visual gastric lesions: Gastric score was calculated by method of Chan et al [14]. After 4 hr of dosing, animals were sacrificed and stomach was excised along its greater curvature. After rinsing with normal saline, the mucosa was examined for the presence of petechiae or frank hemorrhage lesions. Petechiae were assigned a score of 1, and lesions were scored according to their length (a score of 5 for lesions with length between 1 and 3 mm; a score of 10 for lesions greater than 3 mm). The sum of total scores was used for comparison. All treatment groups were coded to prevent measurement bias.

Intravital microscopic measurement of neutrophil adhesion in the rat mesenteric venules: After 60 min of single acute/last chronic dose, the rats were anesthetized with thiopental sodium (25 mg/kg, ip) and were placed on a heated (37°C) platform used to adapt a microscope for intravital microscopy. A midline laparotomy was performed and a segment of mid-jejunum was exteriorized and placed over an optically clear saline-coated cover slip in such a way that a clear area of mesentery was within the focal area. The tissue was covered with heated (37°C) phosphate buffered saline (PBS) and saline moistened gauze was placed over the exposed intestine to prevent the tissue from dehydrating and to hold the tissue in the position. Single unbranched postcapillary venules approximately 25-35mm in diameter were used for these studies, since they are transparent enough to observe blood flow and leukocyte adhering to the endothelial wall of the vessel[15]. The preparation was allowed to stabilize for 8-10 min and mesenteric circulation was observed using an microscope (Nikon Eclipse E600). A camera (Nikon DMX 1200F) mounted on the microscope projected the image on the monitor. The area of normal blood flow and that with leukocyte adherence in mesentery was traced and photographed.

Measurement of lipid peroxides and LTB_4 in rat gastric mucosa: Animals were administered vehicle or test compounds once and killed by cervical dislocation 60 min post-treatment. The gastric mucosa was removed from each stomach and placed in a glass tissue homogenizer. Tissue homogenate was prepared in a ratio of 1g of wet tissue to 9 ml 1.15% KC1 for lipid peroxides and in methanol for LTB_4 estimation. Different group of animals were used for lipid peroxide and LTB_4 measurements. The lipid peroxides (thiobarbituric acid reactive substances; (TBARS) were measured by method of Wills[16]. For LTB_4 measurements

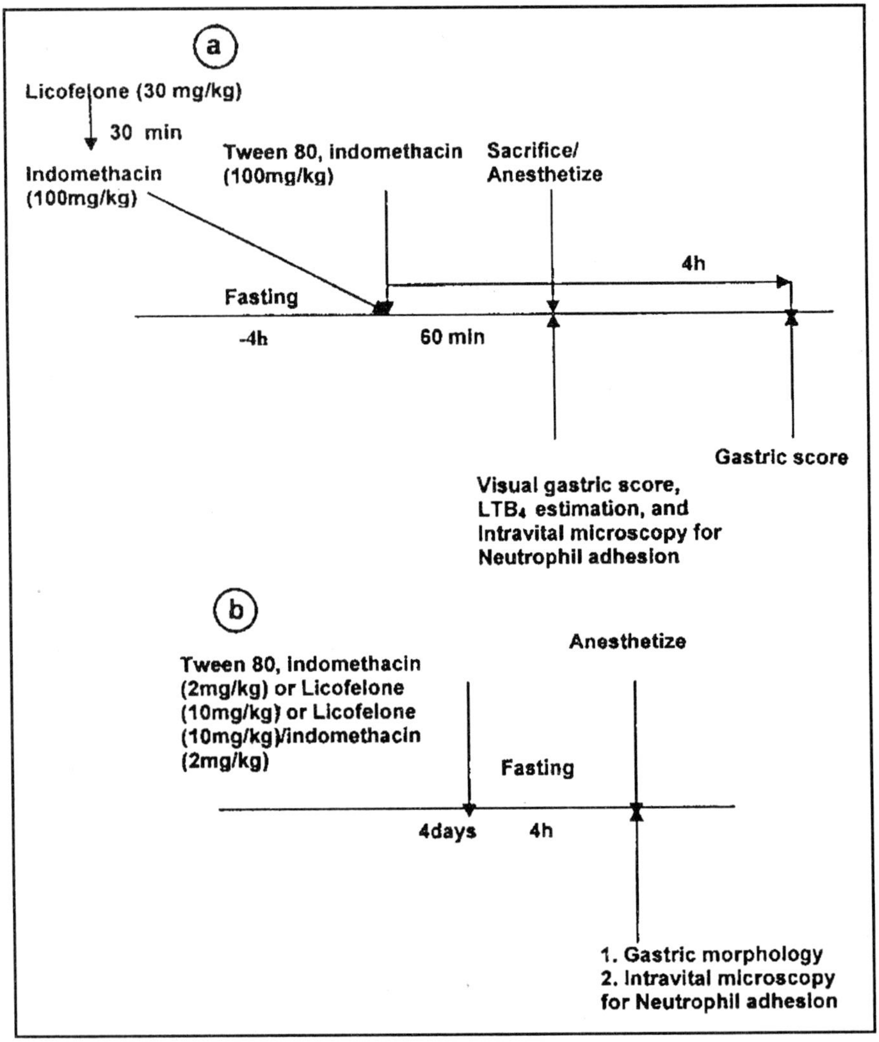

Fig. 1. Schematic drawings representing the experimental design and drug regimen to study (a) early events (b) late events associated with indomethacin-induced gastric damage.

the methanol homogenate was centrifuged (-13°C, 11,000 rpm, 20 min), and supernatant separated. The LTB_4 content was determined using LCMS/MS (API 3000: PE SCIEX, using turbo ion spray as ion source. Column C18/5cm/Novopak, mobile phase: 0.001% ammonium acetate and acetonitrile in ratio 65:35, flow rate 0.2ml/min, injection volume: 50 μl). A linearity upto 500 g concentration was observed. Neutrophil count in blood was carried out at time interval parallel to intravital microscopy. The neutrophil count in blood was determined using autocell-counter (Swelab, Sweden).

Gastric vascular permeability in mice: The effect on vascularity was assessed by the formation of vascular casts incorporating supra allura red in mouse stomach[17]. Briefly, mice were fasted for 4 hr and administered indomethacin (10 mg/kg, po) or licofelone (10 mg/kg, po)/ indomethacin (10 mg/kg, po). Indomethacin was administered 30 min after licofelone. After 30 min of indomethacin, mice were anesthetized with thiopental sodium (25 mg/kg, i.p) and peripheral vasodilation was achieved by placing in an heated jacket at 40°C for 10 min. The induction of peripheral vasodilation in the mice is important in overcoming alterations in peripheral vasomotor tone and tissue perfusion related to anesthesia and ambient temperature that may invalidate the results[18]. The cast was formed by iv injection of 1 ml of 5% supra allura red in 10% gelatin at 40°C into the warmed mice. The carcasses were chilled and the stomach isolated. The tissue was oven dried at 56°C for 48 hr and weighed. To overcome dye bleaching by the digestion of tissue in sodium hydroxide, the dried tissue was instead papain digested for 24 hr at 56°C in 0.9ml of digestive buffer (dithiothreitol 2 mM, disodium hydrogen orthophosphate 20 mM, EDTA 1 mM, papain 12 U/ml) according to method of Farndale et al[19]. The dye was then dissolved by the addition of 0.1 ml of 5M sodium hydroxide, and the digest were centrifuged at 2000 g for 10 min and filtered through a 0.45 mm nitrocellulose filter. The dye content of the filtered samples was spectrophotometrically determined at 504 nm. The result was expressed as either mg of dye content per sample or vascularity (V.I) as mg dye/mg dry weight of tissue.

Statistical analysis: Data presented as mean ± SE was analyzed using one-way ANOVA followed by post hoc Dunnett's test. $P<0.05$ was accepted as the level of significant difference compared to time matched controls.

Results

Effect of chronic administration of indomethacin, and its modification by licofelone of gross morphology of stomach and neutrophil adhesion in the rat mesenteric venules: Chronic administration of indomethacin (2 mg/kg, po) for 4 consecutive days was associated with mortality (40%) and intestinal perforations (100%) in surviving rats. Licofelone (10 mg/kg, po) administered daily 30 min prior to indomethacin prevented any death and completely inhibited the intestinal perforation. In earlier studies, licofelone (10mg/kg, po) per se is reported to be free from any gastric side effects in rats[20]. Further, rats chronically treated with indomethacin showed a marked cellular infiltration within the mesenteric venules (Fig 2).

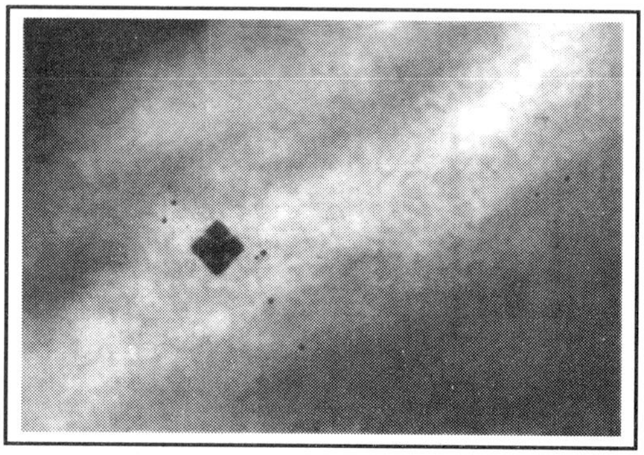

Fig. 2. Intravital microscope photography of rat mesenteric venules (40x) taken after 4 days treatment with indomethacin (2 mg/kg). (cellular infiltration).

Intravital microscopic evaluation of effects of COX, or dual COX 1/5-LOX inhibitor on the neutrophil adhesion in the rat mesenteric venules: Single oral administration of indomethacin (100mg/kg), produced significant number of gastric lesions at 4hr after dosing. In comparison, 30 min prior administration of licofelone (30 mg/kg, po) was able to significantly reduce the indomethacin-induced gastric lesion score (Fig3).

In another group, 1 hr after oral administration of indomethacin (100 mg/kg, po) neutrophil adherence to mesentery venules was microscopically recorded. Indomethacin induced a significant adherence of neutrophils when compared to the control group (Fig 4a and b). To study the effect of dual COX and LOX inhibition, on indomethacin-induced neutrophil adhesion, rats were pretreated with licofelone (30 mg/kg, po). Licofelone pretreated animals showed response similar to that of control group (Fig 4c). Licofelone per se did not induce any neutrophil adhesion administered upto 100 mg/kg, po. Pretreatment with another NSAID, naproxen (100 mg/kg, po) also did not produce any significant increase in adhesion when compared with indomethacin treatment alone (data not shown).

Pretreatment with licofelone (30 mg/kg, po) also significantly inhibited the indomethacin-induced increase in blood neutrophil count ($1.45 \pm 0.72 \times 10^3/\mu l$ vs. $4.72 \pm 0.98 \times 10^3/\mu l$ in indomethacin group)

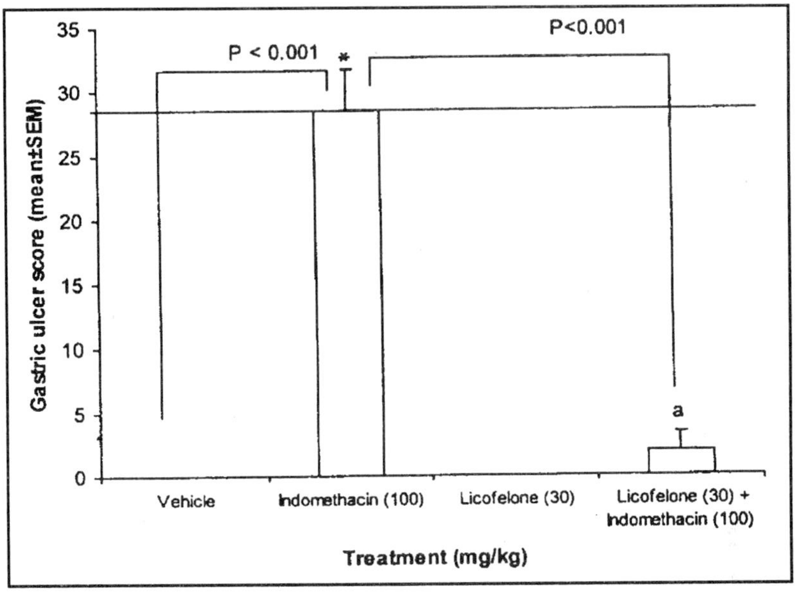

Fig. 3. Mean gastric lesion scores in rats following acute administration of indomethacin, licofelone or pretreatment with licofelone. P<0.001* as compared to vehicle control; [a]as compared to indomethacin *per se* treatment. Vertical lines represent mean ± SE (n=5-6).

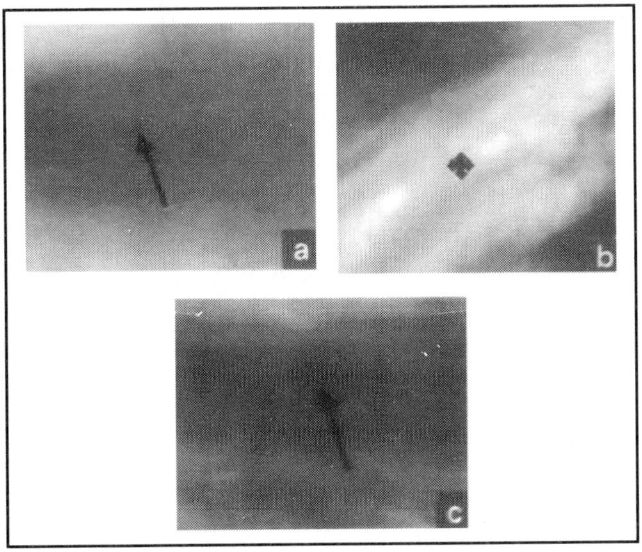

Fig. 4. Intravital microscope photography of rat mesenteric venules (40x) taken after 60 min treatment with a) vehicle, b) indomethacin (100 mg/kg), and c) licofelone(30)/indomethacin (100). [Straight arrow: ® clear blood flow through mesenteric venule; (accumulated neutrophils seen as white debris)].

Effect of orally administered indomethacin, or licofelone on LTB_4 concentration and lipid peroxide in gastric mucosa: LTB_4 levels were elevated after indomethacin (100 mg/kg, po) administration, but not in licofelone (30 mg/kg, po) or licofelone pretreated group (Table 1).

Table 1. Effect of indomethacin, licofelone and licofelone/indomethacin on gastric LTB_4 levels [Values are mean ± SE]

Treatment (mg/kg)	LTB_4 ng/g tissue
Vehicle	25.9 ± 3.0
Indomethacin (100)	40.2 ± 2.1*
Licofelone (30)	23.2 ± 4.1
Licofelone (30)/Indomethacin (100)	28 .0 ± 4.21[a]

P values: <0.05* as compared to vehicle control; [a]as compared to indomethacin

The level of thiobarbituric acid reactive substances (TBARS, index of lipid peroxidation) of gastric mucosa was 0.529 ± 0.05 nmol/mg protein in indomethacin group vs. 0.303 ± 0.03 nmol/mg protein in control group. Licofelone per se did not alter the TBARS level (0.295 ± 0.04 nmol/mg protein). Pretreatment with licofelone significantly reduced the generation of TBARS (0.319 ± 0.02 nmol/mg protein vs. 0.529 ± 0.05 nmol/mg protein in indomethacin group) (Figs 5,6).

Effect of licofelone pretreatment against indomethacin-induced vascular permeability: The vascularity (VI) of stomach derived from supra allura red administered with 10% gelatin (iv), was assessed after acute administration of indomethacin (10 mg/kg, po), and pretreatment with licofelone (10 mg/kg, po). Indomethacin resulted in significant ($P<0.05$) increase in VI when treated to control animals which was significantly reversed by pretreatment with licofelone. Licofelone per se did not affect the VI of mice stomach (Table 2).

Discussion

In the present study pretreatment with licofelone reversed the indomethacin-induced morphological changes, gastric ulceration, neutrophil adhesion in mesentery venules. Prior administration of licofelone also caused a significant reduction of blood neutrophil count, and lipid peroxides in rats. In addition, a reduction in mice stomach vascularity was observed.

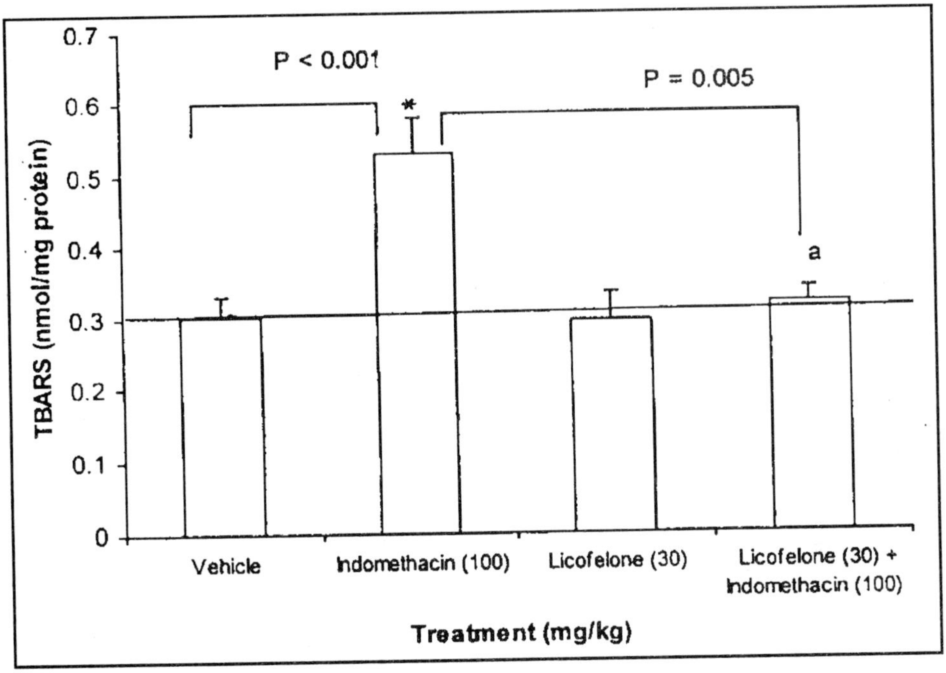

Fig. 5. Effect of different treatments on thiobarbituric acid reactive substances (TBARS) in rat gastric mucosa. P<0.001* as compared to vehicle control; P=0.005 [a]as compared to indomethacin *per se* treatment. Vertical lines represent mean ± SE (n=5-6).

Table 2. The effect of indomethacin, and pretreatment with licofelone on the tissue vascularity derived from supra allura red dye in mice gastric mucosa [Values are mean ± SE]

Treatment (mg/kg)	Concentration of dye (µg)	Vascularity index (V.I) Amount of dye (µg/mg tissue)
Vehicle	0.975 ± 0.08	0.0285 ± 0.003
Indomethacin (10)	4.56 ± 0.23*	0.071 ± 0.003*
Licofelone (10)	1.20 ± 0.05	0.030 ± 0.005
Licofelone (10)/Indomethacin (10)	2.8 ± 0.49[a]	0.037 ± 0.004[a]

P values : <0.05* as compared to vehicle control; [a]as compared to indomethacin

Further, indomethacin treatment caused an elevation in LTB_4 levels in gastric mucosa, which was prevented with licofelone pretreatment. It is suggested that inhibition of COX enzyme by NSAIDs leads to increased flux of AA through lipoxygenase pathway with a concomitant increase in LTs (LTB_4, and peptidoleukotrienes: LTC_4) production[1]. LTB_4, a very potent chemotaxin can promote leukocyte recruitment by upregulating expression of β2 integrins on these cells[21].

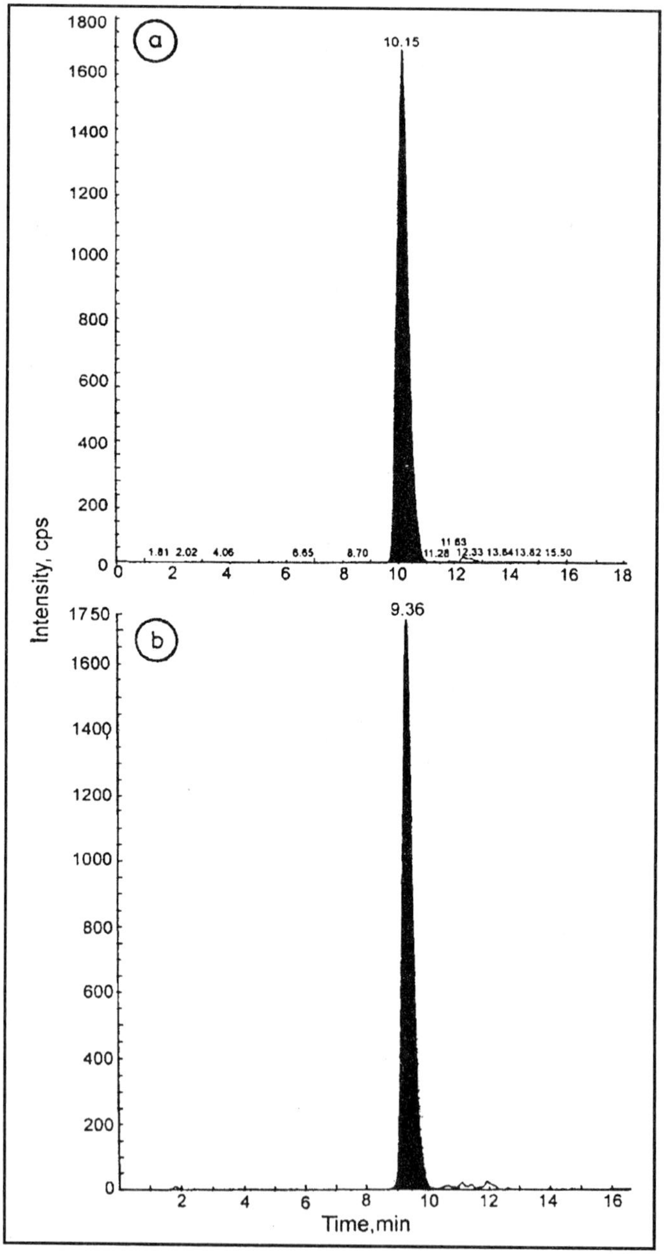

Fig. 6. LCMS/MS chromatogram of (a) leukotriene B_4 (RT 10.15 min, Mass selection 337.5 to 249.5) (b), leukotriene internal standard (RT 9.36 min, Mass selection 411.1 to 380.1).

Licofelone, a dual inhibitor is reported to suppress *in vitro* both 5-LOX (IC50 = 0.18μM) and COX (IC50 = 0.21 μM) activity [12], reduce LTB_4 levels in rat paw[22] and did not increase the gastric mucosal damage in aspirin treated rats[23]. In the present study licofelone also attenuated indomethacin-induced increased gastric vascularity in mice. Licofelone is reported to inhibit LTC_4 formation in polymorphonuclear cells (IC50 = 3.8 μM)[24]. Peptido-leukotrienes are known to increase the permeability of the vascular endothelium and increase P-selectin expression on these cells thereby promoting the rolling of leukocytes[21]. This indicated that licofelone conferred gastroprotection by inhibiting the indomethacin-induced increase in 5-LOX effectors. Since neutrophils are the major source of LTB_4[21] and extravasated neutrophils are implicated in the pathogenesis of gastric damage-induced by NSAIDs[9], effect of licofelone on neutrophils was also studied.

The effect on neutrophils was observed parallel to the effect on LTB_4 levels. Indomethacin caused significant neutrophil accumulation in postcapillary mesenteric venules, and increased neutrophil count in blood, which was completely inhibited following pretreatment with licofelone. Neutrophils by several possible mechanism contribute to NSAID-induced gastric ulceration. Neutrophils generated free radicals significantly contribute by a (i) direct tissue necrotic effect[25,26] (ii) and indirectly via oxygen free radicals. These free radicals influence the inactivation of endothelium-derived relaxing factor and alters the resistance of gastric mucosa to damage[27]. Also, neutrophils can release protease and lipid mediators that contribute to gastrointestinal ulceration, changes in mucosal permeability and affect the vascular tone and permeability, respectively[28]. In the present study, licofelone while inhibiting the indomethacin-induced neutrophil adhesion also significantly reduced the corresponding increase in TBARS levels. LTB_4 can stimulate the release of reactive oxygen metabolites from neutrophils. Lipid peroxidation (TBARS) degrades polyunsaturated fatty acids of the cellular membranes with subsequent disruption of membrane integrity and its role in pathogenesis of indomethacin-induced gastric ulceration is reported[29,30]. Indeed, licofelone is shown to inhibit generation of reactive oxygen species, and release of elastase by polymorphonuclear cells[31].

Thus, the results of the present study further indicates the role of 5-LOX metabolites in NSAIDs-induced gastroinflammation and suggests that licofelone counteracted the indomethacin-induced gastropathy by a combination of its effect on LTB_4 levels, inhibition of neutrophil adherence in postcapillary mesenteric venules and through decrease in related production of free radicals that disrupts integrity of stomach mucosa.

However, the role of LTs in the pathogenesis of NSAIDs-induced GI damage is controversial. There are evidences both in support and contrary to this hypothesis. Various studies have demonstrated no inhibition while others have demonstrated the amelioration of NSAIDs-induced gastric irritant effect by selective 5-LOX inhibitor and dual inhibitors[3-7]. Inhibition of ulcerogenic events by licofelone within the dose range of its reported 5-LOX activity is suggestive of an important balance between cyclooxygenase and 5-lipoxygenase products. A marginal shift towards 5-LOX metabolite can induce diapedesis of inflammatory cells during NSAID therapy. However, as observed here and earlier by Wallace et al.[13] that licofelone per se did not change gastric leukotriene contents raises the possibilities that 5-LOX could have other likely implication viz. (i) formation of oxygenation products, and/or (ii) direct oxygenation of membrane phospholipids without participation of phospholipase during gastric injury.

Recently, Smolka et al.[32] reported that licofelone inhibits gastric H, K-ATPase enzyme and interleukin-8 secretion. This could also be an important mechanism in licofelone-persuaded amelioration of NSAIDs-induced gastropathy.

Acknowledgement

Grant support provided by Panacea Biotec Ltd., New Delhi, India to one of the authors (VPS) as Research Associate (RA) and for LCMS/MS facility is appreciated.

REFERENCES

1. Whittle B J R, Arachidonic acid metabolites and the gastrointestinal toxicity of anti-inflammatory agents, *Prostaglandins*, 21 (Suppl.) (1981) 113.
2. Rainsford K D, The effects of 5-lipoxygeanase inhibitors and leukotriene antagonists on the development of gastric lesions induced by non-steroidal antiinflammatory drugs in mice, *Agents Actions*, 21 (1987) 316.
3. Rainsford K D, Leukotrienes in the pathogenesis of NSAID induced gastric and intestinal damage, *Agents Actions*, 39 (1993) C24.
4. Konturek S J, Brzozwski T, Drozdowicz, Garlicki J & Beck G, Role of leukotrienes and platelet activating factor in acute gastric mucosal lesions in rats, *Eur J Pharmacol*, 164 (1989) 285.

5. Kirchner T, Aparicio B, Argentieri D C, Lau C Y & Ritchie D M, Effects of tepoxalin, a dual inhibitor of cyclooxygenase/5-lipoxygenase, on events associated with NSAID-induced gastric inflammation, *Prostaglandins Leukot Essent Fatty Acids,* 56 (1997) 417.

6. Rainsford K D, Mechanism of arachidonic acid ulceration from non-steroidal antiinflammatory drugs: A basis for use and development of protective agents, in: Side effects of antiinflammatory drugs, edited by KD Rainsfrord, GP Velo (Kluwer, Lancaster) 1992, 97.

7. Cho C H & Ogle C W, Potentiation of indomethacin-induced gastric ulcers in rats by nordihydroguaiaretic acid (NDGA), an inhibitor of lipoxygenase, *Asia Pacific J Pharmacol,* 2 (1987) 49.

8. Poff C D & Balazy M, Drugs that target lipoxygenases and leukotrienes as emerging therapy for asthma and cancer, *Current Drug Targets: Inflammation Allergy,* 3 (2004) 19.

9. Wallace J H, Keeman C M & Granger D N, Gastric ulceration induced by nonsteroidal antiinflammatory drugs is a neutrophil-dependent process, Am *J Physiol,* 259 (1990) G462.

10. Wallace J L & Granger D N, Pathogenesis of NSAID-gastropathy: Are neutrophils the culprit? *TIPS,* 13 (1992) 129.

11. Naito Y, Yoshikawa T, Matsuyama K, Nishimura S, Yagi N & Kondo M, Effects of free radicals on indomethacin-induced aggravation of gastric ulcers in rats, *Dig Dis Sci,* 40 (1995) 2019.

12. Ding C & Cicutttini F, Licofelone Merckle, *Drugs* 6 (2003) 803.

13. Bias P, Buchner A, Klesser B, & Laufer S, The gastrotolearbility of the LOX/COX inhibitor, licofelone is similar to placebo and superior to naproxen therapy in healthy volunteers, *Am J Gastroenterol,* 99 (2004) 611.

14. Chan C C, Boyee J, Brideau C, Ford-Hutchinson A W, Gordon R, Guay D, Hill R G, Li C S, & Manicincni J, Pharmacology of selective cyclooxygenase-2 inhibitor L745,337, a novel non-steroidal anti inflammatory agent with ulcerogenic sparing effect in rat and non human primate stomach, *J Pharmacol Exp Ther,* 271 (1995) 1531.

15. Asako H, Kubes P, Wallace J L, Gaginella T, Wolf R E & Granger D N, Indomethacin-induced leukocyte adhesion in mesenteric venules: role of lipoxygenase products, *Am J Physiol,* 259 (1992) G903.

16. Wills E D, Mechanism of lipid peroxide formation in animal tissues, *Biochem J,* 99 (1966) 667.

17. Kimura M, Amemiya K, Yamada T & Suzuki J, Quantitative method for measuring adjuvant-induced angiogenesis in insulin treated diabetic mice, *J Pharmacobiodyn,* 9 (1986) 442.

18. Orlandi C, Dunn C J & Cutshaw L G, Evaluation of angiogenesis in chronic inflammation by laser-doppler flowmetry, *Clin Sci*, 74 (1988) 119.

19. Farndale R W, Buttle D J & Barret A J, Improved quantitation and discrimination of glycosaminoglycan by use of dimethylmethylene blue, *Biochim Biophys Acta*, 883(1986) 173.

20. Wallace J L, Carter L, McKnight W, Tries S, & Laufer S, ML 3000 reduces gastric prostaglandin synthesis without causing mucosal injury, *Eur J Pharmacol*, 271 (1994) 525.

21. Wallace J L & Ma Li, Inflammatory mediators in GI defense and injury. *Exp Biol Med*, 226 (2001) 1003.

22. Tries S, Neupert W & Laufer S, ML 3000, a novel antiinflammatory compound without the potential for causing gastric damage, *Inflamm Res*, 50 (2001) S203.

23. Pelletier J M, Lajeunesse D, Reboul P & Pelletier J P, Therapeutic role of dual inhibitiors of 5-LOX and COX, selective and non-selective non-steroidal antinflammatory drugs, *Ann Rheum Dis*, 62 (2003) 501.

24. Tries S, Neupert W & Laufer S, The mechanism of action of new antiinflammatory compound ML 3000, inhibition of 5-LOX and COX1/2, *Inflamm Res*, 51 (2002) 135.

25. Parks D A, Bulkley G B, Granger D N, Hamilton S R & McCord J M, Ischemic injury in cat small intestinal : role of superoxide radicals, *Gastroenterology* 82 (1982) 9.

26. Parks D A & Granger D N, Ischemic-induced vascular changes: role of xanthine oxidase and hydroxyl radicals, *Am J Physiol*, 245 (1983) G285.

27. Gryglewski R J, Palmer M J & Moncada S, Superoxide anions are involved in the breakdown of endothelium-derived vascular relaxing factor, *Nature Lond*, 320 (1986) 454.

28. Parks D A, Granger D N, Bulkley G B, & Shah A K, Soybean trypsin inhibitor attenuates ischemic injury to the feline small intestine, *Gastroenterology*, 89 (1985) 6.

29. Mead J F, Free radical mechanisms of lipid damage and consequences for cellular memberanes, in: Free radicals in biology edited by WA Proyr: (Academic Press, New York) 1976, 51.

30. Yoshikawa T, Naito Y, Kishi A, Tomii T, Koaneko T, Linuma S, Ichikawa H, Yasuda M, Takashi S & Kondo M, Role of active oxygen, lipid peroxidation, and antioxidants in the pathogenesis of gastric mucosal injury in rats, *Gut*, 34 (1993) 732.

31. Rotondo S, Dell'Elba G, Krauze-Brzoskok, Manarini S, Martelli N, Pecce R, Evangelista V & Cerletti C, Licofelone a dual lipoxygenase-cyclooxygenase

inhibitor downregulates polymorphonuclear leukocyte and platelet function, *Eur J Pharmacol*, 453 (2002) 131.

32. Smolka A J, Goldenring J R, Gupta S & Hammond C E, Inhibition of gastric H K ATPase activity and gastric epithelial cell IL-8 secretion by pyrrolizine derivative ML3000, *BMC Gastroenterol*, 10 (2004) 4.

Paper Published In:
I.J.E.B. (Vol. 43, March 2005, pp.247-253)

25

Possible analgesic and anti-inflammatory interactions of aspartame with opioids and NSAIDs

SAMEER SHARMA, N.K. JAIN AND S.K. KULKARNI
Pharmacology Division, University Institute of Pharmaceutical Sciences,
Panjab University, Chandigarh 160 014, India

The purpose of the present study was to investigate analgesic and anti-inflammatory properties of aspartame, an artificial sweetner and its combination with various opioids and NSAIDs for a possible synergistic response. The oral administration of aspartame (2-16mg/kg, po) significantly increased the pain threshold against acetic acid-induced writhes in mice. Co-administration of aspartame (2mg/kg, po) with nimesulide (2 mg/kg, po) and naproxen (5 mg/kg, po) significantly reduced acetic acid-induced wriths as compared to effects *per se* of individual drugs. Similarly when morphine (1 mg/kg, po) or pentazocine (1 mg/kg, po) was co-administered with aspartame it reduced the number of wriths as compared to their effects *per se*. Aspartame (4,8,16 mg/kg, po) significantly decreased carrageenan-induced increase in paw volume and also reversed the hyperalgesic effects in rats in combination with nimesulide (2 mg/kg, po).The study indicated that aspartame exerted analgesic and anti-inflammatory effects on its own and have a synergistic analgesic response with conventional analgesics of opioid and non-opioid type, respectively.

Keywords: Aspartame, NSAIDs, Opioids, Synergism

Aspartame (N-L-alpha-aspartyl-L-phenylalanine-l-methyl ester), a non-caloric compound is widely used as an artificial sweetener in various food preparations and beverages. Sweetening agents have been known to have food-drug interactions, particularly with commonly used drugs like analgesics[1]. However, exact mechanism of action of sweetening agents-induced antinociception remains uncertain. Previous research suggested a connection between the intake of palatable foods and endogenous opioid peptide system. Several studies with animals also suggest that aspartame may possess antinociceptive properties. The anti-inflammatory and analgesic actions of aspartame may involve similar mechanisms of action as aspirin possibly through the interference of prostaglandin (PG) synthesis[2,3]. The co-administration of aspartame with opiates or non-steroidal antiinflammatory drugs (NSAIDs) may have clinical significance both in terms of desired and undesired consequences. In the present study, attempts have been made to study the interactions between aspartame and opioids and NSAIDs in animals for its effect on antinociception caused by these agents.

Materials and Methods

Animals: Laca mice and Wistar rats of either sex (bred in Central Animal House, Panjab University, Chandigarh), weighing 18-25 g and 150-200g, respectively were used. They were housed in plastic cages maintained at 25°±0.5°C 12/12 hour natural light/dark cycle and were given food and water *ad libitum.* All experiments were carried out between 1000 and 1700 hrs. The experimental protocols were approved by the Institutional Animal Ethics Committee.

Drugs and regimen: Aspartame, naproxen, rofecoxib, nimesulide (Panacea Biotec Ltd., New Delhi, India), pentazocin (Ranbaxy Labs Ltd., AP), morphine (Govt. Labs, Chandigarh), naloxone, carrageenan (type IV), (Sigma, USA), saccharin, and acetic acid (S.D. fine Chemicals, Biosar) were used. All the drugs used were dissolved in distilled water except nimesulide and naproxen which were suspended in 0.25% sodium CMC. Drugs were injected intraperitoneally 60 min before acetic acid injection in the writhing test. Carrageenan (type IV, 1% w/v) was injected (0.1 ml per paw) in the plantar region of the paw for anti-inflammatory test.

Writhing test (acetic acid induced writhing): Antinociceptive response was assessed by counting the number of writhes (constriction of abdomen, turning of trunk (twist) and extension of hind limbs) in mice as described by Koster *et al*[4]. Acetic acid solution (1%, 1 ml/ 100g) was used to produce writhing response in mice. Number of writhes per animal was counted during a 20 min test period, beginning 3 min after the injection of acetic acid[4].

Carrageenan-induced paw edema: Acute edema was induced in the hind right paw of rats by injecting 0. 1 ml of freshly prepared 1 %

solution of carrageenan (type IV). The left paw (non-inflamed paw) served as control for comparison (0.9%, 0.1 ml saline injected). The carrageenan was injected under the planter region of right hind paw and paw volumes were measured using plethysmometer (Ugo Basil, Italy) at 30, 60, 120, 180, 240 and 300 min after carrageenan challenge. Percent change in paw volume was calculated and expressed as amount of inflammation[5].

Antihyperalgesic activity: Acute edema was induced in the right hind paw of rats by injecting 0.1 ml of freshly prepared 1 % solution of carrageenan (type IV). The left paw served as control (non-inflamed paw) for comparison (0.9% 0.1 ml saline injected). Each paw was dipped alternatively in the water bath maintained at 47° ± 0.3°C and paw withdrawal latencies were noted at 30, 60, 120, 180, 240 and 300 min after carrageenan challenge. Three trials were recorded for each animal for calculating the mean basal paw withdrawal latencies. A reduction (time) in the paw withdrawal latency (sec) from the basal reaction time is referred to as the hyperalgesic effect[6].

Statistical analysis: Results are expressed as mean ± S.E. Data were analysed statistically using analysis of variance (ANOVA) followed by Dunnett's t-test to assess the significance. $P<0.05$ was considered as statistically significant.

Results

Effect of aspartame against acetic acid-induced writhing in mice: Oral administration of aspartame dose dependently decreased the number of wriths in acetic acid-induced writhing assay in mice (Fig. la). Saccharin (4, 8, 16 mg/kg, po) did not alter the number of wriths as compared to the control (Fig. l b). Aspartame (4 mg/kg, po) however, significantly reduced the number of wriths at 15, 30 and 60 minutes and the maximum analgesic effect was observed at 60 min (Fig. 2).

Effect of aspartame on NSAIDs-induced analgesia in acetic acid-induced writhing in mice: Nimesulide (1 and 2 mg/kg, po) and naproxen (5 mg/kg, po) significantly ($P<0.05$) reduced the number of wriths in mice as compared to the control group (Fig. 3). Naproxen also significantly ($P< 0.05$) reduced the number of wriths in mice as compared to control animals (Fig. 3). The co-administration of aspartame (2 mg/kg, po) with nimesulide (2 mg/kg) or naproxen (5 mg/kg, po) significantly ($P<0.05$) decreased the number of wriths in mice when compared to the effect *per se* of individual drugs (Fig. 3).

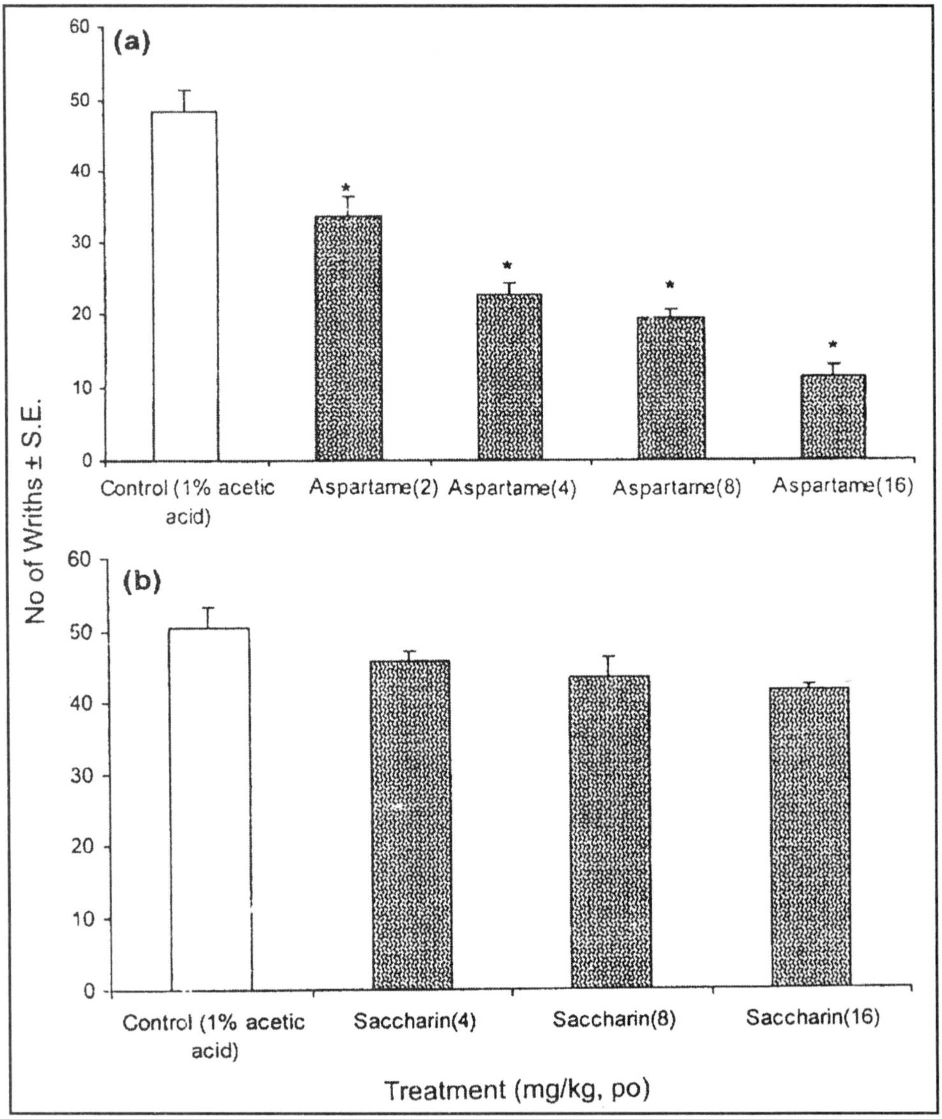

Fig. 1. Effect of (a) aspartame (2-16 mg/kg) and (b) saccharin against acetic acid-induced writhing in mice. [Vertical lines shows SEM. **P*<0.05 compared with control.]

Effect of aspartame on opioid-induced analgesia in acetic acid-induced writhing in mice: Morphine (1 mg/kg, po) significantly reduced the number of wriths as compared to control and pentazocine (1 mg/kg, po) had no significant analgesic effect in this pain assay. However, co-administration of morphine (1 mg/kg, po) or pentazocine (1 mg/kg,

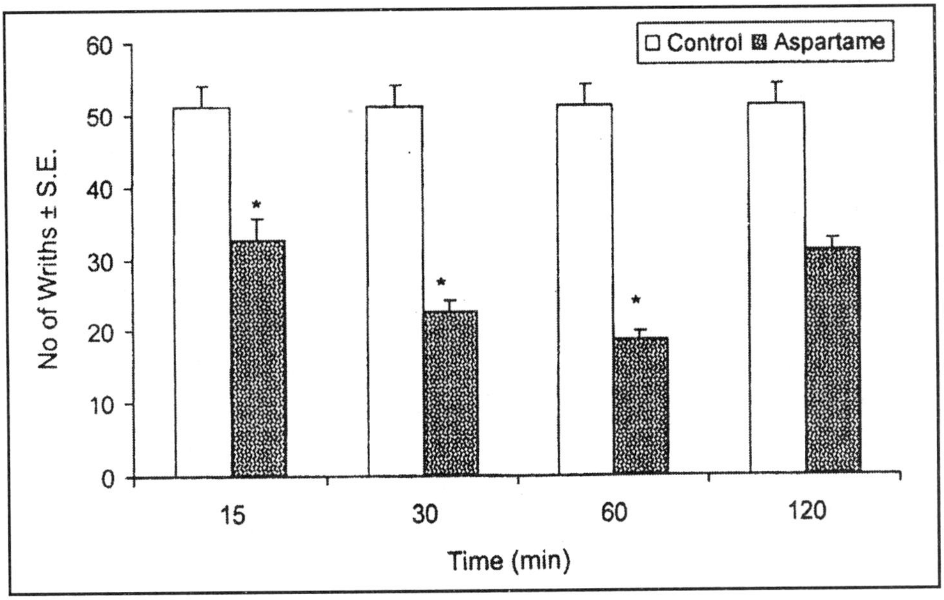

Fig. 2. Time dependent effect of aspartame (4mg/kg) against acetic acid - induced wriths in mice. [Vertical lines show SEM. **P*<0.05 compared with control]

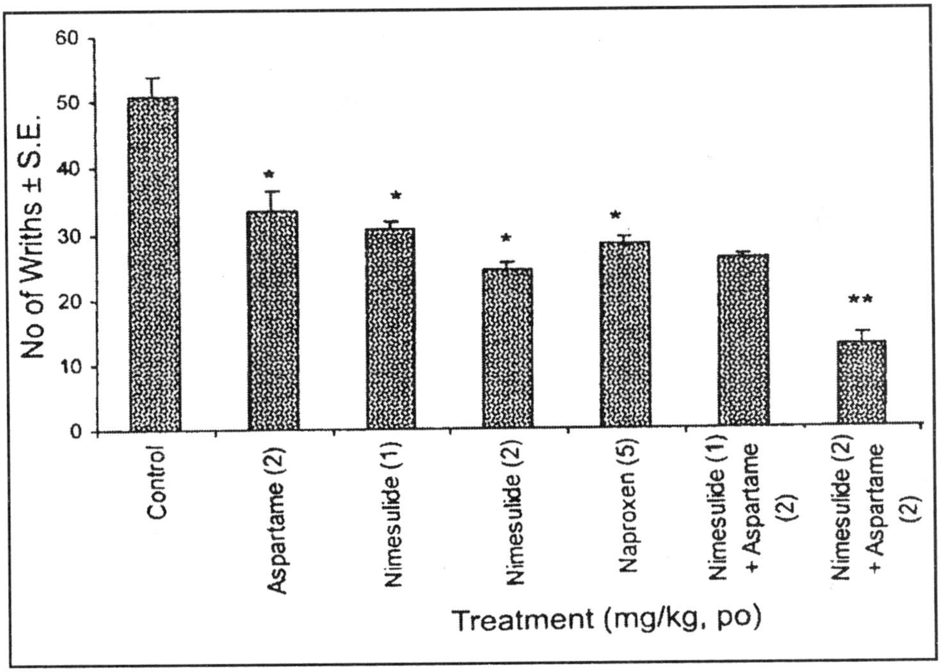

Fig. 3. Antinociceptive effects of aspartame with NSAIDs in mice. Vertical lines shows SE. **P*<0.05 as compared with control; **<0.05 compared with *per se* effects]

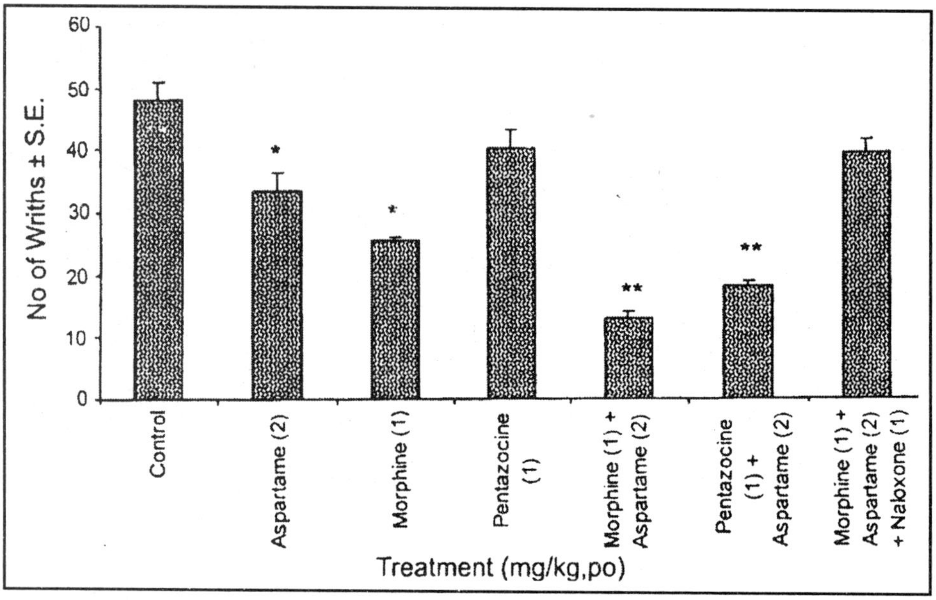

Fig. 4. Interaction of aspartame (2 mg/kg) with morphine (1 mg/kg) and pentazocine (1 mg/kg) and the reversal of antinociceptive effect by naloxone (1 mg/kg) in mice. [Vertical lines show SE. *$P<0.05$ compared with control; **<0.05 compared with *per se* effects]

po) with aspartame (2 mg/kg) significantly (P<0.05) reduced the number of wriths in mice as compared to their effects *per se* (Fig. 4). Naloxone (1 mg/kg) when coadministered with aspartame (2 mg/kg) and morphine (1 mg/kg), significantly (P<0.05) reversed the facilitatory effect of morphine but not that of aspartame (2 mg/kg) (Fig. 4). The analgesic response of aspartame (4mg/kg, po) in the wriths-test was not altered by naloxone (1 mg/kg; Fig. 5).

Effect of aspartame in carrageenan-induced paw oedema and hyperalgesia in rats: Carrageenan (1%) produced significant increase in paw edema in control group. Aspartame (4, 8 and 16 mg/kg, po) significantly (P<0.05) decreased the carrageenan-induced increase in paw volume as compared to the control rats (P<0.05) (Fig. 6). Aspartame (4 mg/kg, po) also significantly reversed the carrageenan-induced hyperalgesia in rats (Fig. 7).

Modification of aspartame-induced antiinflammatory and anti-hyperalgesic effect by opioids or NSAIDs: Both morphine (0.5 mg/kg) and nimesulide (2 mg/kg, po) failed to alter the aspartame-induced (4 mg/kg) anti-hyperalgesic effect in rats (Fig. 7). Co-administration of nimesulide (2 mg/kg, po) but not morphine significantly enhanced the antiinflammatory effect of aspartame (4 mg/kg, po) (Fig. 8).

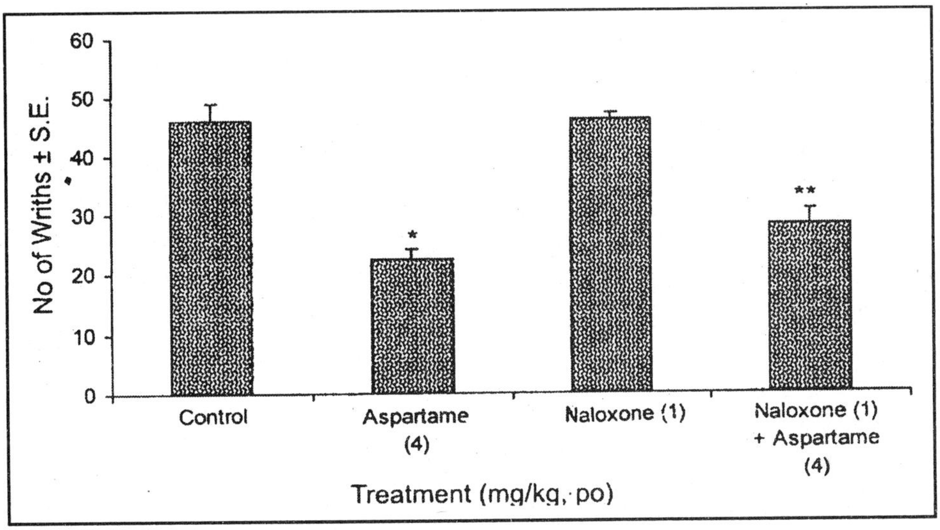

Fig. 5. Effects of naloxone (1 mg/kg) on aspartame (4 mg/kg) induced analgesia in mice. [Vertical lines show SE. *P<0.05 compared with control; **<0.05 compared with *per se* effects]

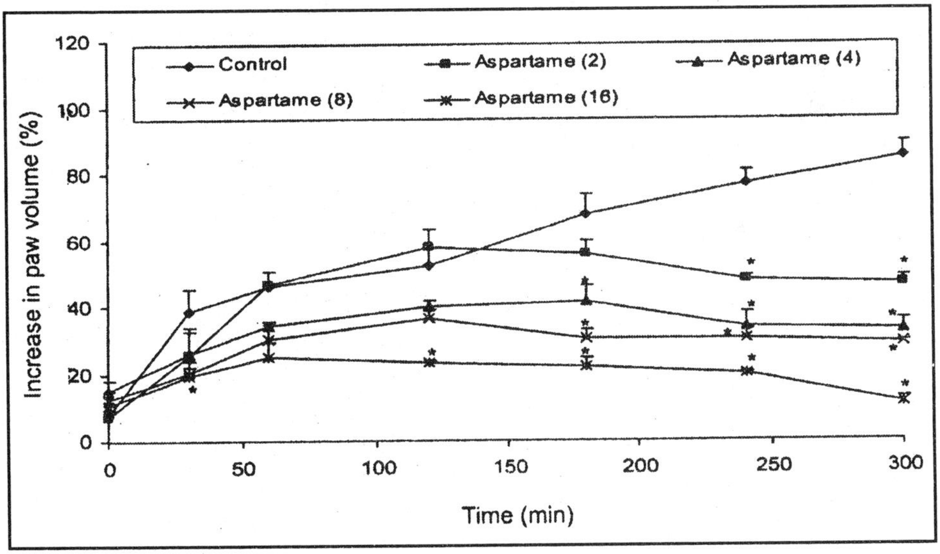

Fig. 6. Anti-inflammatory effect of aspartame (2-16 mg/kg, po) against carrageenan-induced paw edema.[Vertical lines show SE. *P<0.05 compared with control]

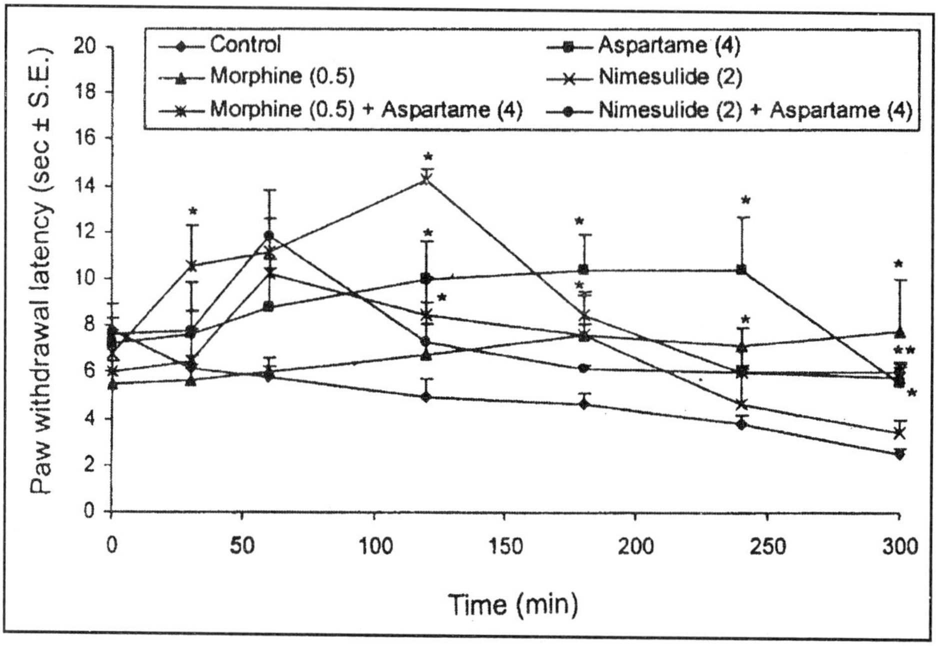

Fig.7. Anti-hyperalgesic effect of morphine and NSAIDs on aspartame. [Vertical lines show SE. **P*<0.05 compared with control, ** p<0.05 compared with aspartame]

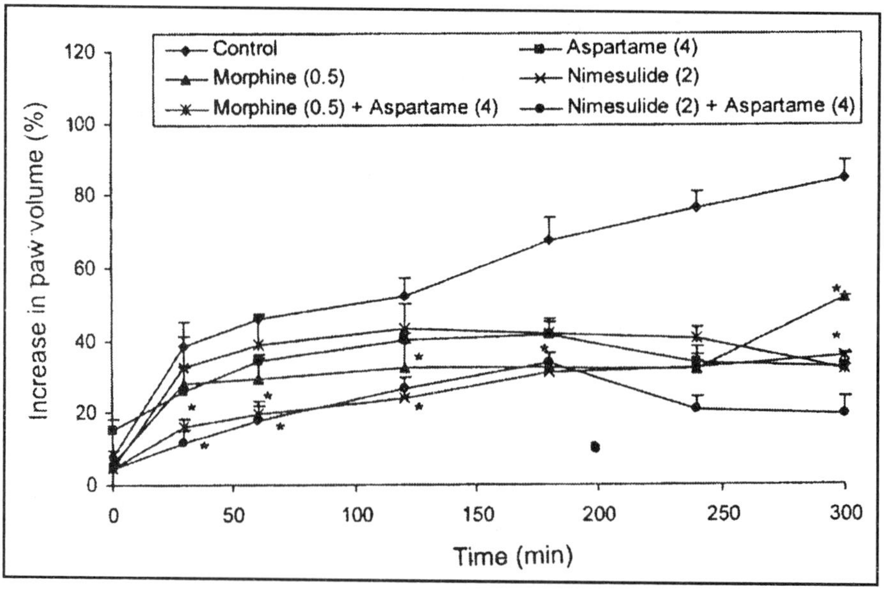

Fig. 8. Anti-inflammatory effect of morphine and NSAIDs on aspartame. [Vertical lines show SE. **P*<0.05 compared with control, ** p<0.05 compared with aspartame.]

Discussion

Aspartame is a widely known artificial sweetener and is about 160 times sweeter than sucrose in aqueous solutions. There have been reports in recent times that aspartame may possess biological response and help in maintaining homeostasis and bone mass regeneration. Aspartame is known to promote calcium deposition in bones, lowers fever in animal models and has also been found to prolong bleeding time in humans[7].

In the present study, the analgesic and antiinflammatory effects of aspartame and saccharin were investigated. Aspartame significantly and dose dependently (2-16 mg/kg) increased the pain threshold in acetic acid-induced chemonociception, whereas saccharin did not have any such property which correlates with the previous data[4-7].

Aspartame is speculated to interact with NSAIDs and endogenous opioid systems and increases levels of β-endorphin in hypothalamus[2]. The antiinflammatory and analgesic actions of aspartame may involve similar mechanisms of action as aspirin, possibly through the interference of prostaglandin (PG) synthesis. Aspartame's effect on PG synthesis has not been empirically substantiated, but computer-assisted modeling suggests an action similar to aspirin's inhibition of cyclooxygenase activity[7]. In the present study, saccharin and sucrose decreased the antinociceptive effect of morphine while aspartame increased the effect of morphine-induced analgesia. Nikfar *et al.*[8] have also shown that aspartame increases the analgesic effect of morphine and naloxone only reversed the action of opioids but had no effect on aspartame.

Aspartame (2 mg/kg) was used in combination with nimesulide (a preferential COX-2 inhibitor) and a conventional NSAID, naproxen, the combination exhibited a synergistic activity. The study showed that besides the interaction of aspartame with opioids and NMDA receptor antagonists it could also interact with some NSAIDs such as nimesulide and naproxen in a sub maximal dose to show a synergistic effect[9,10].

Although there is no direct evidence available, to support the present data it can be speculated that aspartame and NSAIDs may act through a central nociceptive mechanism. Another speculation could be that this interaction may influence the pharmacokinetic parameters of the drugs in combination or may reduce the renal clearance of drugs thereby acting at the site of action for a longer duration of time and thus showing synergistic effect.

Aspartame also possessed a significant antiinflammatory action against carrageenan-induced paw oedema but it was found to be not effective in combination with opioids/NSAIDs in inflammatory and hyperalgesic pain models. The interaction between these drugs is highly speculative at the present and further studies are needed to find out the possible therapeutic implications of such interactions in humans.

REFERENCES

1. Nikfar S, Abdollahi M, Sarkarati F & Etemad F, Interaction between calcium channel blockers and sweetening agents on morphine- induced analgesia in mice by formalin test, *Gen Pharmacol*, 3 (1998) 431.
2. Bergmann F, Lieblich L, Cohen E & Ganchrow J R, Influences of intake of sweet solutions on the analgesic effect of a low dose of morphine in randomly bred rats, *Behav Neural Biol*, 44 (1985) 347.
3. Kanarek R B, White E S, Biegen M T & Marks-Kaufman R, Dietary influences on morphine-induced analgesia in rats, *Pharmac Biochem Behav*, 38 (1991) 681.
4. Koster R, Anderson M & DeBeer E J, Acetic acid for analgesic screening, *Fed Proc*, 18 (1959) 4.
5. Kulkarni S K, Mehta A K & Kunchandy J, Antiinflammatory actions of clonidine, guanfacine and B-HT920 against various inflammagen-induced acute paw edema in rats. *Arch Int Pharmacodyn Ther*, 279 (1986) 324.
6. Aley K O, Green P G & Levine J D, Opioid and adenosine peripheral antinociception are subject to tolerance and withdrawal, *J Neurosci*, 15 (1995) 8031.
7. Labuda C J & Fuchs P N, A comparison of chronic aspartame exposure to aspirin on inflammation, hyperalgesia and open field activity following carrageenan-induced monoarthritis, *Life Sci*, 69 (2001) 443.
8. Nikfar S, Abdollahi M, Etemad F & Sharifzadeh M, Effects of sweetening agents on morphine induced analgesia in mice by formalin test, *Gen Pharmacol*, 29 (1997) 583.
9. Edmundson A B & Manion C V, Treatment of osteoarthritis with aspartame. *Clin Pharmacol Ther*, 63 (1998) 580.
10. Abdollahi M, Sarrafzadeh J, Nikfar S & Roshanzamir F, Mechanism of aspartame-induced antinociception in mice. *Indian J Pharmacol*, 35 (2003) 37.

Paper Published In:
I.J.E.B. (Vol. 43, June 2005, pp.498-502)

26

Cholinergic-NO-cGMP mediation of sildenafil-induced antinociception

CHANDRASHEKHAR S PATIL[A], NAVEEN K. JAIN[B], VIJAY PAL SINGH[B] AND S.K. KULKARNI[A]
[A]Pharmacology Division, University Institute of Pharmaceutical Sciences
Panjab University, Chandigarh 160 014, India
[B]R&D Division, Panacea Biotec Ltd., Chandigarh Road, Lalru, 140 501, India

Acetylcholine and cholinomimetic agents with predominant muscarinic action are known to increase the concentration of cGMP by activation of nitric oxide signaling pathway in the nociceptive conditions. The present study was aimed to investigate the NO-cGMP-PDE_5 pathway in nociceptive conditions in the experimental animals. Nociceptive threshold was assessed by acetic acid-induced writhing assay (chemonociception) or carrageenan-induced hyperalgesia. Sildenafil [1-5 mg/kg, ip, 50-200 mg/paw, intraplantar (ipl)] produced dose dependent antinociception in both the tested models. Coadministration of acetylcholine (50 mcg/paw, ipl) or cholinomimetic agent, neostigmine (0.1 mcg/kg, ip and 25 ng/paw, ipl) augmented the peripheral antinociceptive effect of sildenafil. This effect was sensitive to blockade by L-NAME (20 mg/kg, ip, 100 μg/paw, ipl), a non-selective NOS inhibitor and methylene blue (MB) (1 mg/kg, ip), a guanylate cyclase inhibitor,which *per se* had little or no effect in both the models of nociception. Further, the *per se* analgesic effect of acetylcholine and neostigmine was blocked by both L-NAME and methylene blue in the models of nociception, suggesting the activation of NO-cGMP pathway. Also, both L-NAME and methylene blue blocked the *per se* analgesic effect of sildenafil. These results indicate the peripheral accumulation of cGMP may be responsible for antinociceptive effect, and a possible interaction between cholinergic agents and PDE_5 system in models of nociception.

Keywords: PDE_5 inhibitors, Cholinergic, Cholinomimetic agents; NOS, Nociception

Presence of intrinsic cholinergic inhibitory pathways in modulating pain has been demonstrated[1] as cholinomimetic agents administered centrally or peripherally are known to inhibit nociception by increasing the endogenous acetylcholine. A role for cholinergic system, both central and peripheral, in elicitation of antinociceptive response has been ascribed experimentally as well as clinically [1-5]. Centrally it appears to modulate this effect through nitric oxide synthase (NOS) pathway via enhanced acetylcholine as NOS inhibitor antagonized the antinociceptive response of cholinomimetics[6]. A peripheral analgesic effect of cholinergic agents, as dibutyryl cyclic GMP mimicked acetylcholine induced analgesia, suggesting that cholinergic agents may cause analgesia by altering cyclic GMP at the nociceptor level[7].

The role of NO in the nociception and antinociception is still controversial. The early up-regulation of NOS in the spinal cord and increased production of spinal NO after nerve constriction and tissue inflammation[8-11] during acute and chronic pain favours a pronociceptive action of NO. In contrast, recent studies where systemic administration of NO precursor, L-arginine has been shown to produce analgesia in mice[12,13]. Besides, peripheral activation of NO-cGMP pathway in antinociception in animal models [14] provide supportive evidence that spinal NO plays a role in antinociception.

Phosphodiesterases (PDEs) are the large group of structurally related enzymes that catalyse the hydrolysis of 3',5'-cyclic nucleotides to corresponding inactive nucleosides, 5'-monophosphate. Eleven families (PDE 1-11) of PDEs have been identified with each family being the product of a separate gene and usually comprise several isoforms[15]. PDE_5 is predominant cGMP-specific PDE expressed in skeletal, cardiac and smooth muscle[16] and is responsible for the hydrolysis of cGMP[16,17]. Sildenafil is a potent selective and reversible phosphodiesterase 5 inhibitor that blocks cyclic GMP hydrolysis (ki = 3 nM). Recently Jain *et al.* [14], have reported the peripheral analgesic effect of sildenafil in the animal models of nociception on systemic and local administration. This effect was found to be mediated through inhibition of cyclic GMP specific phosphopdiesterase type 5 (PDE_5). In the present study the possible interaction between PDE_5 and cholinergic system was explored in the animal models of nociception and the possible participation of NO-cGMP-PDE_5 pathway.

Materials and Methods

Animals: Albino mice (Swiss strain, 20-30 g) and rats (Wistar strain, 150-200 g) of either sex (Central Animal House, Panjab University,

Chandigarh, India) were housed under standard laboratory conditions and kept under a 12:12 hr L:D cycle. Experiments were carried out between 0900 and 1800 hrs. All the experimental protocols were approved by the Institutional Animal Ethics Committee.

Antinociceptive study: Writhing test (acetic acid assay): A 1% acetic acid solution (10 mg/kg, ip) was used to produce writhing in mice. The number of wriths (constriction of abdomen, turning of the trunk (twist) and extension of the hind limbs) due to acetic acid[18] was expressed as the pain response. The number of wriths per animal was counted during a 20 min session, beginning 3 min after the injection of acetic acid.

Induction and assessment of carrageenan-induced hyperalgesia: Acute inflammation was induced in the right hind paw by injecting, ipl, 0.1 ml of freshly prepared solution of 1% carrageenan. The left paw received 0.1 ml of saline which served as control. The response to inflammatory pain was determined by measuring the mechanical nociceptive pressure by the paw pressure test[19] via a commercially available analgesiometer (Ugo Basile, Italy). The apparatus was set up to apply a force of 0-1000 g, increasing from zero. The nociceptive threshold was taken as the end point at which the rat vocalized or struggled vigorously.

The test drug sildenafil and acetylcholine and/or neostigmine were injected in the volume of 50 µl intraplantarly in right hind paw 30 min prior to the carrageenan challenge and the pressure threshold was observed at 15, 30, 60, and 120 min. The time selection was made on the basis of the preliminary studies.

Locomotor activity test: The animal locomotor behavioural pattern was monitored using activity meter (IMCORP, India). The animals were individually placed in a plexiglass cage (40x15x15 cm) and the total activity count registered for 5 min. The locomotor activity was expressed in terms of total photo beam counts/5 min/animal[20].

Drugs: Sildenafil citrate (Panacea Biotec. Ltd), L-NAME and carrageenan IV (Sigma, U.S.A.), methylene blue, acetylcholine chloride and acetic acid (S D Fine Chemicals), neostigmine (Neon Labs, Mumbai) were obtained commercially.

Statistical analysis: Results are expressed as mean ± S E. The significance of the difference in the responses of treatment groups in comparison to the, control was determined by one-way analysis of variance (ANOVA) followed by Dunnet's test. A level of P < 0.05 was considered statistically significant.

Results

Antinociceptive activity of sildenafil in mice and rats: Systemic administration of sildenafil (1-5 mg/kg, ip) showed a dose-dependent decrease in the number of wriths indicating an increase in pain threshold (Fig. la). In carrageenan-induced hyperalgesia ipsilateral, but not contralateral administration of sildenafil (50-200 mcg/paw, ipl) exhibited a dose-dependent increase in pain threshold (Fig. 2). The antinociceptive effect of sildenafil (1 mg/kg, ip and 50 mg/paw, ipl) was blocked by L-NAME (20 mg/kg, ip, 100 mg/paw, ipl) and methylene blue (1 mg/kg, ip) in both the tests of nociception (Fig. 3).

Antinociceptive activity of acetylcholine and/or neostigmine in mice and rats: Neostigmine (0.1-0.5 mg/kg, ip) produced a dose-dependent increase in nociceptive threshold in writhing assay in mice (Fig. lb). Acetylcholine (50-200 mg/paw, ipl) and neostigmine (25-100 mg/paw) produced a dose-dependent antinociceptive effect against carrageenan-induced hyperalgesia in rats (Fig. 4). The antinociceptive effect of acetylcholine (50 mg/paw, ipl) was blocked by L-NAME (100 mg/paw, ipl) and methylene blue (1 mg/kg, ip) in carrageenan-induced hyperalgesia. Also, the antinociceptive effect of neostigmine (0.1 mg/kg, ip and 25 mg/paw, ipl) was blocked by L-NAME (20 mg/kg, ip, 100 mg/paw, ipl) and methylene blue (1 mg/kg, ip) in both the tests of nociception (Fig. 7).

Effect of acetylcholine and/or neostigmine on sildenafil-induced antinociception in mice and rats: The lowest effective dose of acetylcholine (50 mcg/paw, ipl) potentiated the antinociceptive effect of sildenafil (50 mcg/paw, ipl) in carrageenan-induced hyperalgesia and the effect was blocked by L-NAME (100 mcg/paw, ipl) and methylene blue (1 mg/kg, ip) (Fig. 5). Similarly, neostigmine (0.1 mg/kg, ip, and 25 ng/paw, ipl) enhanced the antinociceptive effect of sildenafil (1 mg/kg, ip, 50 mg/paw, ipl) in both the tests of nociception and the effect was blocked by L-NAME (20 mg/kg, ip, 100 μg/paw, ipl) and methylene blue (1 mg/kg, ip) (Figs lc and 6).

Effect of neostigmine, sildenafil and their combinations on locomotor activity in mice: No significant behavioural or motor dysfunctions were observed on treatment of sildenafil (1-5 mg/kg, ip), neostigmine (0.1-0.5 mg/kg, ip), or their combination in mice (Table 1).

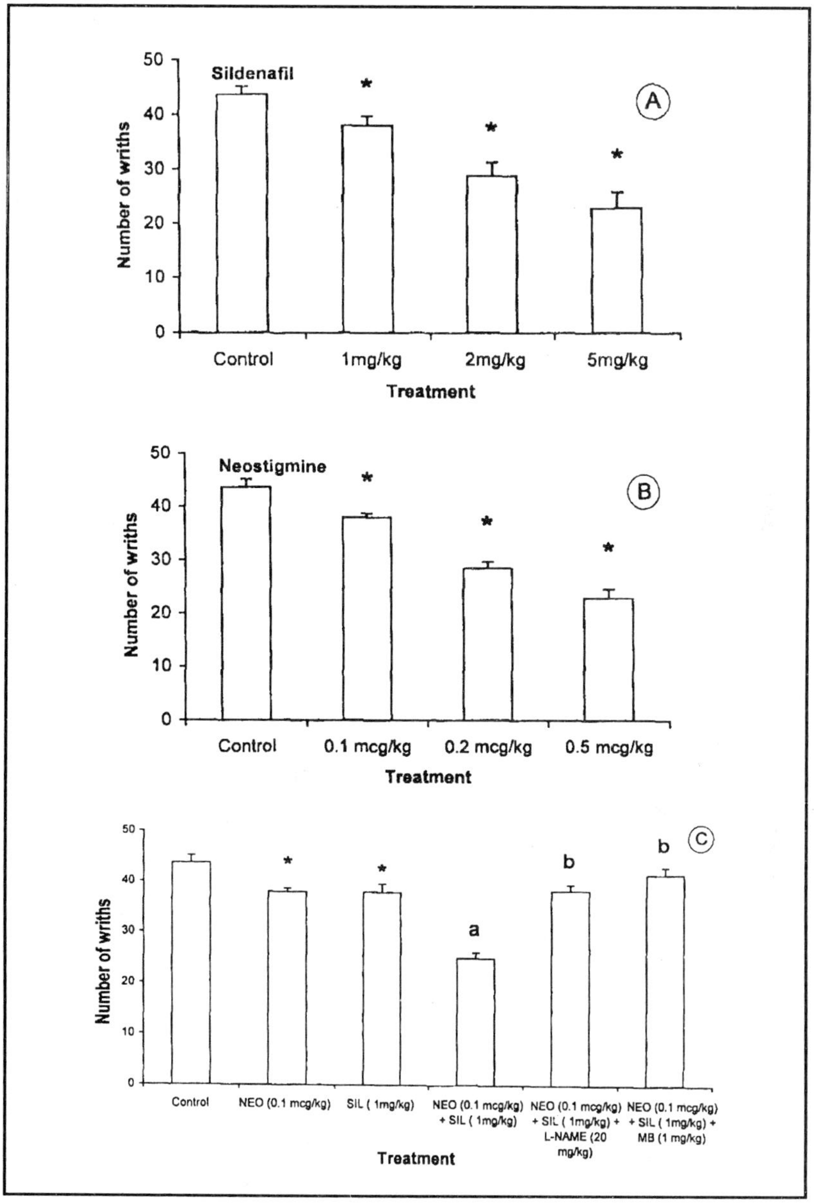

Fig. 1. Antinociceptive effect of (A) sildenafil (SIL) (1-5 mg/kg, ip), (B) neostigmine (NEO) (0.1-0.5 mcg/kg, ip), and (C) their combination and its reversal by L-NAME (20 mg/kg, ip) and methylene blue (1 mg/kg, ip) in the mouse writhing test. Data are expressed as mean ± S.E. (n = 6 or 8 mice per group). *P < 0.05 as compared with control, [a]P < 0.05 as compared with sildenafil (1 mg/kg, ip) and neostigmine (0.1 mg/kg, ip) *per se*, [b]P < 0.05 as compared with sildenafil and neostigmine combination.

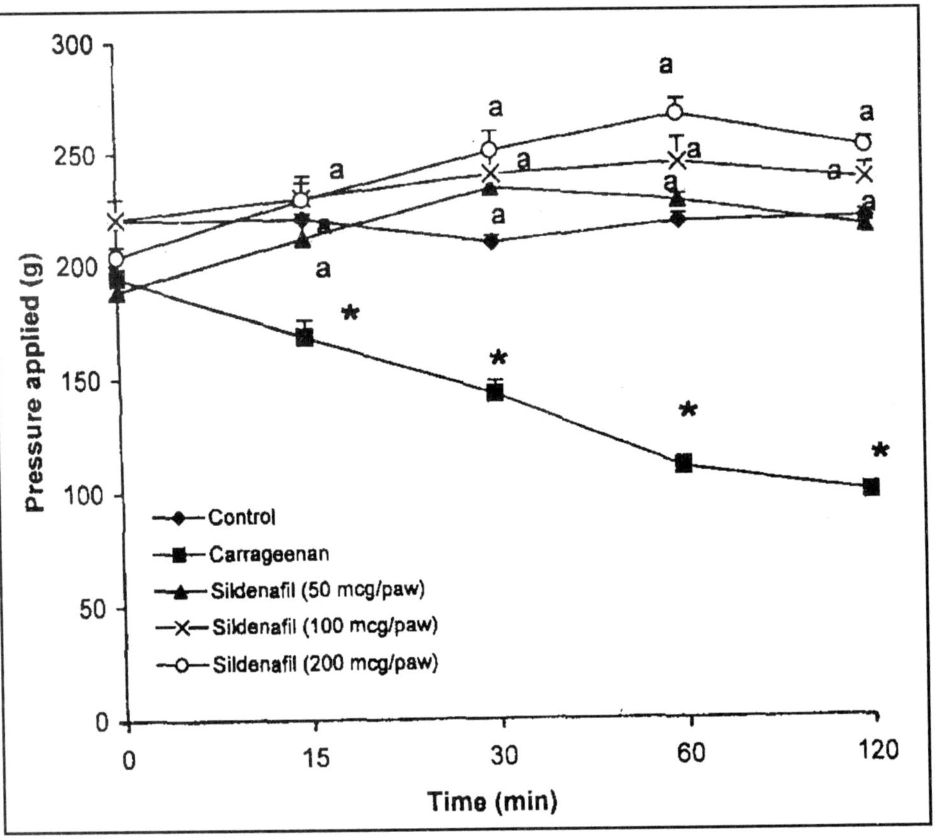

Fig. 2. Effect of sildenafil (50-200 mg/paw, ipl) against carrageenan-induced hyperalgesia (paw pressure test) in rats. Data are expressed as mean ± S.E. (n = 6 or 8 rats per group). *P < 0.05 as compared with control, ^{a}P < 0.05 as compared with carrageenan treated group.

Discussion

Antinociceptive action of sildenafil– Findings of present study indicate that sildenafil on systemic (1-5 mg/kg, ip) and local (50-100 mg/paw) administration produced dose-dependent antinociceptive effect in animal models of nociception. This effect appears to be a local action, as the contralateral administration of the drug was ineffective to reduce nociception. This is suggestive of a major contribution by peripheral PDE 5 and NO-cGMP pathways in sildenafil-induced peripheral antinociception. The sildenafil produces antinociception probably through the inhibition of cyclic GMP degradation by PDE_5 enzyme, suggesting the major participation of peripheral PDE_5 and NO-cGMP pathway[14,21,22].

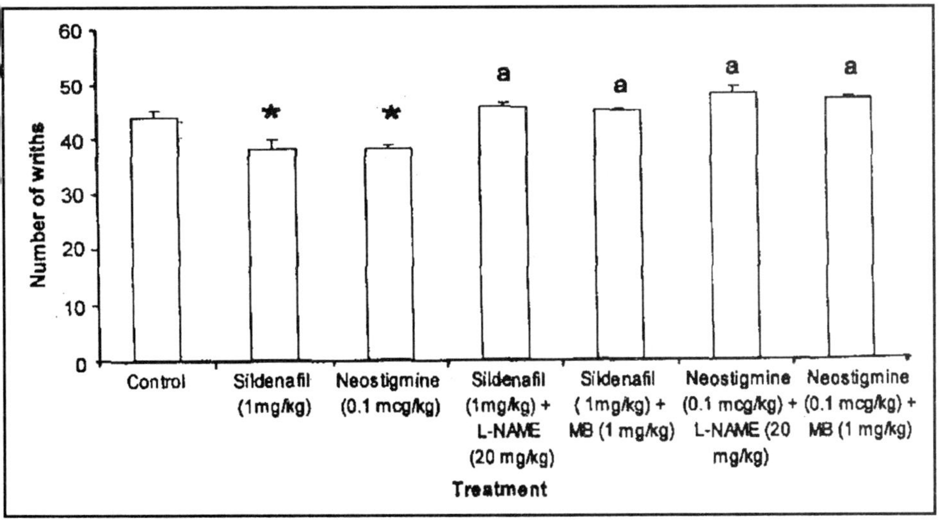

Fig. 3. Effect of L-NAME (20 mg/kg, ip) and methylene blue (MB) (1 mg/kg, ip) on sildenafil (1 mg/kg, ip) and neostigmine (0.1 mg/kg, i.p.) in the mouse writhing test. Data are expressed as mean ± S.E. (n = 6 or 8 mice per group). *P < 0.05 as compared with control, [a]P < 0.05 as compared with sildenafil (1 mg/kg, ip) and neostigmine (0.1 mg/kg, ip) per se.

It has been postulated that the administration of anticholinesterase neostigmine, modulated central and peripheral sites of intrinsic cholinergic inhibitory pathway of pain perception[1]. This involves hyperpolarization of neurons, reduction in the release of pronociceptive neurotransmitters and activation of the NO-cGMP pathway mediate cholinergic antinociception by elevating endogenous acetylcholine[23-25].

In the present study acetylcholine (50-200 mg/paw, ipl) and neostigmine (0.1 mg/kg, ip and 25 -100 ng/paw, ipl) produced a dose-dependent analgesic effect in models of nociception. This effect may be due to spinal or peripheral accumulation of acetylcholine as observed by Duarte *et al*[26]. Further, the antagonism of the effects of acetylcholine and neostigmine by L-NAME and methylene blue indicate a role for NO-cGMP pathway.

This is supported by the observation that potentiated response was recorded when lowest effective dose of sildenafil and cholinomimetic agents was used. Additionally, this enhancement was reversed by L-NAME and MB. These data favour the contention of role for nitric oxide synthase in the antinociceptive response of

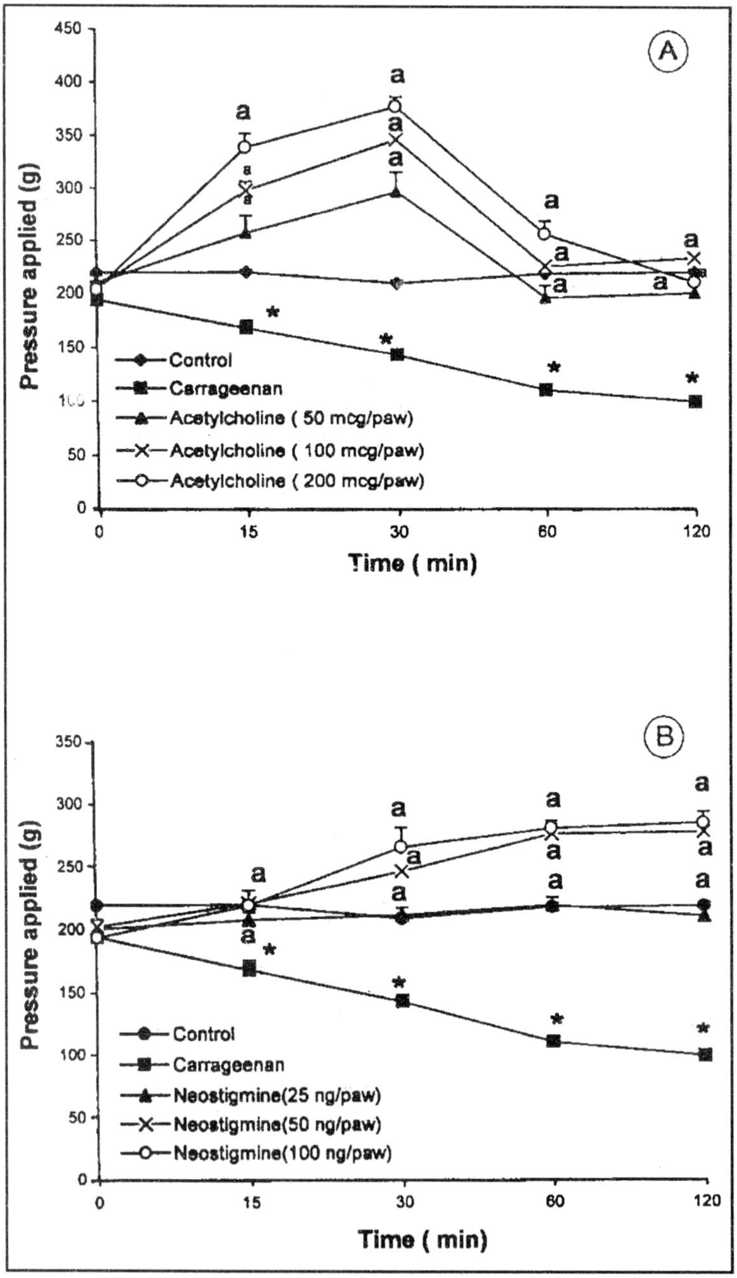

Fig. 4. Effect of (A) acetylcholine (50-200 mg/paw, ipl) and (B) neostigmine (25-100 mg/paw, ipl) against carrageenan-induced hyperalgesia (paw pressure test) in rats. Data are expressed as mean ± S.E. (n = 6 or 8 rats per group). *P < 0.05 as compared with control, [a]p < 0.05 as compared with carrageenan treated group.

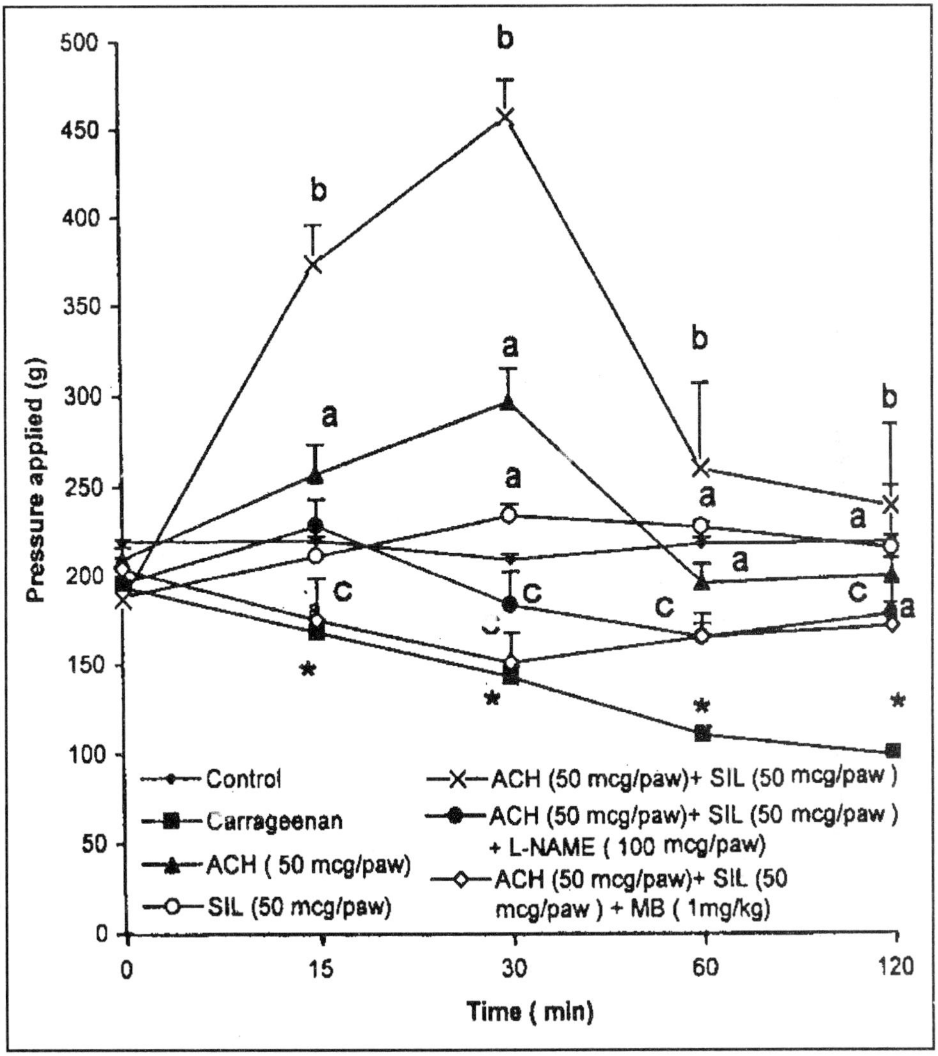

Fig. 5. Effect of acetylcholine (ACH: 50 mg/paw, ipl) on sildenafil (SIL: 50 mg/paw, ipl)-induced antinociception and its modification by L-NAME (100 mg/paw, ipl) and methylene blue (MB) (1 mg/kg, ip) in carrageenan-induced hyperalgesia (aw pressure test) in rats. Data are expressed as mean ± S.E. (n = 6 or 8 rats per group). *P < 0.05 as compared with control, [a]P < 0.05 as compared with carrageenan treated group, [b]P < 0.05 as compared with sildenafil (50 pg/paw) and acetylcholine (50 mg/paw) *per se*, [c]P < 0.05 as compared with sildenafil and acetylcholine combination.

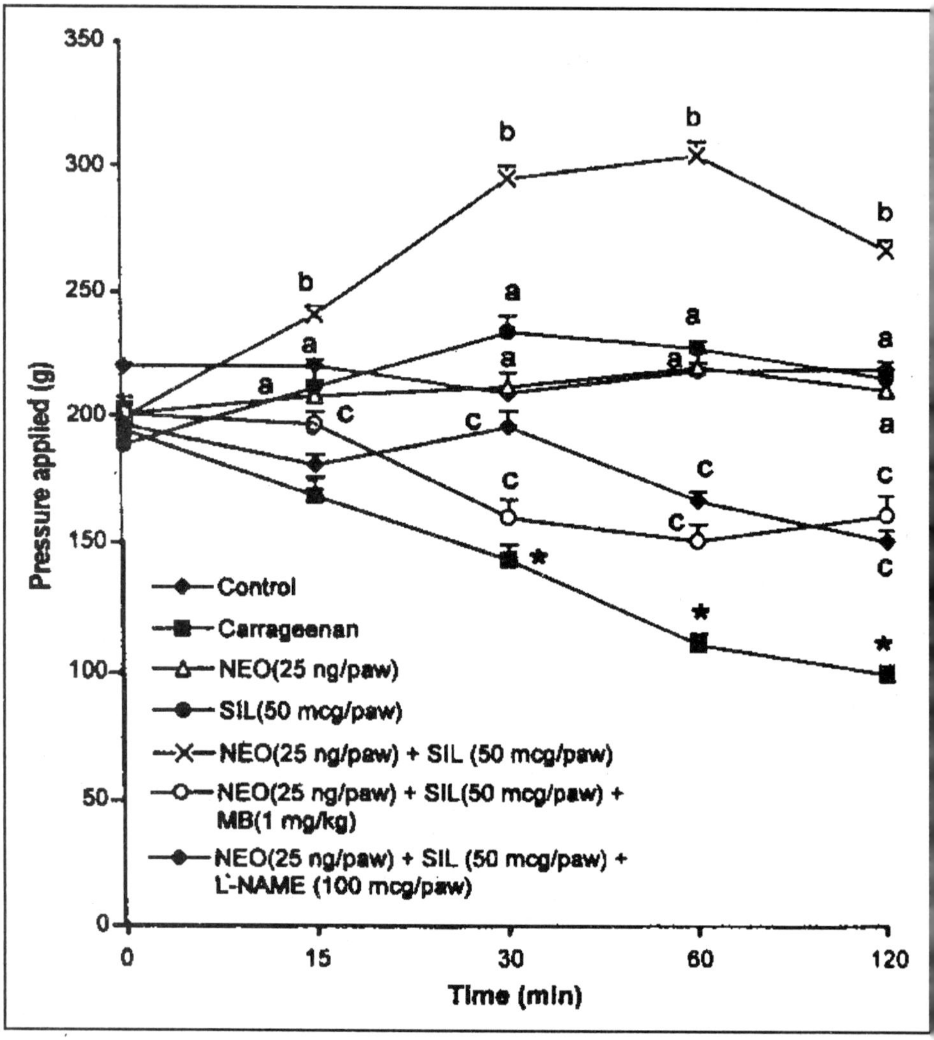

Fig. 6. Effect of neostigmine (NEO: 25 mg/paw, ipl) on sildenafil (SIL: 50 mg/paw, ipl)-induced antinociception and its modification by L-NAME (100 mg/paw, ipl) and methylene blue (MB) (1 mg/kg, ip) in carrageenan-induced hyperalgesia (paw pressure test) in rats. Data are expressed as mean ± S.E. (n = 6 or 8 rats per group). *P < 0.05 as compared with control, [a]P < 0.05 as compared with carrageenan treated group, [b]P < 0.05 as compared with sildenafil (50 mg/paw) and neostigmine (25 mg/paw) *per se*, [c]P < 0.05 as compared with sildenafil and neostigmine combination.

acetylcholine. A hypothetical schematic diagram is present in Fig. 8. A similar role in acetylcholine-induced vasodilation has been reported[27].

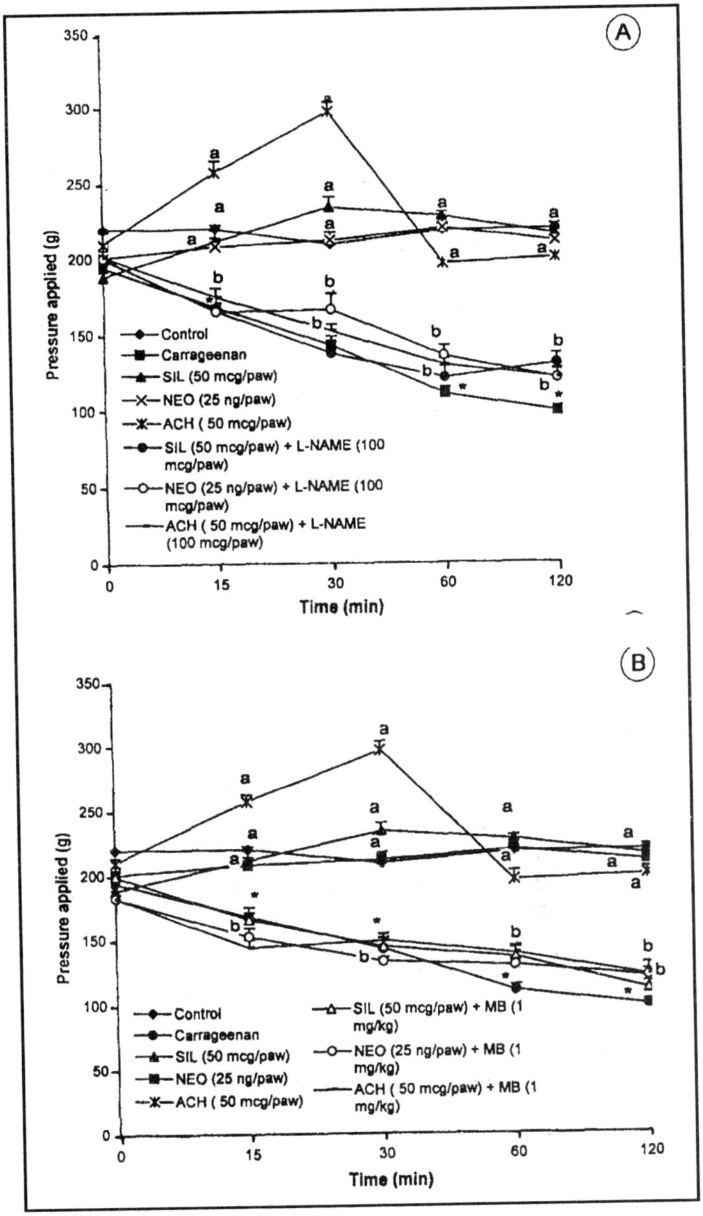

Fig. 7. Effect of (A) L-NAME (100 mg/paw) and (B) methylene blue (MB:1 mg/kg, ip) on sildenafil (SIL: 50 mg/paw, ipl), neostigmine (NEO: 25 mg/paw, ipl) and acetylcholine (ACH: 50 mg/paw, ipl) in carrageenan-induced hyperalgesia (paw pressure test) in rats. Data are expressed as mean ± S.E. (n = 6 or 8 rats per group). *P < 0.05 as compared with control, [a]P < 0.05 as compared with carrageenan treated group, [b]P < 0.05 as compared with sildenafil (50 mg/paw), neostigmine (25 mg/paw) and acetylcholine (50 mg/paw) *per se*.

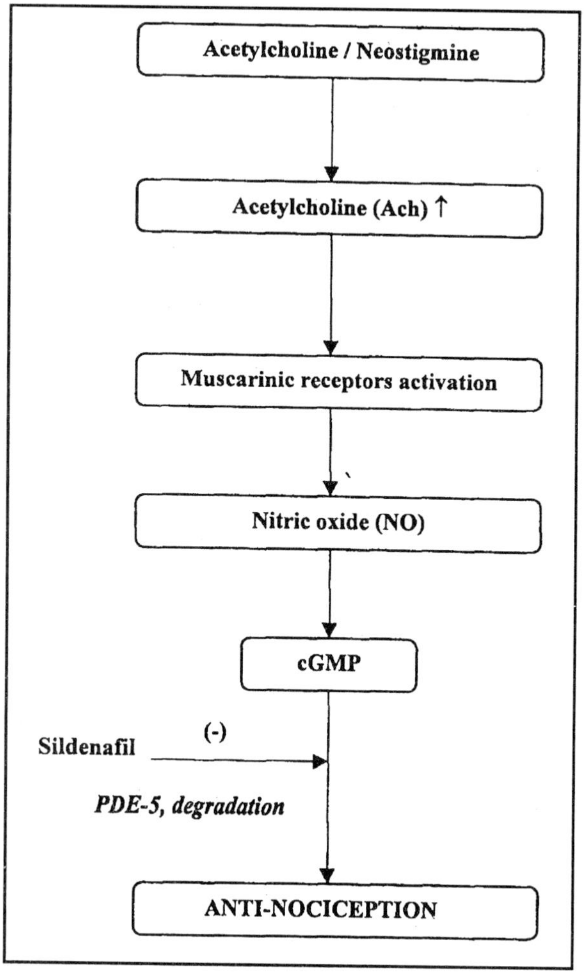

Fig. 8. Possible mechanism for cholinergic-NO-cGMP induced antinociception.

Table 1. Effect of sildenafil, neostigmine and its combination on locomotor activity in mice [Values are mean ± SE from 5 animals in each group]

Treatment (ip)		Locomotor activity (photobeams/5 min)
Control		156.6 ± 3.69
Sildenafil	1 mg/kg	161.9 ± 5.61
	2 mg/kg	149.8 ± 4.88
	5 mg/kg	159.9 ± 9.39
Neostigmine	0.1 mcg/kg	144.9 ± 10.2
	0.25 mcg/kg	150.3 ± 6.6
	0.5 mcg/kg	166.9 ± 5.59
Sildenafil neostigmine	1 mg/kg + 0.1 mcg/kg	161.6 ± 9.99

The possibility that the drugs used in the present study are known to cause hypotension by increasing the levels of cGMP[28] thereby may alter the ability of the animals to respond to nociceptive stimuli is unlikely as, acetylcholine and neostigmine *per se* and in combination with sildenafil neither produced a significant change in blood pressure (data not shown) nor altered its locomotion. Besides other classical cholinergic symptoms viz lacrimation and salivation was observed at the tested doses. Considering together, the findings of the present study clearly defines a significant role for NO and cGMP in cholinergic mechanisms involved in the elicitation of antinociception.

In summary, the current study provides the evidence that sildenafil and cholinergic/cholinomimetic agents produced antinociceptive effect in the models of nociception. In addition sildenafil increased the antinociceptive effect of cholinergic/cholinomimetic agents, which may be due to the peripheral accumulation of cGMP and a possible interaction between cholinergic agents and PDE 5 system.

REFERENCES

1. Buekle H, Boschin M, Marcus M A, Brodner G, Wusten R & Aken H, Central and peripheral analgesia mediated by the acetylcholinesterase-inhibitor neostigmine in the rat inflamed knee joint model, *Anesth Analg,* 86 (1998) 1027.
2. Pedigo W, Determination and characterization of the antinociceptive effect of intraventricularily administered acetylcholine in mice, *J Pharamacol Exp Ther,* 193 (1975) 845.
3. Naguib M & Yaksh T L, Antinociceptive effect of spinal cholinesterase inhibition and isobolographic analysis of the interaction with mu and alpha 2 receptor systems, *Anesthesiology,* 80 (1994) 1338.
4. Hood D D, Elsenach J C & Tong C, Cardiorespiratory and spinal cord blood flow effects of intrathecal neostigmine methylsulfate, clonidine, and their combination in sheep, *Anesthesiology,* 82 (1995a) 428.
5. Hood D D, Elsenach J C & Tuttle R, Phase I safety assessment of intrathecal neostigmine methylsulfate in humans, *Anesthesiology,* 82 (1995b) 331.
6. Xu Z, Tong C & Eisenach J C, Acetylcholine stimulates release of nitric oxide from rat spinal cord, *Anesthesiolgy,* 85 (1996) 107.
7. Ferreira S H & Nakamura M, Prostaglandin hyperalgesia, A cAMP/Ca^{2+} dependent process, *Prostaglandins,* 18 (1979) 179.
8. Meller S T, Cummings C P, Traub R J & Gebhart G F, The role of nitric oxide in the development and maintenance of the hyperalgesia produced by intraplantar injection of carrageenan in the rat, *Neuroscience,* 60 (1994) 367.

9. Meller S T & Gebhart G F, Nitric oxide (NO) and nociceptive processing in the spinal cord, *Pain,* 52 (1993) 127.

10. Yang L C, Marsala M & Yaksh T L, Charecterization of time course of spinal amino acids, citrulline and PGE2 release after carrageenan/kaolin-induced knee joint inflammation: A chronic microdialysis study, *Pain,* 67 (1996) 545.

11. Gordh T, Sharma H S, Alm P & Westman J, Spinal cord nerve lesion in the upregulation of neuronal nitric oxide synthase in the spinal cord- an immunohistochemical investigation in the rat, *Amino Acids,* 14 (1998) 105.

12. Kawabata A, Nishimura Y & Takagi H, L-leucyl-L-arginine, naltrindole and D-arginine block antinociception elicited by L-arginine in mice with carrageenan-induced hyperalgesia, *Br J Pharmacol,* 107 (1992) 1096.

13. Kamei J, Iwamoto Y, Misawa M, Nagase H & Kasuya Y, Antinociceptive effect of L-arginine in diabetic mice, *Eur J Pharmacol,* 254 (1994) 113.

14. Jain N K, Patil C S, Singh A & Kulkarni S K, Sildenafil induced peripheral analgesia and activation of the nitric oxide-cyclic GMP pathway, *Brain Res,* 909 (2001) 170.

15. Terrett N K, Bell A S, Brown D & Ellis P, Sildenafil (Viagra R) a potent and selective inhibitor of type 5 cGMP phosphodiesterase with utility for treatment of male erectile dysfunction, *Bioorg Med Chem Lett,* 6 (1996) 1819.

16. Moreland R B, Goldstein I, Kim N N & Traish A, Sildenafil citrate, a selective phosphodiesterase type 5 inhibitor: research and clinical implications in erectile dysfunction, *Trends Endocrinol Metab,* 10 (1999) 97.

17. Beavo J A, Cyclic nucleotide phosphodiesterases, functional implications of multiple isoforms, *Physiol Rev,* 75 (1995) 725.

18. Jain N K, Singh A & Kulkarni S K, Analgesic, antiinflammatory and ulcerogenic activity of a zinc-naproxen complex in mice and rats, *Pharmacol Commun,* 5 (1999) 599.

19. Randall L O & Selitto J J, A method for measurement of analgesic activity on inflammation tissue, *Arch Int Pharmacodyn,* 111 (1957) 409.

20. Reddy D S & Kulkarni S K, Possible role of nitric oxide in the nootropic and antiamnesic effects of neurosteroids on aging- and dizocilipine- induced learning impairment, *Brain Res,* 799 (1998) 215.

21. Mixcoatl Z T, Aguirre B P & Granadosn S V, Sildenafil produces anti-nociception and increases morphine antinociception in the formalin test, *Eur J Pharmacol,* 400 (2000) 81.

22. Asomoza-Espinosa R, Alonso-Lopez R, Mixcoatl-Zecuatl T, Aguirre-Banuelos P, Torres-Lopez J E & Granados-Soto V, Sildenafil increases diclofenac antinociception in the formalin test, *Eur J Pharmacol,* 27 (2001) 195.

23. Bernardini N, Sauer S K, Haberberberger R, Fischer M J & Reeh P W, Excitatory nicotinic and muscarinic (M2) effects on C-nociceptors in isolated heart skin, *J Neurosci*, 21 (2001) 3295.

24. Yang L C, Chen L M, Wang C J & Buerkle H, Postoperative analgesia by intra-articular neostigmine in patients undergoing knee arthroscopy, *Anesthesiology*, 88 (1998) 334.

25. Hugo F M, Fernando S & Gianni P, Neostigmine interactions with nonsteroidal anti-inflammatory drugs, *Br J Pharmacol*, 135 (2002) 1591.

26. Duarte I D G, Lorenzetti B B & Ferreira S H, Peripheral analgesia and activation of the nitric oxide-cyclic GMP pathway, *Eur J Pharmacol*, 186 (1990) 289.

27. Pan H L, Chen S R & Eisenach J C, Role of spinal NO in antiallodynic effect of intrathecal clonidine in neuropathic rats, *Anesthesiology*, 89 (1998) 1518.

28. Rees D D,.Palmer R M J & Moncada S, Role of endotheliumderived nitric oxide in the regulation of blood pressure, *Proc Natl Acad Sci USA*, 86 (1989) 3375.

Paper Published In:

I.J.E.B. (Vol. 42, January 2004, pp.361-367)

27

Effect of 5-lipoxygenase inhibition on events associated with inflammatory bowel disease in rats

VIJAY PAL SINGH, CHANDRASHEKHAR S. PATIL AND S.K. KULKARNI

Pharmacology Division, University Institute of Pharmaceutical Sciences, Panjab University, Chandigarh 160 014, India

Leukotrienes play a part in inflammatory response. The unique role of the enzyme 5-lipoxygenase (5-LOX) in the production of leukotrienes makes it a likely therapeutic target for inflammatory conditions like asthma, rheumatoid arthritis, psoriasis, and inflammatory bowel disease (IBD). The aim of the present study was to evaluate the effect of zileuton, an orally active selective 5-LOX inhibitor against the events associated with dextran sodium sulphate-induced colitis in a rat model of IBD. The animals werę administered simultaneously zileuton (100 mg/kg) or sulphasalazine (100 mg/kg) orally for 7 days. On day eight, rats were sacrificed, and distal colon isolated to determine myeloperoxidase activity, *in vivo* superoxide dismutase activity, prostaglandin E_2 levels and histological examination. Both zileuton and sulphasalazine significantly prevented the development of inflammatory events associated with colitis. The effect of zileuton was more pronounced towards reducing myeloperoxidase activity and increasing PGE_2 levels in distal colon. The results show that chemotactic leukotrienes are responsible for inflammatory surge in damaged colon and, zileuton, significantly improved healing by inhibition of neutrophil recruitment and indirectly through increase in prostaglandins at the site of inflammation. It is suggested that inhibitors of 5-LOX enzyme may have useful therapeutic role in the treatment of chronic intestinal inflammation.

Keywords: Inflammatory bowel disease, 5-Lipoxygenase: 5-LOX, Colitis, Zileuton

Inflammatory bowel disease (IBD) is a general term for a group of chronic inflammatory disorders of gastrointestinal tract [Ulcerative colitis (UC) and Crohn's disease (CD)][1]. The pathological hallmark of

IBD is marked by the presence of mucosal ulceration, infiltration of the mucosa with neutrophils and abdominal discomfort or pain with altered bowel habits (diarrhea, constipation or alternating episodes of diarrhea and constipation)[2]. Though etiologic agents as well as the chemical mediators to this multifactorial disorder are unknown and largely undefined, role of numerous inflammatory mediators in both acute and chronic forms is recognized. Products of arachidonic acid (AA) metabolism (prostaglandins: PGs and leukotrienes: LTs) are mediators of intestinal inflammatory response that initiate and maintain the sequence of pathological events of IBD[3,4].

Leukotrienes, the lipoxygenase product of AA, are one of the vital mediators highlighted in inflammatory cascade allied to IBD[5]. Leukotrienes (mainly leukotriene B_4: LTB_4) have been found in inflamed colon mucosa in concentration known to induce deleterious effects (chemokinesis, cell aggregation, increasing vascular permeability)[4]. These concentrations are similar to those seen in human IBD[6]. In addition, drugs known to be effective in the treatment of IBD are capable of reducing intestinal leukotriene production in both experimental models of colitis and human IBD[7-11]. Consequently, the 5-lipoxygenase (LOX) enzyme responsible for the synthesis of leukotrienes has become a target for the development of new potential anti-inflammatory drug in ulcerative colitis and other inflammatory conditions[12].

Zileuton, an orally effective 5-LOX inhibitor has been shown to selectively inhibit *in vitro* synthesis of LTB_4 in a variety of intact cell and cell free systems[13]. In patients with active ulcerative colitis, zileuton 600 mg, qid has shown to reduce the local release of leukotrienes into rectal dialysates[14]. However, lipoxygenase inhibitors such as benoxaprofen and MK-591 did not offer meaningful advantage in relieving the IBD symptoms[15,16]. Hendel *et al.*, demonstrated no significant relationship with IBD activity and alteration in mRNA for 5-LOX in colonic biopsies[17]. This suggests a further scrutiny of potential of 5-LOX inhibitors in IBD.

The present study has been aimed to evaluate the effect of zileuton in comparison to sulphasalazine in an experimental model of dextran sodium sulfate (DSS)-induced colitis in rats.

Materials and Methods

Animals: Wistar rats weighing 150-200 g body weight (Central Animal House, Panacea Biotec Ltd., Lalru) of either sex were used.

They were housed in plastic cages in a room at 25°±0.5° C and 12:12 hr L:D cycle. Animals were given food and water *ad libitum*. Experiments were carried out between 0900 and 1500 hrs. The experimental protocols were approved by the Institutional Animal Ethics Committee.

Drugs and regimen: Sulphasalazine (Panacea Biotec Ltd., New Delhi, India), zileuton (Archechem, Mumbai India), dextran sodium sulphate (DSS, mol wt 5000) and nitro blue tetrazolium (NBT, Himedia Laboratories Ltd, India) were used. Sulphasalazine (100 mg/kg) and zileuton (100 mg/kg) was suspended in tween 80 and administered orally once daily in the dose volume of 10 ml/kg, 24 hr before the induction of colitis until the day of sacrifice. DSS (5%w/v) was administered in drinking water.

Induction of inflammatory bowel disease/experimental colitis in rats and drug regimen: For the induction of experimental colitis, rats received standard meal with normal drinking water replaced with water containing 5% w/v DSS for 7 days. Sulphasalazine and zileuton treated group received standard meal, DSS containing water, and respective drugs orally, once a day. Control rats were given same food, plain water without DSS, and 0.5% CMC orally.

Histopathological evaluations: The distal colon segments from 0.5% CMC, DSS, sulphasalazine, and zileuton treated animals were isolated and immersed in 10% neutral buffered formalin till further processing. Sections were stained with hemotoxylin-eosin and investigated by light microscopy for the presence of inflammatory changes. At least three specimens per treatment were viewed to study the histopathological changes.

Myeloperoxidase (MPO) activity: Myeloperoxidase activity was determined following technique reported earlier by Singh *et al.*[18]. The isolated segments from different treatment groups were individually homogenized in 5 ml of phosphate buffer (0.01 M). Homogenized tissue was centrifuged at 10,000 rpm. Supernatant was mixed with o-phenylenediamine (600 µg/ml in phosphate buffer) and 300 mM of H_2O_2 was added to initiate the reaction. Absorbance was observed at 492 nm at an interval of 30 sec for 5 min. Change in the optical density per minute was calculated and the results were expressed as percentage increase of myeloperoxidase activity over the control.

In situ detection of superoxide (levels of oxidative stress): Tissue superoxide estimation was performed as per Hagen *et al.*[19] using Nitro

Blue Tetrazolium (NBT) perfusion. In the presence of superoxide, NBT forms an insoluble blue formazan precipitate within the tissues. The method was adapted as follows. The animals from different treatment groups were anesthetized (thiopental sodium 25 mg/kg ip), a midline laprotomy was performed and a solution of 5ml 1% NBT in 0.9 % sodium chloride (NaCl) at 37°C containing 0.2 mg/ml heparin was slowly (within 2 min) perfused in the dorsal aorta. This was followed by perfusion of 5 ml 0.9 % NaCl at 37°C. The animals were killed immediately, the distal colon regions isolated and placed on a non-absorbent surface. They were then flushed with 0.9 % NaCl (4°C) and fixed in neutral buffered formalin till further processing. Sections were stained with hemotoxylin-eosin for histological examination. The number of formazan precipitates in a total of ~270 mm^2 colonic mucosa was counted and expressed as number of cells containing formazan precipitates/100 mm^2 of the mucosa.

PGE_2 levels in distal colon: The PGE_2 were determined by modification in the method reported earlier by Tries *et al.*[20] for determination of eicosanoids in the inflamed paw. Briefly, seven days after DSS or drug treatment the distal colon was isolated, and homogenized in ice cold buffer containing 33% (v/v) acetonitrile and 67% (v/v) of disodium hydrogen orthophosphate (Na_2HPO_4). The final solution was brought to pH 3 with 100 *mM* of-phosphoric acid. After centrifugation for 30 min (4000 g, 4°C), the supernatants were collected and kept at -13°C until extraction of eicosanoids. Extraction of eicosanoids was performed using C18 columns (Orochem Technologies, USA). The columns were initially saturated with the mobile phase, sample applied and then washed with water, ethanol 10% and hexane successively twice and finally eicosanoids were eluted with methylformate. The solvent was evaporated with N_2 under pressure and the residual thus obtained was resolved using reverse phase HPLC (Agilent Technologies, USA) and PGE_2 levels were quantified. The results are expressed as ng/gm of colon weight.

Statistical analysis: Data presented as mean ± S.E. were analyzed using one-way ANOVA followed by post hoc Dunnett's test. $P<0.05$ was accepted as the level of significant difference compared to time matched controls.

Results

Morphological changes and histopathological examination: All the rats treated with DSS developed noticeable inflammation in the distal colon; the middle and the proximal colon had fewer lesions. DSS-evoked colitis was characterized by thickening of muscles, shortening of crypts, edema, a massive immune cells infiltration, ulceration and significant areas of complete epithelial rupture (Fig. 1 a,b).

Following sulphasalazine or zileuton treatment for 7 days, the hyperemic and ulcerative changes were almost normal. The crypts length was normalized with absence of inflammatory changes (Fig. 1 c,d).

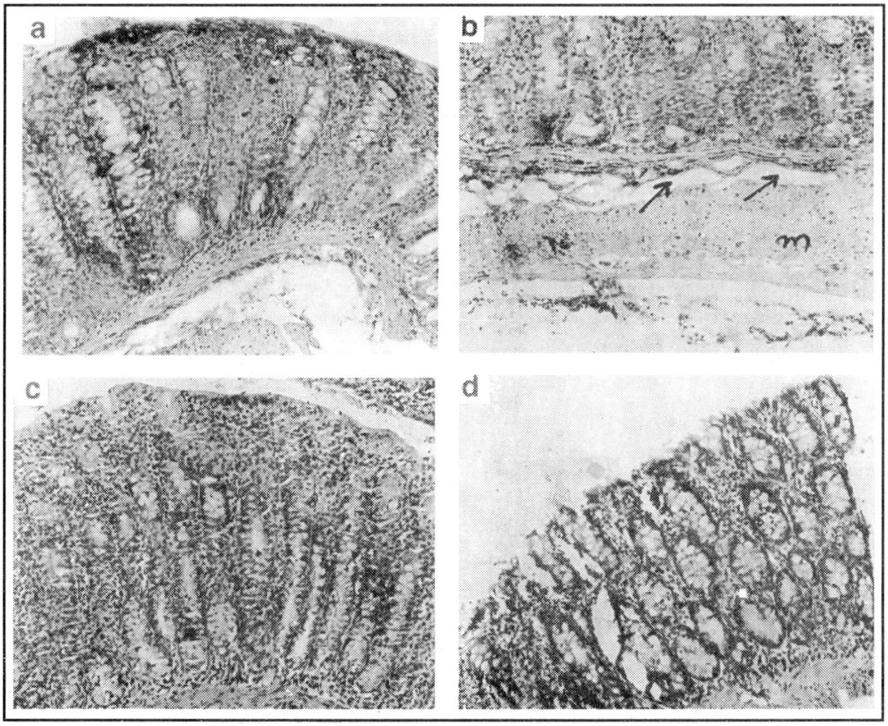

Fig. 1. Microphotographs of distal colonic segments from (a) control rats, (b) rats treated with DSS, (c) DSS and sulphasalazine (100 mg/kg), and (d) DSS and zileuton (100 mg/kg), [m: muscle, small arrow heads denote edema, large arrow heads indicate inflammatory infiltrate x 125].

MPO activity and oxidative stress–Myeloperoxidase activity in animals with DSS was found to be 2.5 times higher than the control value. The increase in the myeloperoxidase activity was significantly ($P < 0.05$) reduced in zileuton (100 mg/kg) or sulphasalazine (100 mg/kg) treatments. However, zileuton was more effective in reducing MPO activity when compared to sulphasalazine (Fig. 2).

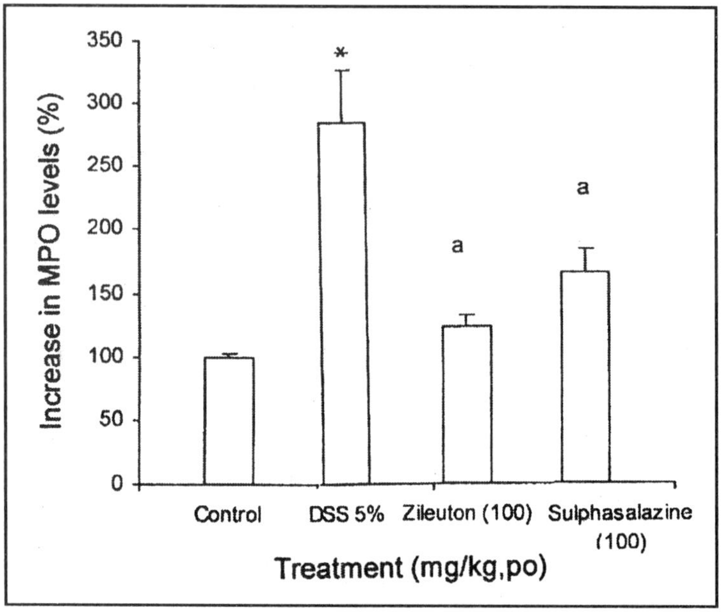

Fig. 2. Effect of DSS and co-administration of sulphasalazine and zileuton on myeloperoxidase activity (MPO) in distal colon segment. *$p<0.05$ as compared to plain water (control) group, [a]$p< 0.05$ as compared to DSS-treated group. The numbers in the parenthesis are dose in mg/kg body weight (Basal MPO levels considered 100%).

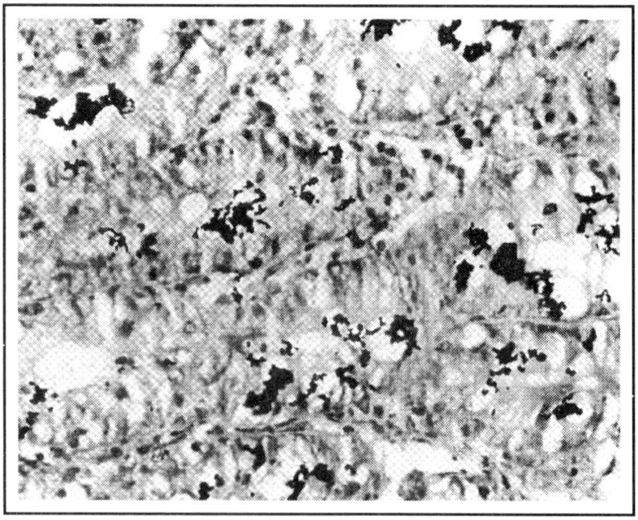

Fig. 3. Formazan blue precipitates after 7 days in distal colonic mucosa of rats treated with DSS. [The anesthetized animals were perfused with a solution contain 1% NBT before being killed x 250].

NBT especially forms insoluble formazan precipitates in presence of superoxide[19]. NBT perfusion led to the formation of formazan precipitates in the distal colon segment of DSS-treated rats. These precipitates were strictly localized inside the goblet cells of the colonic mucosal (Fig. 3). Formazan precipitates were increased twice the control value with DSS. Co-administration of sulphasalazine significantly prevented the increased formation of formazan precipitates by NBT, whereas zileuton had no significant effect as compared to DSS-treated group (Table 1).

Eicosanoid levels: PGE_2 levels were estimated in the distal colon segments isolated after 7 days. Coadministration of zileuton significantly increased PGE_2 levels to 132.25±8.80 ng/g tissue (vs. DSS treated rats; 99.22 ± 3.32 ng/g tissue). The change in the PGE_2 levels with co-administration of sulphasalazine was not significant (106.28 ± 6.03 ng/g tissue vs. DSS-treated rats 99.22 ± 3.32 ng/g tissue) (Fig.4).

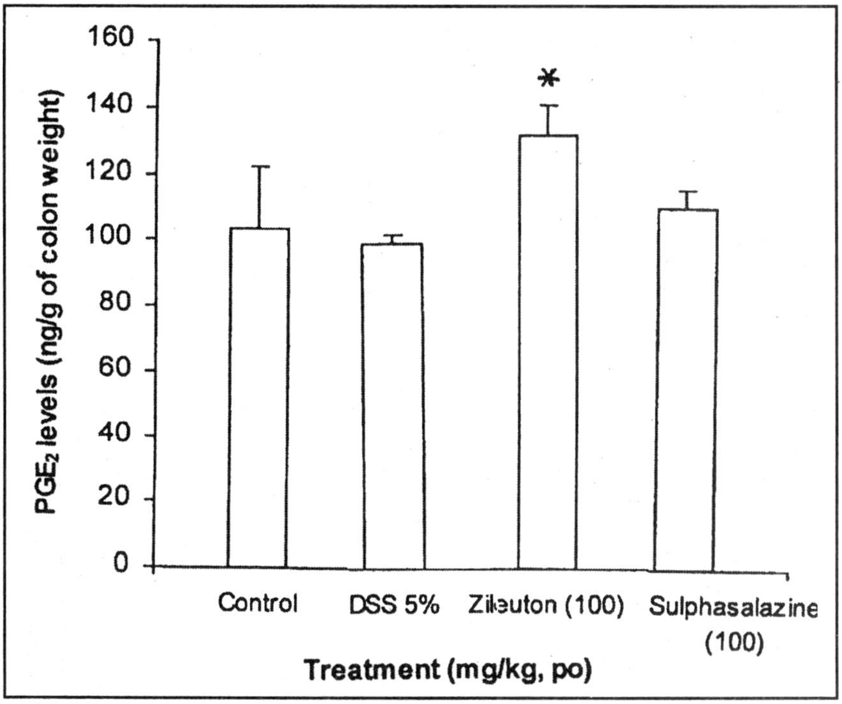

Fig. 4. Effect of sulphasalazine, and zileuton on PGE_2 levels (n = 5-6). [Vertical lines show mean ± S.E. *P < 0.05 as compared to DSS-treated group. The numbers in the parenthesis indicate dose in mg/kg body weight.]

Table 1. Number of formazan precipitates per 100mm^2 of colonic mucosa [values are mean ± S.E.]

Treatment	No. formazan precipitates per 100 mm^2 of colonic mucosa
Control	438.2± 67.33
DSS	840.6 ± 82.44*
Zileuton (100 mg/kg, po)	616.0 ± 55.89
Sulphasalazine (100 mg/kg, po)	457.0 ±49.87^a

**P*: <0.05 as compared to control, ^{a}p<0.05 as compared to DSS treated rats

Discussion

The etiology of inflammatory bowel disease remains undefined, but it is recognized that during IBD, inflammatory mediators (prostaglandins, thromboxanes and leukotrienes) are generated within the colonic mucosa[2,3]. Recent experimental studies have demonstrated the role of 5-LOX enzyme metabolites in IBD because of their potent stimulatory activity on inflammatory cells. Indeed, elevated concentration is detected in dialysates and biopsies of patients with active ulcerative colitis[20,21]. In particular, LTB_4 has been reported to account for majority of chemotactic activities detected in rectal dialysis[4]. Therefore, in the present study zileuton, a specific 5-LOX inhibitor was evaluated in well-characterized model of DSS-induced colitis in rats. This model shares many of the histopathological features of human ulcerative colitis and Crohn's disease. Oral administration of DSS to rodents results in overt inflammation in the mid distal colon that is reminiscent of human IBD[22].

In the present study, chronic administration of zileuton normalized the colonic tissue architecture and significantly reduced MPO without significantly affecting SOD activity. The assessment of MPO activity as an index to quantify intestinal inflammation and leukocyte accumulation has been proposed[23]. MPO is an enzyme found in the neutrophils and in smaller quantities in the monocytes and macrophages. It has been reported that MPO activity is directly proportional to the number of neutrophils seen in histological sections[24]. The reduction in the MPO activity by zileuton suggests a reduction in neutrophil infiltration in the colon. In fact, neutrophils appear to be affected by increased concentration of the powerful chemotactic LTs (most notably LTB_4)[24]. Therefore, it appears that zileuton ameliorates inflammation in colitic rats through down-regulating the recruitment of neutrophils to colon via inhibiting production of 5-LOX pathway metabolites.

However, chronic administration of zileuton also caused an increase in colon PGE_2 concentration. It therefore appears that zileuton treatment leads to a shift in arachidonic metabolism towards production of prostaglandins (PGs), which in addition to reduction in MPO activity, may have played a role in the accelerated mucosal healing seen with this agent. A role of prostaglandins (namely PGE_2) has been indicated in DSS-induced colitis[25]. The PGs play a key role in the maintenance of the mucosal integrity. Administration of minute quantities of prostaglandins has been shown to provide protection against several experimental colitis models, which is suggestive of protective role of PGs in mucosal defense[26,27]. This shift of AA metabolism with 5-LOX inhibitor has been identified in some of the studies[28,29] but not significantly in others[30,31]. This discrepancy in reports may relate to the time period at which eicosanoid levels were measured. Furthermore, whether this represents a true shift in AA metabolism or stimulation of other enzymes by zileuton further along AA biosynthesis cascade remains to be determined.

To further confirm the hypothesis that a relation exists between leukotrienes and leukocyte recruitment in IBD, rats were subjected to DSS colitis and sulphasalazine, which is well established in the management of human IBD. It acts as an inhibitor of prostaglandin synthase, 5-LOX and as a free radical scavenger[32,33]. In the present study sulphasalazine significantly reduced MPO and SOD activity and increased PGE_2 contents. However, the effect of sulphasalazine was less marked for MPO activity and PGE_2 contents than that of zileuton. These findings further support the notion that the main effect of zileuton is on the synthesis of LTs and indirectly on the neutrophil accumulation.

Randomized, double blind clinical trials with zileuton (600 mg qid and 800 mg bid) have shown that the drug is well tolerated and is associated with a trend toward clinical benefit[34]. Zingarelli *et al.* showed zileuton to be effective in attenuating the colitic lesions in trinitrobenzene sulphonic acid (TNBS)-induced IBD in rats[35]. Other studies with zileuton have shown only marginal benefits, which could be due to low doses that were used[36]. Preliminary study with other 5-LOX inhibitor, BWA4C has shown *in vitro* reduction in LTB_4 in colorectal biopsy specimens[37].

In conclusion, the results of the present study clearly show that chemotactic leukotrienes are responsible for inflammatory cascade in damaged colon and, zileuton a 5-LOX inhibitor, significantly improved healing in DSS-induced colitis in rats by inhibition of neutrophil recruitment and indirectly through increase in prostaglandins (which, may be protective) at the site of inflammation.

Therefore, inhibitors of 5-LOX enzyme may be useful therapeutic tools in the treatment of chronic intestinal inflammation.

Acknowledgement

Grant support provided by Panacea Biotec Ltd., New Delhi, India to the author (VPS) as Research Associate (RA) is appreciated.

REFERENCES

1. Ponti F D & Tonini M, Irritable bowel syndrome. *Drugs,* 61 (2001) 31.
2. Riddels R H, Pathology of idiopathic inflammatory bowel disease (Lea and Febiger, Philadelphia) 1988.
3. Wallace J L, Prostaglandin biology in inflammatory bowel disease, *Gastroenterol Clin North Am,* 30 (2001) 971.
4. Sharon P & Stenson W F, Enhanced synthesis of leukotrienes by colonic mucosa in inflammatory bowel disease, *Gastroenterology,* 86 (1984) 453.
5. Donowitz M, Arachidonic acid metabolites and their role in inflammatory bowel disease. An update requiring addition of a pathway, *Gastroenterology,* 88 (1985) 580.
6. Lauritsen K, Laursen L S, Bukhave K & Rask-Nadsen J, Effects of topical 5-aminosalicylic acid and predinisolone on prostaglandin E_2 and leukotriene B_4 levels determined by equilibrium *in vivo* dialysis of rectum in relapsing ulcerative colitis, *Gastroenterology,* 91 (1986) 837.
7. Richard R H, George W C, Randy L B, Jimmie L M & Dee W B, Clinical activity of leukotriene inhibitors, *Int J Immunopharmacol,* 17 (1995) 147.
8. Pesker B M, Dreyling K W, Peskar B A, May B & Goebell H, Enhanced formation of sulfo-peptide leukotrienes in ulcerative colitis and Crohn's disease: Inhibition by sulphasalazine and 5-aminosalicylic acid, *Agents Actions,* 18 (1986) 381.
9. Vilasseca J, Salas A, Guamer F, Rodriguez R & Malagelada J R, Participation of thromboxane and other eicosanoid synthesis in the course of experimental inflammatory colitis, *Gastroenterology,* 98 (1990) 269.

10. Wallace J L, MacNaughton W K, Morris G P & Beck P 1, Inhibition of leukotriene synthesis markedly accelerates the healing in rat model of inflammatory bowel disease, *Gastroenterology,* 98 (1989) 29.

11. Rachmilewitz R, Simon P L, Schwartz L W, Griswold D E, Fondacaro J D & Wasserman M A, Inflammatory mediators of experimental colitis in rats. *Gastroenterology,* 97 (1989) 326.

12. Rask-Nadsen J, Bukhave K, Laursen L S & Lauritsen K, 5-lipoxygenase inhibitors in the treatment of inflammatory bowel disease, *Agents Actions,* (1992) C37.

13. Bell R I & Young P R, The discovery and development of zileuton : an orally active 5-lipoxygenase inhibitor, *Int J Immunopharmacol,* 14 (1992) 505.

14. Laursen L S, Naesdal J, Bukhave K & Rask Madsen J, Selective 5-lipoxygenase inhibition in ulcerative colitis, *Lancet,* 335 (1990) 683.

15. Hawkey C J & Rampton D S, Benoxaprofen in the treatment of active ulcerative colitis, *Prostaglandins Leukot Med,* 10 (1983) 405.

16. Roberts W G, Simon T J, Berlin R G, Haggit R C, Snyder E S, Stenson W F, Hanauer S B, Reagan J E, Cagliola A, Tanaka W K, Simon S & Berger M L, Leukotrienes in ulcerative colitis: Results of a multicenter trial of a leukotriene biosynthesis inhibitor, MK-591, *Gastroenterology* 112 (1997) 725.

17. Hendel J, Ahnfelt R I & Neilson O H, Expression of 5-lipoxygenase mRNA is unchanged in the colon of patients with active inflammatory bowel disease, *Inflamm Res,* 51 (2002) 423.

18. Singh V P, Patil C S, Jain N K, Singh A & Kulkarni S K, Effect of nimesulide against acetic acid-and leukotriene-induced inflammatory bowel disease in rats, *Prostaglandin lipid other med* 71 (2003) 163.

19. Hagen T M, Huang S & Curnette J, Extensive oxidative DNA damage in hepatocytes of transgenic mice with chronic hepatitis destined to develop hepatocellular carcinoma, *Proc Nalt Acad Sci* USA, 91 (1994)12808.

20. Tries S, Neupert W & Laufer S, The mechanism of action of new anti-inflammatory compound ML3000: inhibition of 5-LOX and *COX-1/2, Inflamm Res,* 51 (2002) 135.

21. Nishada T, Miwa H, Shigimatsu M, Yamamoto M, Lida M & Fijishuma M, Increased arachidonic acid composition of phospholipids in colonic mucosa from patients with active ulcerative colitis, *Gut,* 28 (1987) 1002.

22. Granados N D, Howe K & Lu J, Dextran sulfate sodium-induced colonic histopathology, but not altered epithelial ion transport, is reduced by inhibition of phosphodiesterase activity, *Am J Physiol,* 156 (2000) 2169.

23. Krawisz J E, Sharon P & Stenson W F, Quantitative assay for acute intestinal inflammation based on myeloperoxidase activity. Assessment of inflammation in rat and hamster models, *Gastroenterology* 87 (1984) 1344.

24. Lobos E A, Sharon P & Stenson W F, Chemotactic activity in inflammatory bowel disease: Role of leukotrienes, *Dig Dis Sci*, 32 (1987)1380.

25. Hirata I, Murano M & Nitta, Estimation of mucosal inflammatory mediators in DSS-induced colitis. Possible role of PGE_2 in protection against mucosal damage, *Digestion*, 63 (2001) 73.

26. Allgayer H, Deschryver K & Stenson W F, Treatment with 16,16'-dimethyl prostaglandin E_2 before and after induction of colitis with trinitro benzenesulfonic acid in rats decreases inflammation, *Gastroenterology*, 96 (1989) 1290.

27. Fedorak R N, Empey L R & MacArthur, Misprostal provides a colonic mucosal protective effect during acetic acid-induced colitis in rats, *Gastroenterology*, 98(1990) 615.

28. Empey L R, Jewell L D & Garg M L, Fish oil-enriched diet is mucosal protective against acetic acid-induced colitis in rats, *Can J Physiol Pharmacol*, 69 (1991) 480.

29. Empey L R, Walker K & Fedorak R N, Indomethacin worsens and a leukotriene biosynthesis inhibitor accelerates mucosal healing in rat colitis, *Can J Physiol Pharmacol*, 70 (1992) 660.

30. Laursen L S, Naesdal J & Bukhave K, Selective 5-lipoxygenase in ulcerative colitis, *Lancet*, 335 (1990) 683.

31. Wallace J L & Keennan C M, An orally active inhibitor of leukotriene synthesis inhibitor accelerates healing in rat model of colitis, *Am J Physiol*, 258 (1990) G527.

32. Klauritson K J, Hansen P & Baytzer K, Effects of sulphasalazine and disodium azodisalicylate on colonic PGE_2 concentrations determined by equilibrium *in vivo* dialysis of faeces in patients with ulcerative colitis and healthy controls, *Gut*, 25 (1984)1271.

33. Miyachi Y, Yoshioka A, Imamura S & Niwa Y, Effect of sulphasalazine and its metabolites on the generation of reactive oxygen species, *Gut*, 28 (1987) 190.

34. Haweky J H, Dube L M, Rountree L V, Linnen P J & Lancaster J F, A trial of zileuton versus mesalazine or placebo in the maintenance of remission of ulcerative colitis, *Gastroenterology*, 112 (1997) 718.

35. Zingarelli B, Squadrito F, Graziani P, Camerini R & Caputi A P, Effects of zileuton , a new 5-lipoxygenase inhibitor, in experimentally induced colitis in rats, *Agents Action*, 39 (1993)150.

36. Peppercorn M, Das K, Elson C, Geraci K, Robinson M, Rubin A, Salzberg B, Wruble L, Dube L & Rountree L, Zileuton, a 5-lipoxygenase inhibitor in the treatment of ulcerative colitis-A double blind placebo controlled trial (abstr), *Gastroenterology* 106 (1994) A751.

37. Hawthorne A B, Boughton-Smith N K, Whittle B J R & Haweky C J, Colorectal leukotriene B4 *in vitro* in inflammatory bowel disease: Inhibition by the selective 5-lipoxygenase inhibitor BWA4C, *Gut*, 33 (1992) 513.

Paper Published In:
I.J.E.B. (Vol. 42, July 2004, pp.667-673)

28

D_2-dopamine receptor and α_2-adrenoreceptor-mediated analgesic response of quercetin

PATTIPATI S NAIDU, AMANPREET SINGH AND S.K. KULKARNI
Pharmacology Division, University Institute of Pharmaceutical Sciences,
Panjab University, Chandigarh 160 014, India

Quercetin, a bioflavonoid (100-300 mg/kg) produced dose dependent increase in tail-flick latency, the analgesic effect being sensitive to reversal by naloxone (1 mg/kg). Prior treatment with haloperidol (1 mg/kg), D_1/D_2 receptor antagonist haloperidol, sulpiride (50 mg/kg), a selective D_2 receptor antagonist, yohimbine (5 mg/kg), a α_2-adrenoreceptor antagonist but not by SCH 23390 a selective D_1 receptor antagonist blocked this response. Apomorphine (1 mg/kg) a mixed D_1/D_2 dopamine receptor agonist, and quinpirole (0.5 mg/kg), a selective D_2 receptor agonist also produced antinociception, that was reversed by haloperidol (1 mg/kg), sulpiride (50 mg/kg), but not by yohimbine (5 mg/kg). The antinociceptive action of quercetin (200 mg/kg) was potentiated by D_2 agonist quinpirole (0.2 mg/kg). Dopamine D_1 receptor agonist SKF38393 (10 and 15 mg/kg) failed to alter the antinociceptive effect of quercetin (200 mg/kg). Quercetin (200 mg/kg) reversed reserpine (2 mg/kg-4 hr) induced hyperalgesia, which was reversed by sulpiride but not by yohimbine. Thus, a role of dopamine D_2 and α_2-adrenoreceptors is postulated in the antinociceptive action of quercetin.

Keywords : Antinociceptive action, α_2-adrenoreceptors, D_2-dopamine receptors, Pain perception, Quercetin

The complex and multidimensional nature of pain perception necessitates consideration of numerous factors that contribute to it's experience. As nociception involves sensory components and motor responses, a system is required that is capable of sensorimotor integration. The basal ganglia is a group of nuclei involved in the processing and integration of sensory and motor information and may therefore be involved in the processing of nociceptive information[1].

Considerable clinical evidences suggest that dopamine receptor-mediated mechanisms may play an important role in modulating pain in humans. Dopamine receptor stimulation in the spinal cord as well as in the supraspinal structures of the central nervous system evokes an analgesic response[2]. However, the data reported are contradictory and DA agonists have been shown to produce either antinociception[3,4] or hyperalgesia[5]. Non-selective dopamine agonists like Apomorphine[6] and the D_2 selective agonist LY 141865[7] have been shown to have antinociceptive activity whilst the D_1 agonist, SKF 38393[8] was inactive in naive animals[9]. SKF 38393 however enhanced the nociceptive threshold following supersensitization of the dopaminergic system[6]. However,.some dopamine agonists have been reported to suppress the severe pain associated with various states of disease affecting the nervous system, such as the thalamic syndrome, herpes zoster and Parkinson's disease[10-12].

The central noradrenergic system appears to play a modulatory role in the transmission of pain impulses. An interaction between dopaminergic, noradrenergic and opioid system has been suggested in modulation of pain perception[3,13]. Clonidine, B-HT 920 and guanfacine have been shown to evoke analgesic response in a variety of test procedures presumably by acting as agonists at presynaptic α_2-adrenoceptors[14]. Those studies have also indicated the possibility of a link between opioid and noradrenergic systems based on antinociceptive and electroencephalographic data obtained in animals[14,15].

Quercetin (3,5,7,3',4'-pentahydroxyflavone) is a plant polyphenolic compound widely distributed in the plant kingdom and is most abundant of the flavonoid molecules. It is found in many often consumed foods, including apple, onion, tea, berries, and brassica vegetables, as well as many seeds, nuts, flowers, barks and leaves. It is also found in medicinal plants, including *Ginkgo biloba, Hypericium perforatum* (St. John's Wort), *Sambucus canadensis* (Elder) and many others. Quercetin is reported to have many beneficial effects on human health, including cardiovascular protection, anticancer activity, antiulcer effects, anti-allergy activity, cataract prevention, and antiviral activity. Analgesic and antiinflammatory activity of quercetin was reported in a number of recent studies[16-17]. Quercetin is reported to be effective in the treatment of intestinal cystitis[18] and chronic prostatitis[19]. However, the mechanisms underlying the analgesic effect of quercetin remains unclear.

In the present study we have examined the possible involvement of dopaminergic, and noradrenergic systems in the antinociceptive effect of quercetin.

Materials and Methods

Animals: Albino mice (Laka strain) of either sex and 3 months old, bred in Central Animal House facility of the Panjab University, weighing 20-30 g were used. The animals were housed under standard laboratory conditions, maintained on a natural light and dark cycle and had free access to food and water. Animals were acclimatized to laboratory conditions before the test. Each animal was used only once. All experiments were carried out between 0900 and 1700 hrs. The experimental protocols were approved by the Institutional Ethics Committee and conducted according to the Indian National Science Academy guidelines for the use and care of experimental animals.

Antinociceptive activity: The hyperalgesic response in the tail-flick test is usually attributed to central mechanisms[20]. The nociceptive threshold was determined as the tail-flick latencies elicited in response to noxious radiant heat[21]. Baseline latencies to tail withdrawal from the radiant sources (4-6 sec) were established. A cut-off time of 10 s was observed to prevent any injury to the tail. A minimum of three trials, at 2 min intervals, were recorded for each animal before the test.

Drugs and treatment schedule: Quercetin (Sigma, St. Louis, USA), Haloperidol (Searle India, India), SCH23390 maleate (Schering Plough Co., Bloomfield, NJ.), (-) sulpiride hydrochloride (Research Biochemical Inc., Natick, MA.), SKF 38393 (1-phenyl-2,3,4,5-tetrahydro-(1H)-3-benzazepine-7,8-diol hydrochloride; Research Biochemical Inc., MA), Quinpirole (Sigma, USA), apomorphine hydrochloride (Sigma, USA), yohimbine (E-merck, Darmstadt, Germany), naloxone (Sigma, USA), reserpine (Loba Chemicals, India) were used in the present study. All drugs were administered intraperitonially in a constant volume of 1 ml/100g of body weight, either alone or in combination. Quercetin was injected 60 min before the reading and all others were injected 30 min before reading. The antagonists were administered 10 min before agonists. Reserpine (2mg/kg) was administered 4 hr before the experiment[4]. The selection of doses was based on previous reports from our laboratory and from the literature.

Statistical analysis: Values were expressed as mean±SEM. Each group contains 6-8 animals. The data was analyzed using analysis of variance (ANOVA) followed by post hoc comparisons with Tukey's test. In all tests, the criterion for statistical significance was $P < 0.05$.

Results

Effect of quercetin-, apomorphine-, SKF38393-, and quinpirole on reaction time to radiant heat in naive mice: Quercetin (100-300 mg/kg) produced dose dependent increase in antinociception. Lower doses of quercetin (25-50 mg/kg) did not show antinociceptive effect. Apomorphine (1 mg/kg), quinpirole (0.5 mg/kg) displayed significant elevation of tail-flick latency in response to radiant heat. SKF 38393 (10 and 15 mg/kg) failed to alter the tail-flick latency in naive mice (Table1).

Table 1. Effect of quercetin-, apomorphine-, SKF38393-, or quinpirole on reaction time to radiant heat in naïve mice

Group	Treatment (mg/kg)	Tail-flick latency (Mean ± SE)	
		Before	After
1	Vehicle	3.91 ±0.3	4.2±0.34
2	Quercetin (25)	3.9±0.25	4.2±0.33
3	Quercetin (50)	4.09 ±0.2	4.8 ± 0.5
4	Quercetin (100)	3.75 ± 0.25	5.2 ± 0.4[a]
5	Quercetin (200)	4.02 ±0.4	6.4 ± 0.09[a]
6	Quercetin (300)	4.2 ± 0.5	6.96 ± 0.52[a]
7	Apomorphine (1)	4.16±0.15	6.72±0.24[a]
8	Quinpirole (0.5)	3.93 ± 0.23	7.15±0.4[a]
9	SKF38393 (10)	3.99 ± 0.41	4.43 ± 0.52
10	SKF38393 (15)	4.012±0.25	4.5±0.62

[a]$P<0.05$ as compared with the basal value (before treatment) (ANOVA followed by Tukey's test).

Effect of receptor antagonists on quercetin-, apomorphine-, and quinpirole induced increase in reaction time to radiant heat in naive mice: The dopamine D_1/D_2 receptor antagonist haloperidol (1 mg/kg), the selective dopamine D_2 receptor antagonist sulpiride (50 mg/kg), an α_2-adrenoreceptor antagonist yohimbine (5 mg/kg), and an opioid antagonist naloxone (1 mg/kg), but not selective D_1 receptor antagonist SCH23390 (0.5 mg/kg) blocked the increased pain threshold to radiant heat produced by quercetin (200 mg/kg). Haloperidol (1 mg/kg) and sulpiride (50 mg/kg), blocked the antinociceptive action of apomorphine (1 mg/

kg)-, or quinpirole (0.5 mg/kg). Yohimbine (5 mg/kg) failed to modify the increased tail-flick latency produced by apomorphine or quinpirole (Table 2).

Table 2. Effect of receptor antagonists on quercetin-, apomorphine-, or quinpirole induced increase in reaction time to radiant heat in naive mice

Group	Treatment (mg/kg)	Tail-flick latency (Mean ± SE)	
		Before	After
1	Quercetin (200)	3.99 ± 0.4	6.43 ± 0.09
2	Quercetin (200) + Haloperidol (1)	4.10±0.29	5.33±0.23[a]
3	Quercetin (200) + SCH23390 (0.5)	4.13±0.12	6.52±0.16
4	Quercetin (200) + Sulpiride (50)	3.89 ± 0.42	5.01 ± 0.4[a]
5	Quercetin (200) + Yohimbine (5)	3.99 ± 0.35	5.6 ± 0.01[a]
6	Quercetin (200) + Naloxone (1)	4.01 ± 0.40	5.71 ±0.02[a]
7	Apomorphine (1)	4.16 ± 0.15	6.72 ± 0.24
8	Apomorphine (1) + Haloperidol (1)	4.06 ± 0.15	4.72 ± 0.24[b]
9	Apomorphine (1) + SCH23390 (1)	4.12 ± 0.23	6.15 ± 0.5
10	Apomorphine (1) + Sulpiride (1)	4.16 ±0.20	4.90 ± 0.04[b]
11	Apomorphine (1) + Yohimbine (1)	4.25 ± 0.30	6.82 ± 0.31[b]
12	Quinpirole (0.5)	3.93±0.23	7.15±0.4
13	Quinpirole (0.5) + Haloperidol (1)	4.16 ± 0.15	4.82 ± 0.14[c]
14	Quinpirole (0.5) + SCH23390 (1)	4.0 ± 0.13	6.95 ± 0.65
15	Quinpirole (0.5) + Sulpiride (1)	3.96±0.26	4.90±0.04[c]
16	Quinpirole (0.5) + Yohimbine (1)	4.25±0.30	7.25±0.31[c]

[a]$P < 0.05$ as compared to quercetin treated group. [b]$P < 0.05$ as compared to apomorphine treated group. [c]$P < 0.05$ as compared to quinpirole treated group (ANOVA followed by Tukey's test)

Effect of quinpirole- or SKF 38393 on reaction time to radiant heat produced by quercetin in naive mice: Concomitant administration of quinpirole (0.1 and 0.2 mg/kg) but not SKF 38393 (10 and 15 mg/kg) with quercetin (100 mg/kg) dose dependently produced a significant potentiation of quercetin-induced increase in reaction time to the radiant heat in a sulpiride (50 mg/kg) sensitive manner (Table 3).

Effect of sulpiride or yohimbine on antinociceptive action of quercetin or quinpirole in 4 hr reserpinized mice: Reserpine (2 mg/kg) administered 4 hr before the experiment, produced a significant reduction in pain threshold to radiant heat. Quercetin (200 mg/kg), or quinpirole (0.5 mg/kg) reversed the reserpine-induced reduction in tail-flick latency. Sulpiride (50 mg/kg) but not yohimbine (5 mg/kg) antagonized the quercetin-, or quinpirole reversal of reserpine-induced hyperalgesia (Table 4).

Table 3. Effect of quinpirole-, or SKF 38393 on reaction time to radiant heat produced by quercetin

Group	Treatment (mg/kg)	Tail-flick latency (Mean ± SE)	
		Before	After
1	Quercetin (100)	3.95±0.25	5.20±0.40[a]
2	Quinpirole (0.1)	3.93 ±0.23	4.15±0.40[a]
3	Quinpirole (0.2)	4.01 ±0.13	4.70±0.12
4	Quercetin (100) + Quinpirole (0.1)	3.99±0.21	6.33±0.03[b]
5	Quercetin (100) + Quinpirole (0.2)	4.01 ±0.10	8.18±0.23[c]
6	Quercetin (100) + Quinpirole (0.1) + Sulpiride (50)	3.95±0.23	4.96±0.40[d]
7	Quercetin (100) + Quinpirole (0.2) + Sulpiride (50)	4.03 ±0.42	6.10±0.32[e]

[a]$P < 0.05$ as compared to basal values (Before treatment). [b]$P < 0.05$ as compared to group 1 and 2. [c]$P < 0.05$ as compared to group 1 and 3. [d]$P < 0.05$ as compared to group 4. [e]$P < 0.05$ as compared to group 5 (ANOVA followed Tukey's test).

Discussion

Quercetin, a bioflavonoid produced a dose dependent increase of tail-flick latency in naive mice. Of the several putative neurotransmitters that may be involved with basal ganglia modulation of nociceptive information at both spinal and supraspinal levels, dopamine has been proposed to play an important role [22]. Apomorphine, a dopamine D_1/D_2 receptor agonist, quinpirole, a dopamine D_2 receptor agonist also displayed antinociceptive activity. The selective D_1 receptor, agonist however, failed to modify the reaction. This is in accordance with previous reports, where SKF 38393 did not show antinociceptic activity in naïve animals[6,23]. Quinpirole, a D_2 receptor agonist and clonidine an α_2 receptor agonist also displayed antinociceptive activity further supporting the role of dopamine D_2 and α_2 receptors in the pain perception.

Table 4. Effect of sulpiride or yohimbine on antinociceptive action of quercetin or quinpirole in 4 hr reserpinized mice

Group	Treatment (mg/kg)	Tail-flick latency (Mean ± SE)	
		Before	After
1	Reserpine (2)	4.33±0.02	1.98±0.23*
2	Reserpine (2) + Quercetin (200)	4.29±0.25	5.60±0.40^{a}
3	Reserpine (2) + Quinpirole (0.5)	3.93±0.23	5.35±0.40^{a}
4	Reserpine (2) + Quercetin (200) + Sulpiride (50)	3.89 ± 0.05	4.33±0.04^{b}
5	Reserpine (2) + Quercetin (200) + Yohimbine (5)	4.01±0.13	5.40±0.12
6	Reserpine (2) + Quinpirole (0.5) + Sulpiride (50)	3.99±0.21	4.33±0.03^{c}
7	Reserpine (2) + Quinpirole (0.5) + Yohimbine (5)	4.01 ±0.10	5.48±0.23

$^{*}P < 0.05$ as compared to basal latency (before treatment). $^{a}P < 0.05$ as compared to group 1. $^{b}P < 0.05$ as compared to group 2. $^{c}P < 0.05$ as compared to group 3 (ANOVA followed Tukey's test).

Stimulation of D_2 receptors by LY 141865[6] and α_2-arenoceptors by clonidine[24] has also been shown to produce antinociceptive activity. Previous studies showed that D_2 agonists do not show antinociceptive effects at doses, which stimulate presynaptic receptors[25]. Therefore, the possibility of involvement of presynaptic D_2 receptors in the antinociceptive effect is rare.

The combination of quinpirole and quercetin produced a significant increase in the analgesic response due to quercetin. The potentiating response of the combination was blocked by haloperidol, a mixed D_1/D_2 receptor antagonist and D_2 receptor antagonist sulpiride but not D_1 selective antagonist SCH 23390. This suggested that the antinociceptive action of quercetin is mediated by D_2 receptor activation. Further, the antinociceptive action of quercetin was blocked by the α_2-antagonist, yohimbine suggesting the possible role of α_2-adrenergic system in the antinociceptive activity of quercetin. Reserpine, administered 4 hr before the experiment produced hyperalgesia that was accompanied by sedation, ptosis and diarrhoea. Reserpine-induced hyperalgesia was reversed by quercetin. The reversing action was blocked by sulpiride but not by yohimbine. These observations indicated that quercetin-induced antinociception in reserpine-treated animals was D_2 mediated response. The hyperalgesic action of reserpine could be attributed to its ability to deplete catecholamines or 5-hydroxytryptamine[26] and as such be reversed by dopamine agonist like apomorphine. Precursors of catecholamines and 5-hydroxytryptamine have been reported to reverse the behavioral and biochemical changes caused by reserpine[27].

The attenuation of the antinocioceptive action of quercetin by sulpiride a selective D_2 antagonist and yohimbine, an α_2-adrenoreceptor antagonist suggest that quercetin-induced antinociception is mediated by postsynaptic D_2 dopamine as well as α_2-adrenoreceptos. Thus, the antinociceptive effect of quercetin appears to be complex and may involve more than one type of receptors. Moreover, the failure of yohimbine to block antinociceptive effect of quercetin in reserpine treated animals (postsynaptic D_2 receptor mediated) suggests that the antinociceptive action of quercetin could predominantly be a D_2 receptor mediated response. The blockade of the antinociceptive effect of quercetin by naloxone, however, suggests the possible existence of an interaction between dopamine D_2 receptors and opioid receptor system in the antinociceptive action of drugs.

Acknowledgement

One of the authors (PSN) is a recipient of Senior Research Fellowship of CSIR, New Delhi.

REFERENCES

1. Chudler E H, Sugiyama K & Dong W K, Nociceptive responses of neurons in the neostriatum and globus pallidus of the rat, *J Neurophysiol,* 69 (1993)1890.
2. Fleetwood-Walker S M & Hope P J, A selective antinociceptive effect of the diencephalic dopaminecontaining cell group, A11 on dorsal horn neurons in the rats, *J Physiol, 47* (1985) 364.
3. Akil H & Liebeskind J L, Monoaminergic mechanisms of stimulations produced analgesia, *Brain Res,* 94 (1975) 279.
4. Verma A & Kulkarni S K, Modulatory role of D1 and D2 dopamine receptor subtypes in nociception in mice, *J Psychopharmacol, 7* (1993) 270.
5. Tulunay F C, Sparber S B & Takemori A E, The effect of dopaminergic stimulation and blockade on the nociceptive responses in the mice, *Eur J Pharmacol,* 33 (1975) 65.
6. Jensen T S & Yaksh T L, Effects of an intrathecal dopamine agonist apomorphine on the thermal and chemical evoked noxious responses in rats, *Brain Res,* 296 (1984) 285.

7. Barasi S, Ben-sreti M M, Clatworthy A L, Duggal K N, Gonzalez J P, Robertson J, Rooney K F & Sewell R D E, Dopamine receptor-mediated spinal antinociception in the normal and haloperidol pretreated rat: Effects of sulpiride and SCH 23390, *Br J Pharmacol*, 90 (1987) 15.

8. Setler P E, Sarau H M, Zircle C L & Saunders H L, The central effects of a novel dopamine agonist, *Eur J Pharmacol*, 50 (1978) 419.

9. Ben-sreti M M, Gonzalez J P & Sewell R D E, Differential effects of SKF 38393 and LY141865 on nociception and morphine analgesia, *Life Sci*, 33 (1983) 665.

10. Miley D P, Abrams A A, Atkinson J H & Janowsky D S, Successful treatment of thalamic pain with apomorphine, *Am J Psychiat*, 135 (1978) 1230.

11. Kernbaum S & Hauchecome J, Administration of levodopa for relief of herpes zoster pain, *JAMA*, 246 (1981) 132.

12. Nutt J G & Cart J H, Sensory symptoms in parkinsonism related to central dopaminergic function, *Lancet*, 2 (1984) 456.

13. Pollard H, Llorens C & Schwartz J C, Localization of opiate receptors and enkephalins in the rat striatum in relationship with the nigrostriatal dopaminergic system: Lesion studies, *Brain Res*, 151 (1978) 392.

14. Parale M P & Kulkarni S K, Apparent pA_2 estimates for the antinociceptive receptor, *Arch Int Pharmacodyn Ther*, *275* (1985) 59.

15. Kulkarni S K, Parale M P & Nayar U, Morphine-like effects of α_2-adrenoreceptor agonists on cortical EEG pattern of rats, *Indian J Exp Biol*, 24 (1986) 259.

16. Guardia T, Rotelli A E, Juarez A O & Pelzer L E, Antiinflammatory properties of plant flavonoids. Effects of rutin, quercetin and hesperidin on adjuvant arthritis in rat, *Farmaco*, 56 (2001) 683.

17. Sanchez de Medina F, Vera B, Galyez J & Zarzuelo A, Effect of quercetin on the early stages of hapten induced colonic inflammation in the rat, *Life Sci*, 70 (2002) 3097.

18. Katske F, Shoskes D A, Sender M, Poliakin R, Gagliano K & Rajfer J, Treatment of interstitial cystitis with a quercetin supplement, *Tech Urol*, 7 (2001) 44.

19. Shokes D, Use of bioflavonoid quercetin in patients with long-standing chronic prostatitis, *J Am Neutraceut Assoc*, 2 (1999) 18.

20. Kannan S A, Saade N E, Haddad J J, Abdelnoor A M, Atweh S F, Jabbur S J & Garabedian B S, Endotoxin-induced local inflammation and hyperalgesia in rats and mice: A new model for inflammatory pain, *Pain*, 66 (1996) 373.

21. Kulkarni S K, Heat and other physiological stress-induced analgesia: catecholamine mediated naloxone reversible response, *Life Sci, 27* (1980) 185.

22. Chudler E H & Dong W K, The role of the basal ganglia in nociception and pain. *Pain,* 60 (1995) 3.

23. Magnusson J E & Fisher K, The involvement of dopamine in nociception: The role of D_1 and D_2 receptors in the dorsolateral striatum, *Brain Res,* 855 (2000) 260.

24. Kulkarni S K & Verma A, Clonidine analgesia, *Drugs Today,* 30 (1997) 211.

25. Verma A & Kulkarni S K, Differential role of dopamine receptor subtypes in thermoregulation and stereotypic behavior in naive and reserpinized rats, *Arch Int Pharmacodyn Ther,* 324 (1993) 17.

26. Kulkarni S K & Robert R K, Reversal by serotonergic agents of reserpine-induced hyperalgesia in rats, *Eur J Pharmacol,* 83 (1982) 325.

27. Carlson A, Lindquist M & Magnusson T, 3,3-dihydroxy phenylalanine and 5-hydroxytryptamine as reserpine antagonists, *Nature,* 180 (1957)1200.

Paper Published In:
I.J.E.B. (Vol. 41, December 2003, pp.1400-1404)

29

Antinociceptive action of FK506 in mice

AMANPREET SINGH, GAURAV KUMAR, PATTIPATI S. NAIDU, AND S.K. KULKARNI

Pharmacology Division, University Institute of Pharmaceutical Sciences, Panjab University, Chandigarh 160 014, India

Immunophilins are abundantly present in the brain as compared to the immune system. Immunophilin-binding agents like FK506 are known to inactivate neuronal nitric oxide synthase (nNOS) by inhibiting calcineurin and decrease the production of nitric oxide. Nitric oxide is involved in the mediation of nociception at the spinal level. In the present study, the effect of FK506 on the tail flick response in mice and the possible involvement of NO-L-arginine pathway in this paradigm was evaluated. FK506 (0.5, 1 and 3 mg/kg, ip) produced a significant antinociception in the tail flick test. Nitric oxide synthase (NOS) inhibitor L-NAME significantly and dose dependently (10-40 mg/kg, ip) potentiated the FK506 (0.5 mg/kg)-induced antinociception. On the other hand, NOS substrate L-arginine (100, 200 and 400 mg/kg) inhibited the FK506-induced antinociception in a dose-dependent manner. Concomitant administration of L-NAME (20 and 40 mg/kg) with L-arginine (200 mg/kg) blocked the inhibition exerted by L-arginine on the FK506-induced antinociception. Thus, it was concluded that NO-L-arginine pathway may be involved in the FK506-induced antinociception in tail flick test.

Keywords: Antinociception, FK506, Mice

Nitric oxide (NO) is an important mediator of various physiological functions in the central and peripheral nervous systems[1]. It has been demonstrated to have pro-nociceptive activity in the spinal cord[2,3]. NO donors, like L-arginine enhanced the release of substance P and calcineurin gene-related peptide which are involved in nociception in the spinal cord[4]. On the other hand nitric oxide synthase (NOS) inhibitors like L-NAME potentiated the antinociceptive response in tail flick assays[5].

FK506 (tacrolimus), an immunosuppressant drug isolated from *Streptomyces tsukubaensis,* is used worldwide to prevent allograft rejection and with relatively diminished side effects, notably nephrotoxicity[6]. FK506 has shown neuroprotective effect against 6-OHDA-induced toxicity in mice[7] and also reduced the increased level of TNF-alpha level in the nigrostriatal dopaminergic region injured by 6-OHDA in rats[8]. It has been shown that immunophilins protein receptors for immunosuppressant drugs like cyclosporine and FK506, are widely distributed in the brain as compared to immune system[9]. One of the important roles of immunophilins in the neural functions envisaged is the regulation of NO-induced neurotoxicity[10]. FK506 by inhibiting calcineurin[6] indirectly reduces the catalytic activity of nNOS thereby decreasing NO production. Thus it provides neuroprotection like other NOS inhibitors[9].

As stated above NOS plays an important role in both nociception and antinociception. In the present study, the nNOS inactivating property of FK506 was utilized to examine its role in the modulation of tail flick response. Further, the possible involvement of L-arginine NO pathway in this response was evaluated.

Materials and Methods

Animals: Male albino mice (Laka strain) of either sex (20-30g), bred in Central Animal House facility of the Panjab University were used. The animals were housed under standard laboratory conditions, maintained on a natural light and dark cycle and had free access to food and water. Animals were acclimatized to laboratory conditions before the test. All experiments were carried out between 0900 and 1700 hrs. The experimental protocols were approved by the Institutional Ethics Committee and conducted according to the Indian National Science Academy guidelines for the use and care of experimental animals. Each mouse was used only once and each treatment group consisted of 6 animals.

Tail-flick test (radiant heat-induced nociception): The analgesic response was determined by measuring the tail-flick latency to radiant heat[11]. The baseline latency to the tail withdrawal from the radiant heat source (3-5 s) was established. A cut- off time of 10 s was used to prevent any injury to the tail. Three trials were recorded for each animal to calculate the mean basal latency. The increase in latency (nociceptive threshold) was recorded at, 30, 60, 120, 180, 240 and 340 min after drug administration. The observer was unaware of the specific treatment schedule while performing the experiments.

Drugs: The following drugs were used: FK506 (supplied by Archer Chemicals, Mumbai, India), L-arginine (Himedia, Mumbai, India) and L-NAME (Sigma. St. Louis, USA). FK506 was suspended in 0.5% carboxymethyl cellulose. L-arginine, and L-NAME were dissolved in saline. All drugs were administered intraperitoneally (ip). Control animals received corresponding amount of vehicle (0.5% carboxymethyl cellulose) or saline.

Treatment schedule: In the first group of animals, the effect of acute administration of FK506 (0.5-3 mg/kg) on tail flick response was assessed 30, 60, 120, 240 and 300 min after the drug administration. The second group of mice received L-NAME (10, 20 and 40 mg/kg) 30 min before the administration of FK506 (0.5 mg/kg). Third group of mice received L-arginine (50, 100, 200 and 400 mg/kg) 30 min before the administration of FK506 (3 mg/kg). Two other groups received L-NAME (20 and 40 mg/kg) concomitantly with L-arginine 30 min before the administration FK506 (3 mg/kg).

Statistical analysis: Results were expressed as mean ± SE. The significance in the difference in responses to various treatment groups in comparison to the control was determined by one-way analysis of variance (ANOVA) followed by Dunnet's test. $P < 0.05$ was considered statistically significant:

Results

Effect of FK506 on tail flick latency and its modification by L-NAME and L-arginine: Administration of FK506 (0.5-3mg/kg) produced analgesia as it increased the tail flick latency with the maximum effect being observed with 3 mg/kg after 2 hr of drug administration ($P<0.05$) (Fig. 1).

A lower dose (20 mg/kg) of L-NAME, a NOS inhibitor did not produce any significant change in tail flick latency, while a higher dose (40 mg/kg) increased the latency. Pretreatment with L-NAME significantly potentiated the antinociceptive effect of FK506 (0.5 mg/kg) (Fig. 2). L-arginine, a NO donor and a NOS substrate showed a significant nociceptive effect *per se* in doses studied (100, 200 and 400 mg/kg). There was a significant reduction in tail flick latency at 200 and 400 mg/kg doses. Pretreatment with L-arginine also reversed the antinociceptive effect of FK506 (3 mg/kg). At a dose of 200 mg/kg, L-

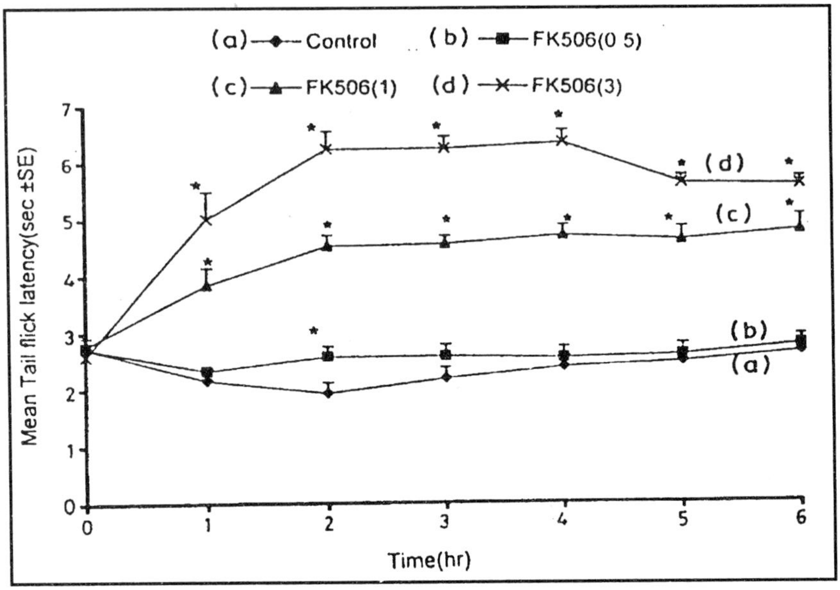

Fig. 1. Time and dose-dependent antinociception induced by acute administration of FK506, (0.5-3 mg/kg, ip). Values are mean±SE. *$P<0.05$ as compared to the vehicle treated group (n=5-8).

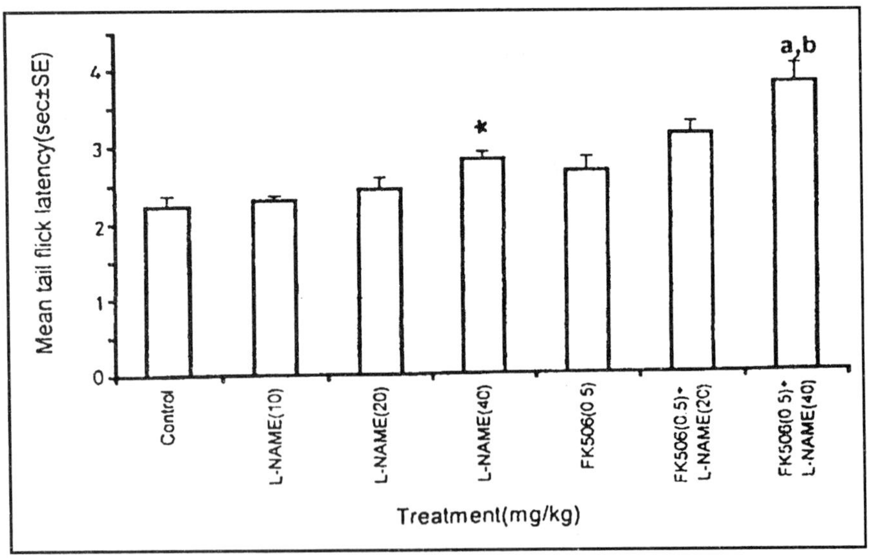

Fig. 2. Effect of L-NAME (10, 20 and 40 mg/kg, ip) on the antinociceptive action of FK506 (0.5 mg/kg. ip). L-NAME was administered 30 min and 150 min before the tail flick test. Values are mean ±SE. *P* values: * <0.05 as compared to the vehicle treated group . [a] <0.05 as compared to the FK506 (0.5 mg/kg) treated group (n= 5-8); [b] <0.05 as compared to the L-NAME (40 mg/kg) treated group.

arginine completely inhibited the FK506-induced antinociception, while the higher dose of L-arginine (400 mg/kg) produced pronociception in FK506 treated animals (Fig. 3). Concomitant administration of L-NAME (20 and 40 mg/kg) with L-arginine (200 mg/kg) reversed the L-arginine-induced inhibition of FK506 (3 mg/kg) antinociception (Fig.4).

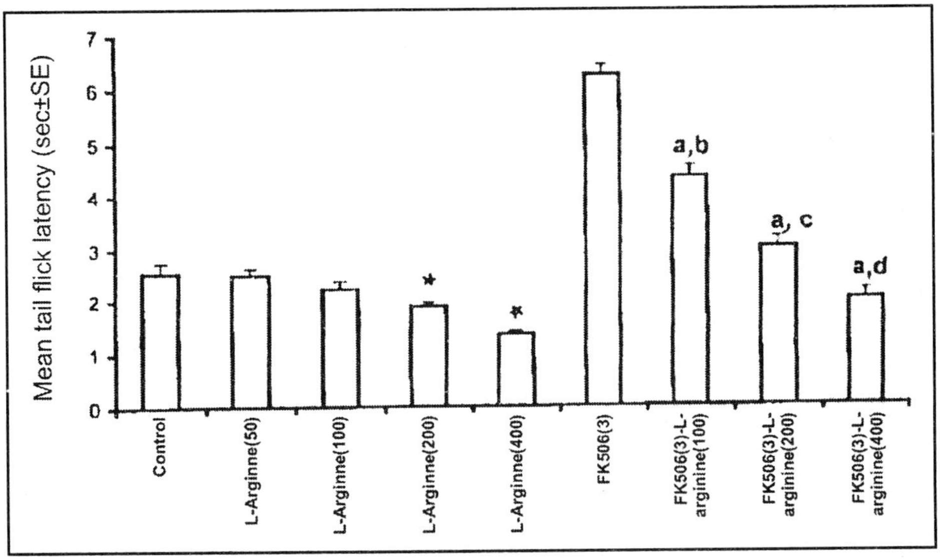

Fig. 3. Effect of L-arginine (50, 100, 200 and 400 mg/kg, ip) on the antinociceptive action of FK506 (3 mg/kg, ip). L-Arginine was administered for 30 min and 150 min before the tail flick test. Values are mean±SE. *P* values: * < 0.05 as compared to the vehicle treated group. [a]<0.05 as compared to the FK506 (3 mg/kg) treated group (n=5-8). [b,c,d]<0.05 as compared to the L-arginine (100, 200, 400 mg/kg) respectively treated group.

Discussion

In acute administration of FK506 produced antinociceptive effect in the tail-flick assay. L-arginine, a NOS substrate completely and dose dependently reversed the antinociceptive effect of FK506, L-NAME, a NOS inhibitor on the other hand potentiated the effect of FK506.

Immunophilins are the receptor proteins for the major immunosuppressant drugs such as cyclosporine A, FK506 and rapamycin[12]. The majority of the research on immunophilins and their ligands has focused on the cells of the immune system, especially lymphocytes, but the findings that immunophilins are abundantly present in the nervous system have lead to the investigations on the role of immunophilins in the neural functions. These include regulation of NO toxicity, neurotransmitter release, intercellular calcium flux, as well as neurotrophic influences with possible therapeutic potentials[13,14].

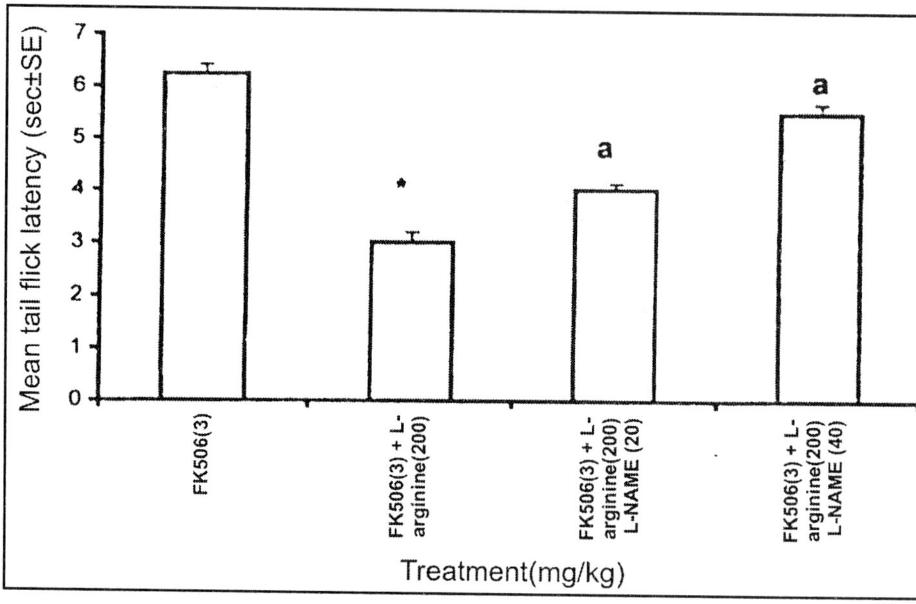

Fig. 4. Effect of concomitant administration of L-NAME (10, 20 and 40 mg/kg) with L-arginine (200 mg/kg, ip) on the antinociceptive action of FK506 (3 mg/kg, ip). L-NAME and L-arginine was administered 30 min and 150 min before the tail flick test. Values are mean±SE. *P* values: *<0.05 as compared to the FK506 treated group: ^{a}<0.05 as compared to the FK506 (3 mg/kg) + L-arginine (200 mg/kg) treated group (n=5-8)

In the nervous system, FK506 by binding to calcineurin, increases the phosphorylated levels of nNOS causing a reduction in the catalytic levels of nNOS; which may contribute to the neuroprotective effect as shown by other NOS inhibitors[9]. The doses employed in the present study have been reported to be insufficient to prevent rejection of neuronal transplants in the rat[15] and hence appears to lack immunosuppressive effects. However, FK506 has been shown to exhibit neuroprotection even in very small doses (% of the immunosuppressive dose) in animal models of neuroprotection[16].

Nociception mechanism(s) known are well reported to involve L-arginine NO pathway. The findings that L-NAME produces antinociception at high doses and L-arginine produces nociception are in accordance with previous reports[17]. The inhibitors of NOS can produce antinociception at high doses and NOS substrates may have *per se* antinociceptive effect, respectively.

Interestingly, in the present study L-NAME dose dependently potentiated the FK506-induced antinociception. A reduction in the activity of the NOS in the nervous system could be the probable mechanism of FK506-induced antinociception. The reversal of FK506-induced antinociception by L-arginine or facilitation further supports this hypothesis. FK506-induced antinociception was abolished by lower dose of L-arginine (100 mg/kg); at this dose it did not produce any nociception *per se.* Thus, the increased NO synthesis due to L-arginine may have compensated for the decreased NOS activity due to FK506.

Concomitant administration of L-NAME with L-arginine blocked the inhibitory effect of L-arginine on FK506-induced antinociception in a dose-dependent manner. This further confirms the hypothesis that FK506 has a modulatory effect on NOS and thus NO synthesis. This is in accordance with the fact that L-NAME in a dose dependent manner reverses the effect of L-arginine in morphine analgesia[18].

FK506 and other non-immunosuppressive derivatives are in clinical trials for their use in CNS disorders such as Parkinson and Alzheimer's diseases but there are no reports till date on the clinical use of FK506 as an antinociceptive agent. Further studies are required to establish the use of FK506 and other nonimmunosuppressive derivates as analgesics clinically. In conclusion, FK506 produces an antinociceptive response in a dose dependent manner on acute systemic administration and the possible involvement of NO L-arginine pathway in its antinociception actions is suggested.

REFERENCES

1. Colasanti M & Suzuki H, The dual personality of NO, *Trends Pharmacol Sci,* 21 (2000) 249.
2. Haley J F, Dickenson A H & Schatcher M, Electrophysiological evidence for a role of nitric oxide in prolonged chemical nociception in rat, *Neuropharmacology,* 31 (1992) 51.
3. Meller S T & Gebhart G F, Nitric oxide (NO) nociceptive processing in the spinal chord, *Pain,* 52 (1993) 123.
4. Garry M G, Richardson J D & Hergreavcs K M. Sodium nitroprusside evokes the release of immunoreactive calcitonin gene related peptide and substance P from dorsal horn slices via nitric oxide dependent and nitric oxide independent mechanism, *J Neurosci,* 14 (1994) 4329.

5. Meller S T, Pechman P S, Gebhart G F & Maves H, Nitric oxide mediates the thermal hyperalgesia produced in the model of neuropathic pain in the rat, *Neuroscience,* 50 (1992) 7.

6. Starzl T E, Todo S, Fung J, Demetris A J, Venkatarantman R & Jain A, FK 506 for liver, kidney, and pancreas transplantation, *Lancet,* 2 (1989) 1000.

7. Tanaka K, Fuiita N, Iligashi Y & Ogawa N, Neuroprotective and antioxidant properties of FKBP-binding inmiunophilin ligands are independent on the FKBP12 pathway in human cells, *Neurosci Lett,* 330(2002)147.

8. Mogi M, Togari A, Tanaka K, Ogawa N, Ichinose H & Nagatsu T, Increase in level of tumor necrosis factor- alpha in 6-hydroxymine striatum lesioned rats is suppressed by immunosuppressant FK506, *Neurosci Lett,* 289 (2000) 165.

9. Synder S H, Sabatini D M, Lai M M, Steiner J P, Hamilton G S & Suzdak P D. Neural actions of immunophilin ligands, *Trends Pharmacol Sci,* 19 (1998) 21.

10. Cameron A M, Nucifora F C, Fung F F, Livingston D J, Aldape R A, Rocs C A & Synder S H, FKBP 12 binds the inositol 1,4,5 triphosphate receptor at leucine-proline (1400-14001) and anchors calcineurin to this FK506 like domain, *J Biol Chem,* 272 (1997) 27582.

11. Jain N K, Kulkarni S K & Singh A, Role of cysteinyl leukotrienes in nociceptive and inflammatory conditions in experimental animals, *Eur J Pharmacol,* 423 (2001) 85.

12. Freman D A, Klee C B, Bierer B E & Burakoff S J, Calcineurin phosphatase activity in T-lymphocyte is inhibited by FK506 and cyclosporine A, *Proc Natl Acad Sci USA.* 89 (1992) 3686

13. Sharkey J & Butcher S P, Immunophilins mediate the immunoprotective effect of FK506 in focal cerebral ischaemia, *Nature,* 371 (1994) 336.

14. Rao M R, Kanji V K, Salahudeen M K, Wang C & Shekhar V, Inhibition of rat brain nitric oxide synthase activity by cyclosporin- A, *Indian J Exp Biol,* 34 (1996) 1265.

15. Sakai K, Date I, Yoshimoto Y, Arisawa T, Nakashima H, Furuta T, Asari S & Ohmoto T, The effect of a new immunosuppressive agent, FK506, on xenogeneic neural transplantation in rodents, *Brain Res, 565* (1991) 167.

16. Kihara M. Kamijo M, Nakasaka Y, Mitsui M. Takahashi M & Schmelzer J, A small dose of the immunosuppressive agent FK506 (Tacrolimus) protects peripheral nerve from ischemic fiber degeneration, *Muscle & Nerve,* 24 (2001) 1601.

17. Houmayoun H, Bahaie A, Gharib B, Etminani A, Khavandgar, S, Mani A & Dehpour A H, The involvement of nitric oxide in the antinociception induced by cyclosporin A in mice, *Pharmacol Biochem Behav,* 72 (2602) 267.

18. Brignola G, Calignano A & Di Rosa M. Modulation of morphine antinociception in the mouse by endogenous nitric oxide, *Br J Pharmacol,* 72 (1994) 74.

—•—

Paper Published In:
I.J.E.B. (Vol. 41, December 2003, pp.1405-1409)

30

Analgesic and anti-inflammatory effects of phosphodiesterase inhibitors

ANIL KUMAR, NAVEEN K. JAIN AND S.K. KULKARNI
Pharmacology Division, University Institute of Pharmaceutical Sciences, Panjab University, Chandigarh 160 014, India

The aim of the present study was to investigate the role of phosphodiesterase (PDE) enzyme inhibitors namely rolipram and theophylline in pain and inflammation in experimental animals. Rolipram, a selective PDE IV inhibitor and theophylline a nonspecific PDE inhibitor exerted dose dependent analgesic and anti-inflamamtory effect against acetic acid-induced writhing in mice and carrageenan-induced paw edema in rats, respectively. Nimesulide (1, 2 mg/kg) produced significant anti-inflammatory effect. Further, nimesulide (0.5 mg/kg) potentiated analgesic effect of rolipram but it failed to modulate the anti-inflammatory effect of PDE inhibitors. Present study suggests that PDE enzymes might be playing a role in nociceptive and inflammatory responses in animals.

Phosphodiesterase (PDE) enzymes occur widely in the biological system and present in the mammalian tissues except in red blood cells[1]. The cyclic nucleotide phosphodiesterases are responsible for degrading the second messenger cyclic nucleotides cAMP and cGMP which are involved in a wide range of physiological processes[2,3]. At least 8 distinct cyclic nucleotide phosphodiesterase isoenzymes (PDE 1-8) have been identified on the basis of their functional characteristics, such as substrate specificity, cellular distribution and susceptibility to selective inhibitors[4]. PDE type 4 (PDE 4) is characterised by cAMP specificity, and sensitivity to inhibition by rolipram[5,6]. PDE 4 inhibitors have shown anti-inflammatory effects due to induction of adenylate cyclase which leads to increase in the intracellular level of cAMP.

Since cAMP suppresses inflammatory cells activities thus inducing relaxation of airway smooth muscle. Furthermore, PDE inhibitors are also able to block production of cytokines i.e. IL-5, IL-6, IL-8 and tumor necrosis factor-α (TNF-α), a proinflammatory mediators which appears to be closely related to inflammatory response[7].

Present study mainly investigate the analgesic, anti-inflammatory effects of selective PDE4 inhibitor rolipram, and nonspecific PDE inhibitor theophylline in acetic acid induced writhing reflex and carrageenan induced paw edema, respectively.

Materials and Methods

Animals: Albino mice (Laka strain, 20-30 g) and rats (Portan strain, 200-250 g) of either sex, bred in Central Animal House, Panjab University, Chandigarh, were housed under standard laboratory conditions with free access to food and water. All experiments were carried out between 0900 and 1700 hr.

Procedure

***Analgesic study**: Writhing test (acetic acid writhing assay)*

1 % acetic acid solution (1 ml/100 g) was used to produce writhing in mice. The severity of pain response (writhing) was assessed by counting number of wriths (constriction of abdomen, turning of trunk (twist) and extension of hind legs) in mice[8]. Number of wriths per animal was counted during a 20 min session beginning 3 min after the injection of acetic acid.

Analgesic activity was calculated as % maximum possible effect (% MPE) using the following relation[9].

$$\% \text{ MPE} = \frac{100 \times (\text{Mean of wriths in control group - Mean of wriths in treated group})}{\text{Mean of wriths in control group}}$$

Anti-inflammatory study–Carrageenan-induced paw edema

Acute edema was induced in the right hind paw of rats by injecting 0.1 ml of freshly prepared 1 % solution of carrageenan (type IV). The left paw served as control (non-inflammed paw) for comparison (0.1 ml of 0.9% w/v saline).

The carrageenan was injected under the planter region of right hind paw and paw volumes were measured using plethysmometer (water displacement, UGO BASILE, Italy) at 15, 30, 60, 90, 120, 150, 180, 210 and 240 min. after carrageenan challenge. Percent increase in paw volumes were calculated and expressed as amount of inflammation[10,11].

$$\% \text{ increase in paw volume} = \frac{100 \times (\text{Paw volume of right paw} - \text{Paw volume of left paw})}{\text{Paw volume of left paw}}$$

Drugs

Rolipram (Schering, Aktiengesellschaft, Berlin), Theophylline (Sigma), Nimesulide (Panacea Biotec, New Delhi), Carrageenan type IV (Sigma), Acetic acid (Sarabhai chemicals, Baroda). Rolipram was suspended in 0.5% carboxymethyl cellulose. Rolipram and theophylline were given intraperiotoneally (ip) 30 min before acetic acid or carrageenan challenge. Carrageenan (1% w/v) was injected in single dose 0.1 ml per paw constantly.

Statistical analysis

Results were expressed as mean ± SEM. and subjected to one way analysis of variance (ANOVA) followed by Student's t-test. $P < 0.05$ were considered significant.

Results

Analgesic activity : *Writhing assay*

Intraperitoneally administered theophylline (2, 4, 8 mg/kg) produced significantly increase ($P < 0.05$) in the pain threshold against acetic acid induced writhing in a dose-dependent manner. Theophylline (8 mg/kg) produced 51.05% MPE.

Rolipram (1, 2 mg/kg ip) also produced significant analgesic effect ($P < 0.05$) against acetic acid-induced writhing response. Nimesulide (0.5, 1 mg/kg) exerted analgesic effect. Co-administration of nimesulide (1 mg/kg) with varying doses of theophylline (4, 8 mg/kg) did not potentiate the analgesic effect of theophylline, however it (nimesulide 0.5 mg/kg) significantly potentiated the analgesic effect of rolipram (1, 2 mg/kg) (Table l, 2).

Anti-inflamamtory activity : *Carrageenan induced paw edema*

Carrageenan (1%) produced significant increase in paw volume in control group. Theophylline (4, 8, 10 mg/kg ip) produced dose dependent (after 90 min) protective effect against carrageenan-induced inflammation as compared to control group (P < 0.05, Fig. 1). Rolipram (2, 5 mg/kg, ip) produced significant anti-inflammatory effect (Fig. 2). Nimesulide (0.5, 1 mg/kg) also produced significant anti-inflammatory effect as compared to control (P < 0.05). When nimesulide (0.5, 1 mg/kg) was given in combination with rolipram (2 mg/kg) or theophylline (8 mg/kg), it failed to modify the antiinflammatory effect of rolipram and theophylline (Fig. 3 and 4).

Table 1. Effect of theophylline, nimesulide and their combinations on acetic acid induced writhing in mice

Treatment	Dose (mg/kg, ip)	n	No. of wriths in 20 min (Mean ± S.E)	Antinociceptive action (% MPE)
Control	(1% acetic acid 10 ml/kg)	24	53.83 ± 1.14	–
Theophylline	2	6	40.50 ± 1.28*	24.76
Theophylline	4	6	31.16 ± 4.88*	42.11
Theophylline	8	6	26.50 ± 0.84*	50.77
Nimesulide	1	6	34.83 ± 4.26*	35.29
Nimesulide + Theophylline	1, 4	6	36.5+ 1.99^{NS}	32.19
Nimesulide + Theophylline	1, 8	6	29.80 ± 3.68^{NS}	44.64

* $P < 0.05$ as compared with control
^{NS} : theophylline *per se.*

Table 2. Effect of rolipram, nimesulide and their combinations on acetic-acid induced writhing in mice

Treatment	Dose (mg/kg, ip)	n	No. of wriths in 20 min (Mean ± S.E)	Antinociceptive action (% MPE)
Control	(1% acetic acid 10 ml/kg)	24	53.83 ± 1.14	–
Rolipram	1	6	38.83 ± 6.04*	27.86
Rolipram	2	6	29.00 ± 4.09*	46.12
Nimesulide	0.5	6	50.33±4.95*	6.50
Nimesulide + Rolipram	0.5, 1	6	24.83±3.44*^{0}	53.87
Nimesulide + Rolipram	0.5, 2	6	15.83 ± 1.04*^{0}	70.59

* $P < 0.05$ as compared with control
$P^{0} < 0.05$ compared with rolipram *per se.*

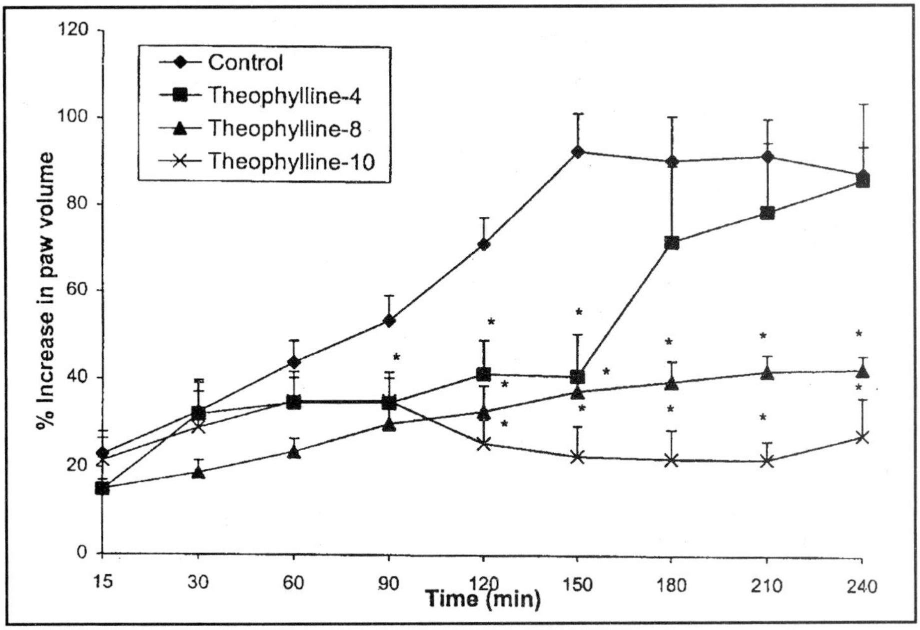

Fig. 1. Effect of various doses (4, 8, 10 mg/kg, i.p) of theophylline on carrageenan-induced paw edema in rats. Vertical lines show mean ± SE * $P < 0.05$ as compared with control. (n = 6)

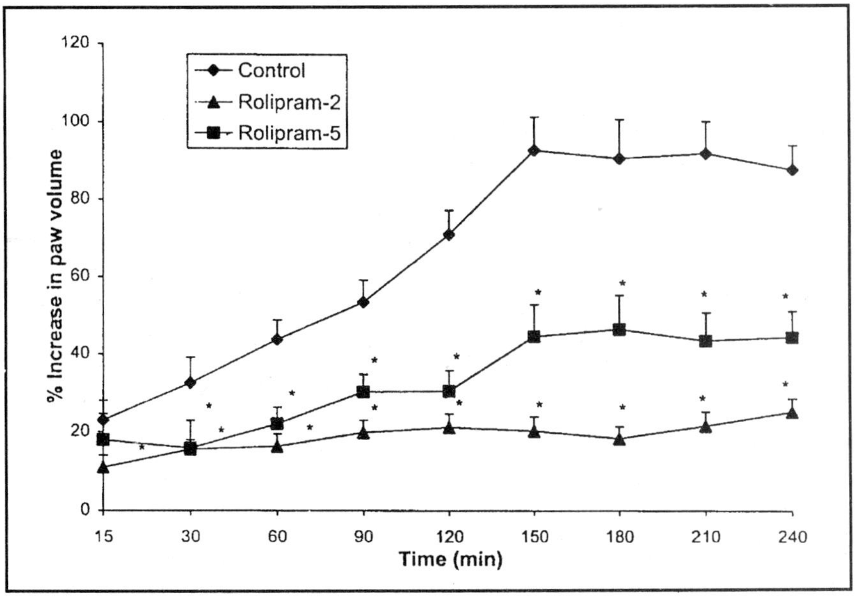

Fig. 2. Effect of rolipram (2, 5 mg/kg, i.p) on carrageenan-induced paw edema in rats. Vertical lines show mean ± SE * $P < 0.05$ as compared with control. (n = 6)

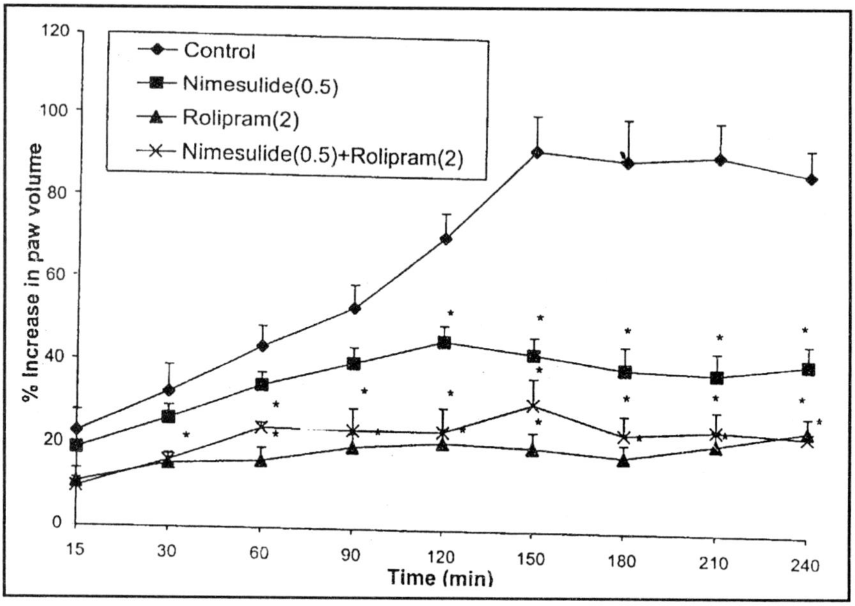

Fig. 3. Effect of rolipram (2 mg/kg, i.p.), nimesulide (0.5 mg/kg) and their combination on carrageenan-induced paw edema in rats. Vertical lines shows mean±SE. *P<0.05 as compared with control (n=6)

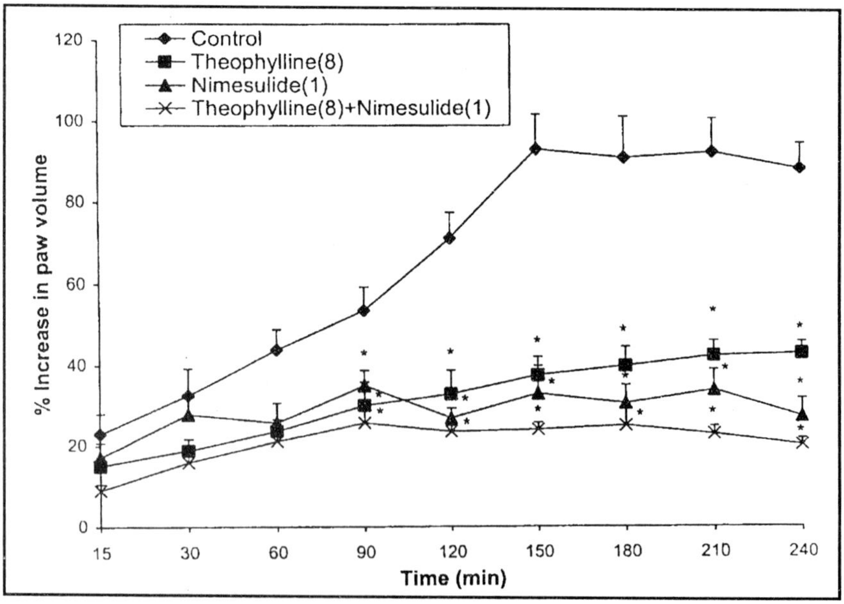

Fig. 4. Effect of theophylline (8 mg/kg, i.p.), nimesulide (1 mg/kg) and their combination on carrageenan-induced paw edema in rats. Vertical lines shows mean±SE. *P<0.05 as compared with control (n=6)

Discussion

Cyclic nucleotide phosphodiesterases play a key role in the metabolism of cAMP and cGMP. Many agents modulate tissue function via stimulation of adenylyl or guanylyl cyclase activity and hence via the elevation of cellular levels of cAMP and cGMP[12].

Rolipram is a selective PDE IV inhibitor which is known as antidepressant and effective in asthma[13] and theophylline a non-specific PDE inhibitor[14], is a one of the most effective drug for the treatment of asthma due to combination of bronchodilatory, pulmonary antiallergic and pulmonary anti-inflammatory activity[15]. The present investigation demonstrated that theophylline (2, 4, 8 mg/kg) and rolipram 1, 2 mg/kg a selective PDE IV inhibitor produced significant analgesic, anti-inflammatory effect against acetic acid induced writhing reflex and carrageenan induced paw edema, respectively. It is reported that PDE IV inhibitors elevate cAMP level in cells that participate in the inflammatory process. The elevation of intracellular cAMP has been associated with inhibition of the function of various types of cells including lymphocytes, monocytes, macrophages neutrophils, eosinophils, mast cells, basophills, endothelial cells and lung epithelial cells[16].

Above mentioned mechanism may be participating in the analgesic and anti-inflammatory effects of rolipram and theophylline, because mediators of these cells could be involved in various painful and inflammatory conditions[17].

Anti-inflammatory effect of theophylline in airway inflammation has been well reported[18] so it may be speculated that theophylline exerted antiinflammatory effect in carrageenan induced paw edema through inhibition of phopshodiesterase activity. Nimesulide, a selective cyclo-oxygenase -2 inhibitor, is also known to have PDE IV inhibiting property[19]. The rationale of combining the nimesulide with theophylline or rolipram was to assess whether nimesulide showed synergestic or potentiating effects in analgesic and anti-inflammatory activity. Coadministration of nimesulide with theophylline did not modify pain threshold and anti-inflammatory activity of theophylline but when nimesulide given with rolipram, it potentiated analgesic activity. It's suggested that nimesulide by PDE IV inhibition potentiates analgesic activity of rolipram.

REFERENCES

1. Beavo, J A & Reifsnyder, D H, *TIPS,* 11 (1990) 150.
2. Bergman, M R & Holygross, B J, *J Pharmacol Exp Ther,* 279 (1996) 247.
3. Verghese, M W, McConnell, R T, Strickland, A B, Gooding, R C, Stimpson, S A, Yarnall, D P. Taylor. J D & Furdon, P J. *J Pharmacol Exp Ther,* 272 (1995) 1313.
4. Ellis, G & Parnham, M J, *D N & P,* 7 (1994) 421.
5. Schwabe, V, Miyake, M, Ohga, Y & Daly, J W, *Molec Pharmacol,* 12 (1976) 900.
6. Christensen, S B, Guider, A & Forster, C J, *J Med Chem,* 41 (1998) 821.
7. Silvestre, J & Graul, J, *Drugs of Future,* 23 (1998) 607.
8. Koster, R, Anderson, M & De Beer, E J, *Fed Proc,* 18 (1959) 112.
9. Cao, B J & Li, W P, *Eur J Pharmacol,* 259 (1994) 75.
10. Winter, C A, Risley, E A & Nuss, G W. *Pros Soc Lip Biol Med,* 111 (1962) 544.
11. Kulkarni, S K, Mehta, A K & Kunchandy J, *J Arch Int Pharmacodyn Ther,* 279 (1986) 324.
12. Nicholson, C D, John R A, Challiss, J & Shahid, M, *TiPS,* 12 (1991) 19.
13. Howell, R E, Sickels, B D & Woeppel, S L, *J Pharmacol Expt Ther,* 264 (1993) 609.
14. Harris, A L, Connell, M J, Ferguson. E W, Wallace, A M, Pagani, E D & Silver P J, *J Pharmacol Expt Ther,* 251 (1989) 199.
15. Pauwels, R, Van Renterghem, D & Vander Straeten, M, *J Allergy Clin Immunol,* 76 (1985) 583.
16. Rabinovici, R et al, *Circ Res,* 78 (1996) 329.
17. Teixeira, M M, Gristwood, R W, Cooper, N & Hcllewell, P G, *TiPS,* 18 (1997) 165.
18. Sullivan, P, Bekir, S, Jaffar, Z, Page, C. Jeffery, P & Costello, J, *Lancet,* 343 (1994) 1006.
19. Bevilacqua, M, Vago, T, Baldi, G, Renesto, E, Dallegri, F & Norbiato, G, *Eur J Pharmacol,* 268 (1994) 415.

Paper Published In:
I.J.E.B. (Vol. 38, January, 2000, pp.26-30)

31

Involvement of dopamine D_2 and $5\text{-}HT_{1A}$ receptors in roxindole-induced antinociception

IPE NINAN AND S.K. KULKARNI
Pharmacology Division, University Institute of Pharmaceutical Sciences, Panjab University, Chandigarh 160 014, India

Roxindole, a DA D_2 receptor agonist (2-16 mg/kg) produced dose-dependent increase in percentage antinociception.The effect which was blocked by DA D_2 antagonist (-)sulpiride (50 mg/kg) and $5\text{-}HT_{IA}$ receptor antagonist (-) pindolol (5 mg/kg). Roxindole (4 and 8 mg/kg) reversed both naloxone (20 mg/kg)-induced hyperalgesia and reserpine (2 mg/kg)-induced hyperalgesia. This reversal was sensitive to blockade by both (-)sulpiride (50 mg/kg) and (-) pindolol (5 mg/kg). The present study suggests that roxindole-induced antinociception is mediated by postsynaptic DA D_2 and $5\text{-}HT_{IA}$ receptors.

Roxindole (EMD 49980) is a representative of a new class of dopaminergic drugs, i.e., the indolyl butylamines, which lack structural similarities with either rigid dopamine (DA) analogs or ergot derivatives[1]. Roxindole exhibits potent, long lasting and highly selective agonistic actions at presynaptic D_2 receptors without stimulating postsynaptic D_2 receptors even at high doses[2]. This selectivity makes roxindole a pre-eminent candidate for a novel type of antipsychotic drug without neurological side effects which limit the usefulness of conventional D_2 receptor blockers. Within the past few years, several new putative, selective DA autoreceptor agonists have been developed, among them are the transfused analog of 3-PPP, (-)-HW 165, the transdihydroergoline terguride and the amino-ergolines SDZ 208-912 (ref. 3-5). Interest in these putative DA autoreceptor agonists derives largely from their potential use as non-classical antipsychotic drugs.

Roxindole, besides its affinity for D_2 receptors, has affinity for the 5-HT_{1A} receptor also[2].

Considerable clinical evidence suggests that DA receptor-mediated mechanisms may play an important role in modulating pain in humans. A number of animal studies have showed that DA is involved in the regulation of nociception. However, the data reported are contradictory and DA agonists have been shown to produce either antinociception[6,7] or hyperalgesia[8,9] or to have both effects[10]. However, some DA agonists have been reported to suppress the severe pain associated with various states of disease affecting the nervous system, such as the thalamic syndrome, herpes zoster and Parkinson's disease[11,12,13,14] and a recent study showed that 8-OH DPAT inhibits nociceptive responses by stimulating postsynaptic 5-HT_{1A} receptors[15].

The present study was undertaken to investigate the role of D_2 and 5-HT_{1A} receptors in the antinociception produced by roxindole in naive and reserpinised mice.

Materials and Methods

Animals: Balb/C mice (bred in Central Animal House facility of Panjab University), weighing 20-25 g, were housed under a standard 12 h light/12 h dark cycle. The animals were acclimatized to the laboratory conditions with free access to food and water for 24 h before the experiment. All experiments were undertaken between 09.00 and 13.00 h.

Technique: The nociceptive threshold was determined as the tail-flick latencies elicited in response to noxious radiant heat[16,17]. Baseline latencies to tail-flick withdrawal from the radiant heat source (3-4 s) were established. A cut off time of 10 s was observed to prevent any injury to the tail. A minimum of three trials, at 2 min intervals, were recorded for each animal before the test. Antinociception was calculated according to the following formula: % antinociception = 100 x (test latency – baseline latency) / (10 – baseline latency).

Drugs: Roxindole mesylate (EMD 49980, Merck KGaA Biomed Res CNS, Germany), (-) sulpiride hydrochloride (Research Biochemicals Inc, MA, USA), naloxone hydrochloride (Sigma, USA), (-) pindolol (Ranbaxy, India) and reserpine (Loba Chemicals, India) were used in the study. The drug solutions were made in distilled water, except reserpine and (-) pindolol. Reserpine was dissolved in a drop of glacial acetic acid while pindolol was dissolved in a drop of dilute HCl, volume made up with distilled water and *p*H adequately adjusted. All the drugs were administered intraperitoneally in a constant volume of 1 ml/100 g of body weight. The selection of doses was based on previous reports from our laboratory. Each group comprised 5-10 mice.

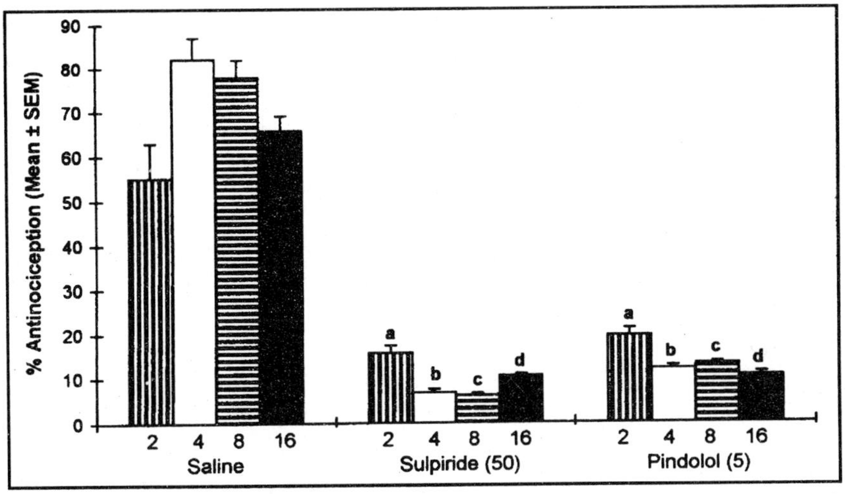

Fig. 1. Antinociceptive effect of roxindole (2-16 mg/kg) and its modification by (-) sulpiride (50 mg/kg) and (-) pindolol (5 mg/kg) in mice. [a,b,c,d]P<0.001 as compared to roxindole (2, 4, 8 and 16 mg/kg) groups, respectively.

Reserpine (2 mg/kg) was administered 4 h prior and naloxone 15 min prior to the experiment. Roxindole was administered 30 min prior to the test. The DA receptor antagonists (-)sulpiride and 5-HT_{1A} antagonist (-) pindolol were administered 30 min prior to the agonists.

Table 2. Reversal of reserpine (4 h post)-induced roxindole and its modification by (-) sulpiride and respectively in mice

No.	Treatment (mg/kg)	% Antinociception (Mean±SE)
1.	Saline	0.88±00
2.	Reserpine (2)	-18.30±0.51
3.	Reserpine (2) + Roxindole (4)	12.46±0.78[a]
4.	Reserpine (2) + Roxindole (8)	23.34±1.36[a]
5.	Reserpine (2) + Sulpiride (50) + Roxindole (4)	-12.93±0.13[b]
6.	Reserpine (2) + Sulpiride (50) + Roxindole (8)	-11.04±0.78[c]
7.	Reserpine (2) + Pindolol (5) + Roxindole (4)	-13.09±0.74[b]
8.	Reserpine (2) + Pindolol (5) + Roxindole (8)	-10.41±0.42[c]

[a]*P*<0.001 as compared to group 2; [b]*P*<0.001 as compared to group 3; [c]*P*<0.001 as compared to group 4

Statistical analysis: The data was analyzed using one way ANOVA followed by student's t-test and P<0.05 was considered statistically significant.

Results

Antinociceptive effect of roxindole and its reversal by (-) sulpiride and (-) pindolol: Roxindole (2-16 mg/kg) produced dose-dependent increase in percentage antinociception with higher doses (8 and 16 mg/kg) showing ceiling effects. Lower doses (0.01-1 mg/kg) of roxindole did not show antinociceptive effect. (-) Sulpiride (50 mg/kg) and (-) pindolol (5 mg/kg) blocked the antinociceptive effect of roxindole (2-16 mg/kg) (P<0.001) (Fig. 1). (-) Sulpiride (50 mg/kg) or (-) pindolol (5 mg/kg) *per se* did not show any effect on nociceptive response.

Effect of roxindole on hyperalgesia induced by naloxone and reserpine: Naloxone (20 mg/kg) produced a significant decrease in percentage antinociception. Roxindole (4 and 8 mg/kg) reversed the naloxone-induced hyperalgesia (P<0.001). Both (-) sulpride (50 mg/kg) and (-) pindolol (5 mg/kg) blocked the reversal of hyperalgesia by roxindole (P<0.001) (Table 1).

Table 1. Reversal of naloxone-induced hyperalgesia by roxindole and its modification by (-) sulpiride and (-) pindolol in mice

No.	Treatment (mg/kg)	% Antinociception (Mean±SE)
1.	Saline	0.88±00
2.	Naloxone (20)	-36.27±4.26
3.	Roxindole (4) + Naloxone (20)	21.60±1.63[a]
4.	Roxindole (8) + Naloxone (20)	8.04±0.87[a]
5.	Sulpiride (50) + Roxindole (4) + Naloxone (20)	0.16±0.10[b]
6.	Sulpiride (50) + Roxindole (8) + Naloxone (20)	-5.68±0.38[c]
7.	Pindolol (5) + Roxindole (4) + Naloxone (20)	-9.15±0.42[b]
8.	Pindolol (5) + Roxindole (8) + Naloxone (20)	-10.4±0.06[c]

[a]*P*<0.001 as compared to group 2; [b]*P*<0.001 as compared to group 3; [c]*P*<0.001 as compared to group 4

Reserpine (2 mg/kg, 4 hr prior) pre-treatment significantly reduced percentage antinociception. The reserpine-induced reduction in the nociceptive threshold was reversed by roxindole (4 and 8 mg/

kg) (P<0.001). Both (-) sulpiride (50 mg/kg) and (-) pindolol (5 mg/kg) blocked the reversal of hyperalgesia by roxindole (P<0.001) (Table2).

Discussion

The present study demonstrates that acute administration of D_2 autoreceptor selective agonist, roxindole produced an antinociceptive response in mice. Previously, Verma and Kulkarni (1993) have reported that DA agonists such as B-HT 920, bromocriptine and apomorphine produced antinociception[7]. The antinociceptive response elicited by roxindole was blocked by (-) sulpiride, a D_2 antagonist and (-) pindolol, a selective 5-HT_{1A} antagonist. The available literature suggests the involvement of postsynaptic D_2 receptors in antinociception[7,18,19]. Previous studies showed that D_2 agonists do not show antinociceptive effect at doses which stimulate autoreceptors[7]. Therefore, the possibility of involvement of presynaptic D_2 receptors in this antinociceptive effect is rare. The antinociceptive effect produced by roxindole was blocked by both (-) sulpiride, a selective D_2 antagonist and (-) pindolol, a 5-HT_{1A} antagonist. It is known that 5-HT_{1A} receptors control DA neurotransmission in several brain areas[20,21,22]. The 5-HT_{1A} agonist, 8-OH DPAT increases locomotor activity in rats[23,24]. It could be possible that roxindole can stimulate DA neurotransmission which inturn might be responsible for the antinociceptive effect. But some recent studies have shown that 5-HT_{1A} agonists including 8-OH DPAT and flesinoxan, have apparent inhibitory actions on dopamine neurotransmission[25].

The reversing effect of reserpine-induced hyperalgesia by roxindole was blocked by (-) sulpiride and (-) pindolol. In reserpinised animals, the consequences of any presynaptic receptor activation are eliminated because of the depletion of various neurotransmitters, and makes it possible to measure postsynaptically mediated effects. This suggests the partial agonistic action of roxindole at postsynaptic D_2 receptors as well as 5-HT_{IA} receptors. Bartoszyk *et al.* (1996) reported that roxindole reverses reserpine-induced hypomotility[26]. Both talipexole and roxindole have been reported to produce psychomotor stimulation and exacerbation of psychosis[27,28]. Recently, we have reported that clozapine, an atypical antipsychotic having partial agonistic action at D_2 receptors in DA depleted animals[28]. Partial agonism of 5-HT_{1A} receptors were recently proposed to contribute to the unique profile of clozapine as compared with classical neuroleptics[29,30]. Similarly, roxindole reversed naloxone-induced hyperalgesia and this effect was reversed by both (-) sulpiride and (-) pindolol. Earlier, Verma and Kulkarni (1993) suggested that there existed an interlink between opioid and DAergic systems in the brain and showed that D_2 agonists reverse naloxone-induced hyperalgesia[7]. Further, recent studies have shown that some possible interaction between $5\text{-}HT_{1A}$-opioid system in antinociceptive response[31,32]. The present study therefore, suggests that roxindole-induced antinociception involved both postsynaptic DA D_2 and $5\text{-}HT_{1A}$ receptors.

Acknowledgement

The Senior Research Fellowship (SRF) of CSIR, New Delhi, is acknowledged. The authors also thank Merck KGaA Biomed Res CNS, Germany for generously donating roxindole mesylate used in this study.

REFERENCES

1. Seyfried CA & Boettcher H, *Drugs of Future*, 15 (1990) 819-832.
2. Seyfried CA, Greiner HE & Haase AF, *Eur J Pharmacol*, 160 (1989) 31.
3. Hjorth S, Svensson K, Carlsson A, Wikstrom H & Andersson B, *Naunyn-Schmiedeberg's Arch Pharmacol*, 333 (1986) 205.
4. Wachtel H & Dorow R, *Life Sci*, 32 (1983) 421.
5. Coward DM, Dixon AK, Urwyler S, White TG, Enz A, Karobath M & Shearman G, *J Pharmacol Exp Ther*, 252 (1990) 279.
6. Akil H & Liebeskind JC, *Brain Res*, 94 (1975) 279.
7. Verma A & Kulkarni SK, *J Psychopharmacol*, 7 (1993) 270.
8. Tulunay FC, Sparber SB & Takemori AE, *Eur J Pharmacol*, 33 (1975) 65.
9. Gonzalez JP, Sewell RDE & Spencer PSJ, *Life Sci*, 28 (1981) 951.
10. Gonzalez JP, Rooney RF, Sewell RDE & Spencer PSJ, *Br J Pharmacol*, 86 (1985) 709.
11. Miley DP, Abrams AA, Atkinson JH & Janowsky DS, *Am J Psychiatry*, 135 (1978) 1230.
12. Grant R & Behan PO, *Br Med J*, 289 (1984) 1272.
13. Kernbaum S & Hauchecorne J, *J Am Med Assoc*, 246 (1981) 132.
14. Nutt JG & Carter JH, *Lancet*, 11 (1984) 456.
15. Cervo L, Rossi C, Tatarczynska E & Samanin R, *Eur J Pharmacol*, 263 (1994)187.
16. D'Armour FE & Smith DL, *J Pharmacol Exp Ther*, 72 (1941) 74.

17. Kulkarni SK, *Life Sci*, 27 (1980)185.

18. Paalzow GHM & Paalzow LK, *Eur J Pharmacol*, 88 (1984) 27.

19. Barasi S, Ben-Sreti MM, Clatworthy AL, Duggal KN, Gonzales JP, Robbertson J, Rooney KF & Sewell RDE, *Br J Pharmacol*, 90 (1987) 15.

20. Hamon M, Fattaccini CM, Adrien J, Gallissot MC, Martin P & Gozlan H, *J Pharmacol Exp Ther*, 246 (1988) 745.

21. Golembiowska K& Wedzony *K, Pol J Pharmacol*, 45 (1993) 299.

22. Rasmussen AM, Goldstein LE, Deutch AY, Bunney BS & Roth RH, *Synapse*, 18 (1994) 299.

23. Dourish CT, Hutson PH & Curzon *G, Psychopharmacology*, 86 (1985) 197.

24. Kalkman HO & Soar J, *Eur J Pharmacol*, 191 (1990) 383.

25. Kleven M, Prinssen EPM & Koek W, *Eur J Pharmacol*, 313 (1996) 25.

26. Bartoszyk GD, Harting J & Minick KO, *J Pharmacol Exp Ther*, 276 (1996) 41.

27. Wetzel H & Benkert O, *Prog Neuropsychopharmacol Biol Psychiatrv*, 17 (1993) 525.

28. Ninan I & Kulkarni SK, *Psychopharmacology*, 135 (1998) 311.

29. Wiedmann K, Benkert 0 & Holsber F, *Pharmacopsychiatry*, 23 (1990) 50.

30. Newman-Tancredi A, Chaput C, Verriele L & Millan MJ, *Neuropharmacology*, 35 (1996) 119.

31. Millan MJ & Colpaert FC, *J Pharmacol Exp Ther*, 256 (1991) 983.

32. Powell KR & Dykstra, LA, *J Pharmacol Exp Ther*, 274 (1995) 1305.

Paper Published In:
I.J.E.B. (Vol. 37, January, 1999, pp.234-237)

32

Antinociceptive effect of sumatriptan in mice

N.K. JAIN AND S.K. KULKARNI
Pharmacology Division, University Institute of Pharmaceutical Sciences, Panjab University, Chandigarh 160 014, India

Antinociceptive effect of the antimigraine drug sumatriptan (5-HT_{IA} agonist) was studied against acetic acid-induced writhing in mice. Sumatriptan produced the effect in a dose-dependent manner (1, 5, 10 and 20 mg/kg, sc). Naloxone (1 mg/kg ip) an opiate antagonist failed to reverse sumatriptan-induced antinociception. Cholinomimetic physostigmine (0.05 mg/kg, ip) potentiated and the muscarinic antagonist atropine (5mg/kg, ip) blocked the antinociceptive effect of sumatriptan, respectively. The antinociceptive effect of sumatriptan was compared with an another 5-HT agonist (5-HT_{1A}) buspirone which also produced antinociception. Like sumatriptan-analgesia, the buspirone response was also potentiated by physostigmine in atropine sensitive way. Further, buspirone potentiated the analgesic effect of sumatriptan. These observations suggest that 5-HT_{1A} agonists produce antinociception possibly by modulating central cholinergic activity.

Sumatriptan is a novel 5-HT_{ID} receptor agonist which is effective in the acute treatment of migraine headache[1,2]. The antimigraine activity has been attributed to the selective vasoconstriction of cranial blood vessels which are dilated during migraine attack[3]. Beside this, sumatriptan also reported to have affinity for 5-HT_{IA} and 5-HT_{1B} receptors[4]. Recently Ghelardini *et al.*[5] reported that sumatriptan by acting at 5-HT_{1A} receptors, produced naloxone resistant cholinergic type of antinociception. Bianchi *et al.*[6] also reported an increase in the acetylcholine efflux from the cerebral cortex of freely moving guinea pigs after administration of 8-hydroxy-2-di-n-propylaminotetralin (8-

OH-DPAT), a 5-HT_{1A} agonist[6]. It is well established that direct or indirect cholinomimetics are able to increase the pain threshold in both humans[7,8] and animals[9]. Therefore, in the present study the possible involvement of cholinergic mechanisms in the antinociceptive effect of sumatriptan was investigated using acetic acid-induced chemonociception and the effect was compared with buspirone, a 5-HT_{1A} partial agonist.

Material and Methods

Animals: Laka mice of either sex (20-30g) obtained from Central Animal House, Panjab University, Chandigarh were used. The animals were kept under 12/12 hr light/dark cycle and had food and water *ad libitum.* All experiments were carried out between 1000hrs to 1700hrs.

Writhing test (Acetic acid writhing assay): A 1% acetic acid solution (1 ml/100 g) used to produce writhing in animals. The number of wriths (constriction of abdomen, turning of trunk (twist) and extension of hind legs) per animal were counted during a 20-min test period beginning 3-min after the injection of acetic acid[10].

Drugs: The following drugs were used. Sumatriptan succinate (Dabur Research Foundation, New Delhi), buspirone hydrochloride (Bristol-Myers Squibb, NJ, USA), atropine (Boehringer-Mannheim), naloxone, physostigmine (Sigma) and acetic acid (S.D. fine chemicals).

Drug administration: Sumatriptan was injected 10 min before acetic acid injection. Atropine and naloxone were injected 15 min before sumatriptan administration. Physostigmine was injected 5 min before sumatriptan. Buspirone was administered 30 min before acetic acid injection. All the drugs were injected intraperitoneally except sumatriptan which was given sc, in a constant volume of 1 ml per 100 g body weight.

Statistical analysis: Results are expressed as mean ± SE. Analysis of variance (ANOVA) followed by Student's t-test of significance level of $P < 0.05$ was used to analyse the data.

Results

Effect on pain threshold: Subcutaneously administered sumatriptan induced a significant increase in the pain threshold against acetic acid writhing in mice, showing a clear antinociception in the dose range of

5-20 mg/kg (Table 1). The antinociceptive effect reached maximum in 20 min and then diminished. Buspirone (5, 10, 20 mg/kg) also produced antinociception and the effect was comparable to that of sumatriptan (Fig. 1) and further it potentiated the antinociceptive action of sumatriptan (Fig. 5). Naloxone (1 mg/kg) failed to reverse the effect of both the drugs (Fig.2).

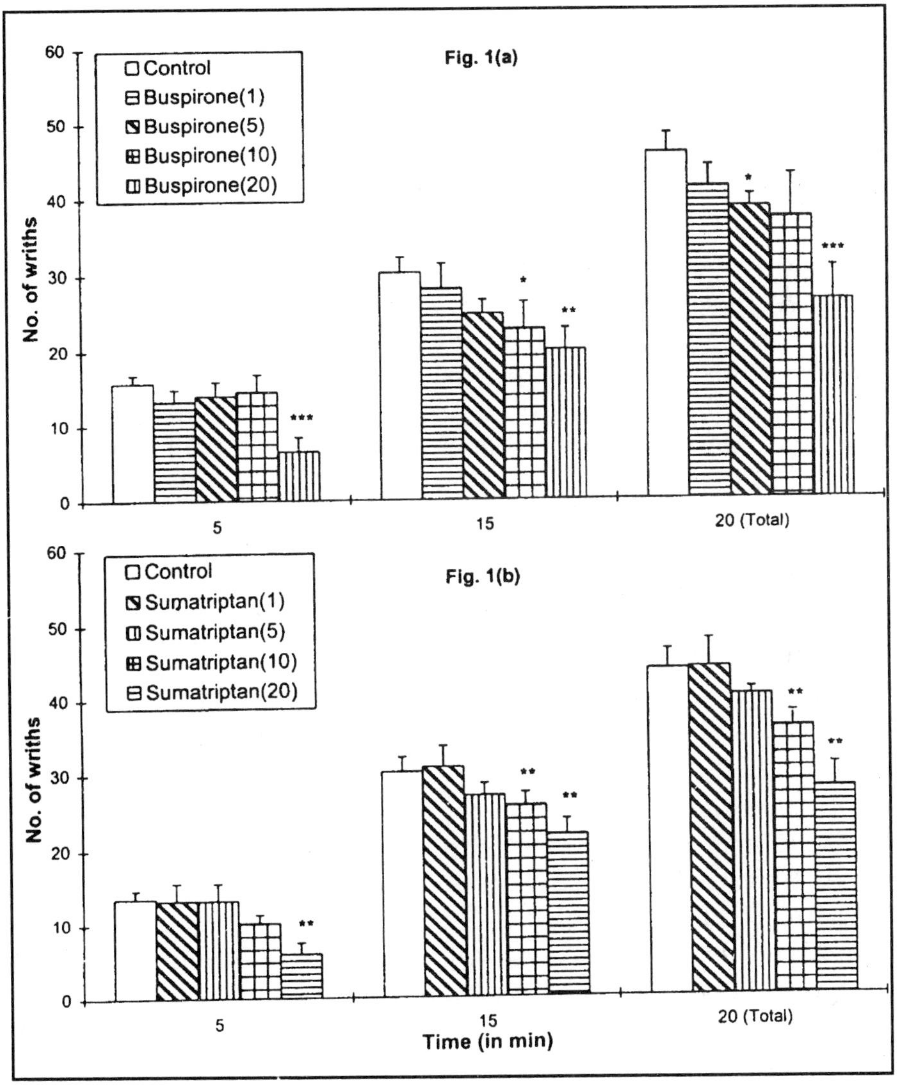

Fig. 1. Comparative antinociceptive profile of buspirone vs sumatriptan in mouse writhing test. The doses are expressed as mg/kg i.p. or s.c. Vertical lines show mean±S.E. **P* <0.01; ***P* <0.05; ****P* <0.001 compared with controls.

Table 1. Effect of various doses of Sumatriptan on acetic acid-induced writhing in mice

Treatment (mg/kg, sc)	n	Number of wriths at		
		5 min	15 min	Total (20 min)
Control	29	13.6±1.15	30.2±1.94	43.82±2.62
Sumatriptan (1)	5	13.2±2.39	30.8±2.85	44.00±3.87
Sumatriptan (5)	5	13.2±2.35	27.0±1.61	40.20±0.970
Sumatriptan (10)	14	10.2±1.0*	25.71±1.69*	35.92±2.05*
Sumatriptan (20)	14	6.0±1.49*	21.85±2.03*	27.85±3.15*

* $P < 0.05$

Interaction of cholinegic drugs with sumatriptan and buspirone- Antinociception induced by sumatriptan or buspirone (20 mg/kg) was significantly increased and prolonged by physostigmine (0.05 mg/kg) (Fig. 3). At this dose, physostigmine neither altered the pain threshold nor exhibited any cholinomimetic property *per se*. Muscarinic antagonist atropine (5 mg/kg) completely blocked sumatriptan or buspirone antinociception (Fig. 4). Sumatriptan neither showed any cholinergic activity by itself nor it potentiated acetylcholine-induced contractions on rat anococcygeus muscle preparations (data not shown).

Discussion

5-HT_{IA} receptors are reported to be located in hippocampus, raphe nuclei, limbic system, hypothalamus, frontal cortex and brain stem areas but they are in high density in the hippocampus[11,12]. Sumatriptan exerts its antinociceptive effect by acting at 5-HT_{IA} receptors[5]. It is well reported that 5-HT (5-hydroxytryptamine) exerted an inhibitory control on the cholinergic system in the brain[6,13]. 5-HT or 5-HT agonists increased acetylcholine content *in vivo* and reduced acetylcholine release from different brain areas *in vitro*[6,13,14]. Muscarinic antagonist atropine completely blocked the sumatriptan and buspirone antinociception. Similarly the antinociceptive effect was potentiated by physostigmine, a cholinomimetic. These observations confirm the possibility of 5-HT_{1A} agonists acting via cholinergic mechanism in inducing antinociception. 5-HT_{1A} agonists may activate somatodendritic autoreceptor in hippocampus, reduce the firing rate of 5-HT neurones and reduce 5-HT release *in vivo*[15,16] but less so *in vitro.* Consequently 5-HT_{IA} activation reduces the tonic inhibitory control on cholinergic cells and that leads to increased hippocampal

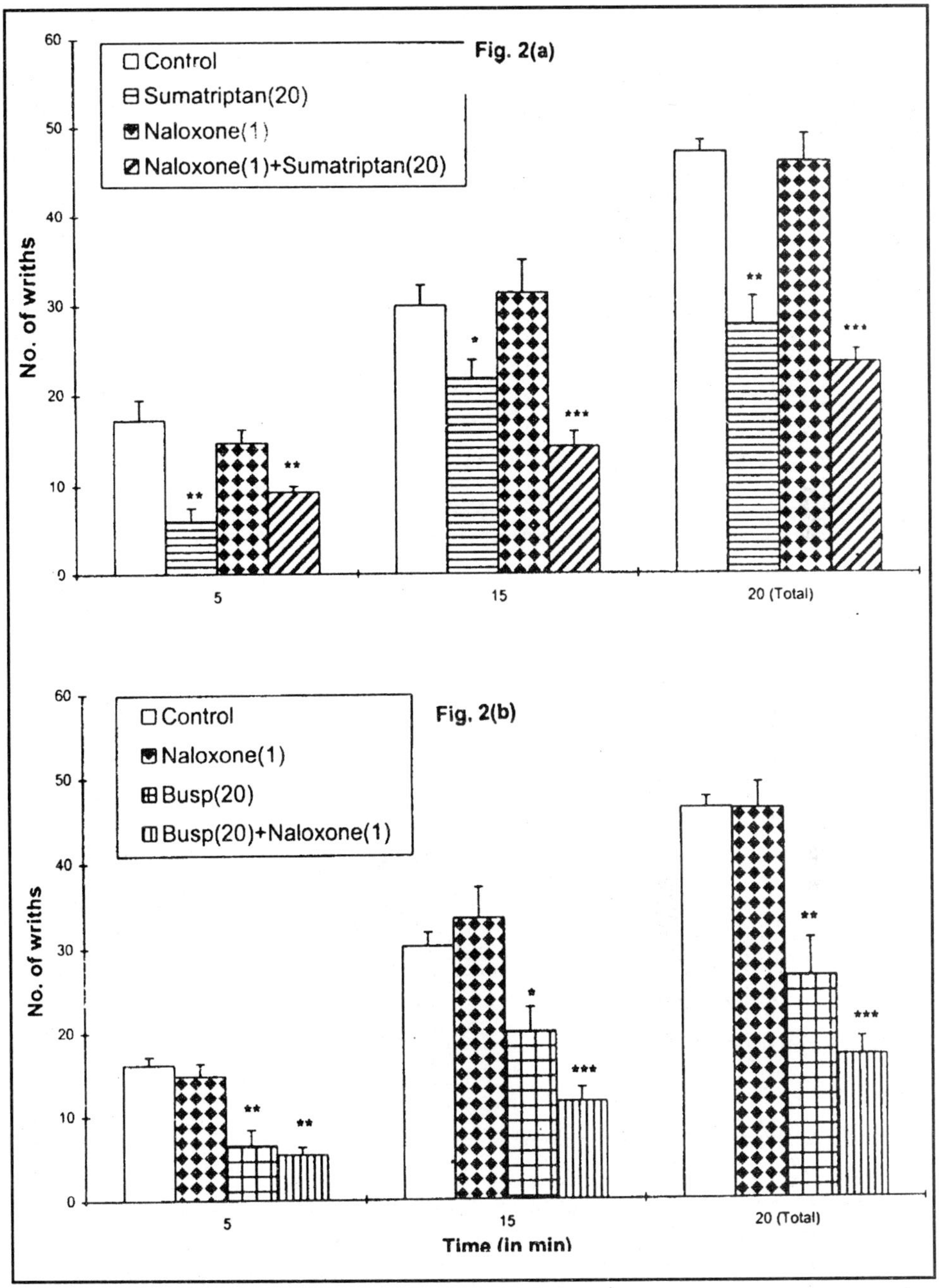

Fig. 2. Effect of naloxone on sumatriptan (a) and buspirone (b) antinociception in the mouse writhing test. The doses are expressed as mg/kg s.c. or i.p. Vertical lines show mean± S.E. $^{*}P < 0.1$; $^{**}P < 0.01$; $^{***}P < 0.001$ compared with controls.

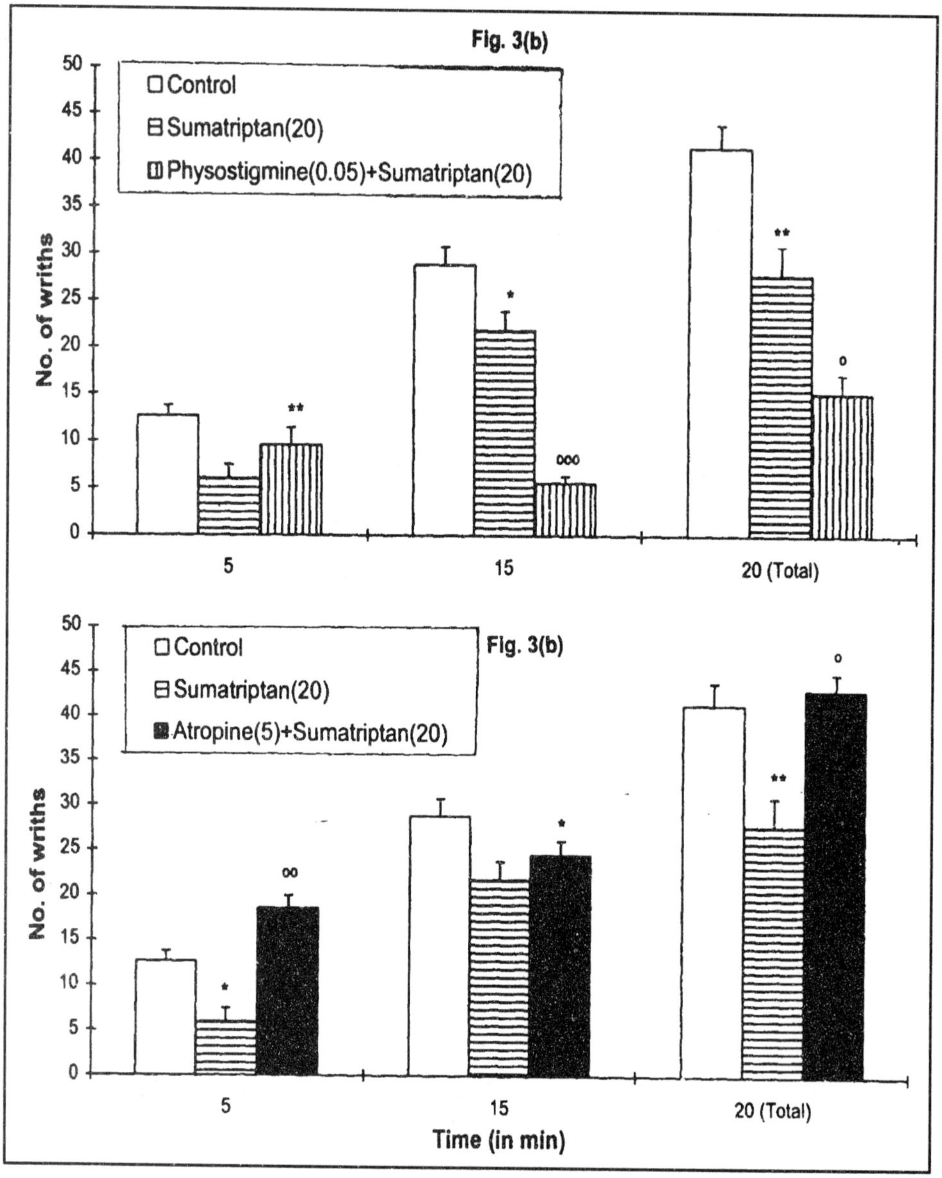

Fig. 3. Effect of Cholinergic drugs on sumatriptan antinociception in the mouse writhing test (a) Potentiation of sumatriptan antinociception by physostigmine (0.05mg) (b) Blockade of sumatriptan antinociception by atropine (5mg). The doses are expressed as mg/kg s.c. or i.p. Vertical lines show mean±S.E. $^{*}P<0.05$; $^{**}P < 0.02$ compared with controls, $^{\circ}P < 0.05$; $^{\circ\circ}P < 0.02$; $^{\circ\circ\circ}P < 0.001$ compared with sumatriptan.

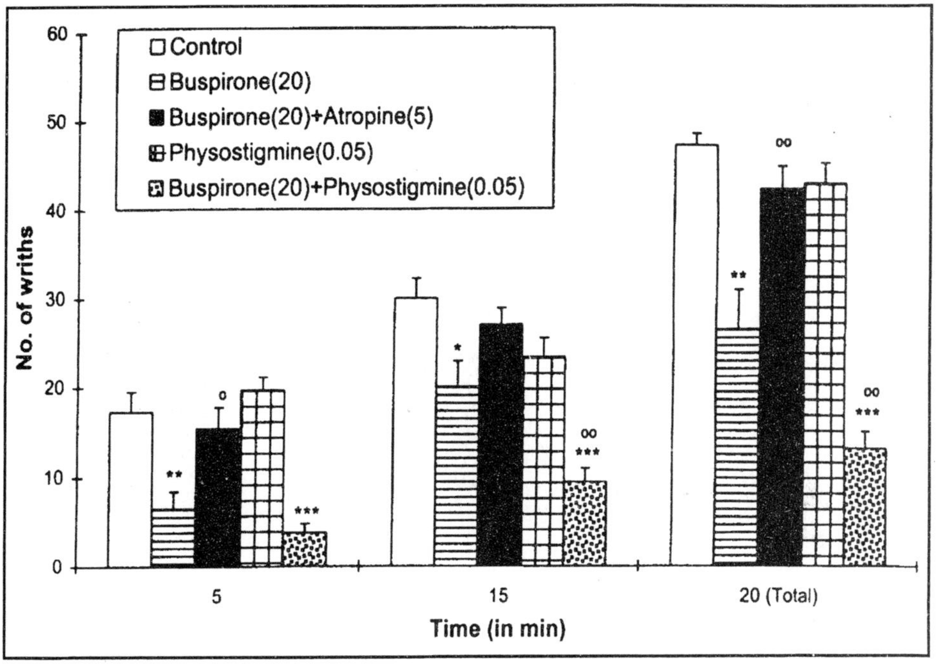

Fig. 4. Effect of Cholinergic drugs (physostigmine, atropine) on buspirone antinociception in the mouse writhing test. The doses are expressed as mg / kg i.p. Vertical lines show mean±S.E. *$P < 0.05$; **$P < 0.01$; ***$P < 0.001$ compared with controls, °P<0.1; °°P<0.05; °°° P < 0.02 compared with buspirone.

acetylcholine release[6,17]. The hippocampus is reported to be rich in muscarinic (M_1) receptors[18] which are responsible for cholinergic antinociception[19,20,21] of sumatriptan and buspirone[22]. The role of opioid system in the sumatriptan antinociception is ruled out as naloxone failed to reverse sumatriptan antinociception.

Sumatriptan antinociception is reported to be not only blocked by 5-HT_{1A} antagonist NAN-190 but also by atropine and acetylcholine depletor HC-3 (Hemicholinium-3)[5]. The antinociceptive action of sumatriptan was comparable with that of buspirone antinociception. The antinociceptive action of buspirone was also sensitive to blockade by atropine[22] and further it potentiated the antinociceptive action of sumatriptan.

It is concluded that sumatriptan produces antinociception by possibly releasing acetycholine via acting on 5-HT_{1A} receptors located on cholinergic nerves in the brain. This action may contribute to its antimigraine as well as to its observed side effects in humans.

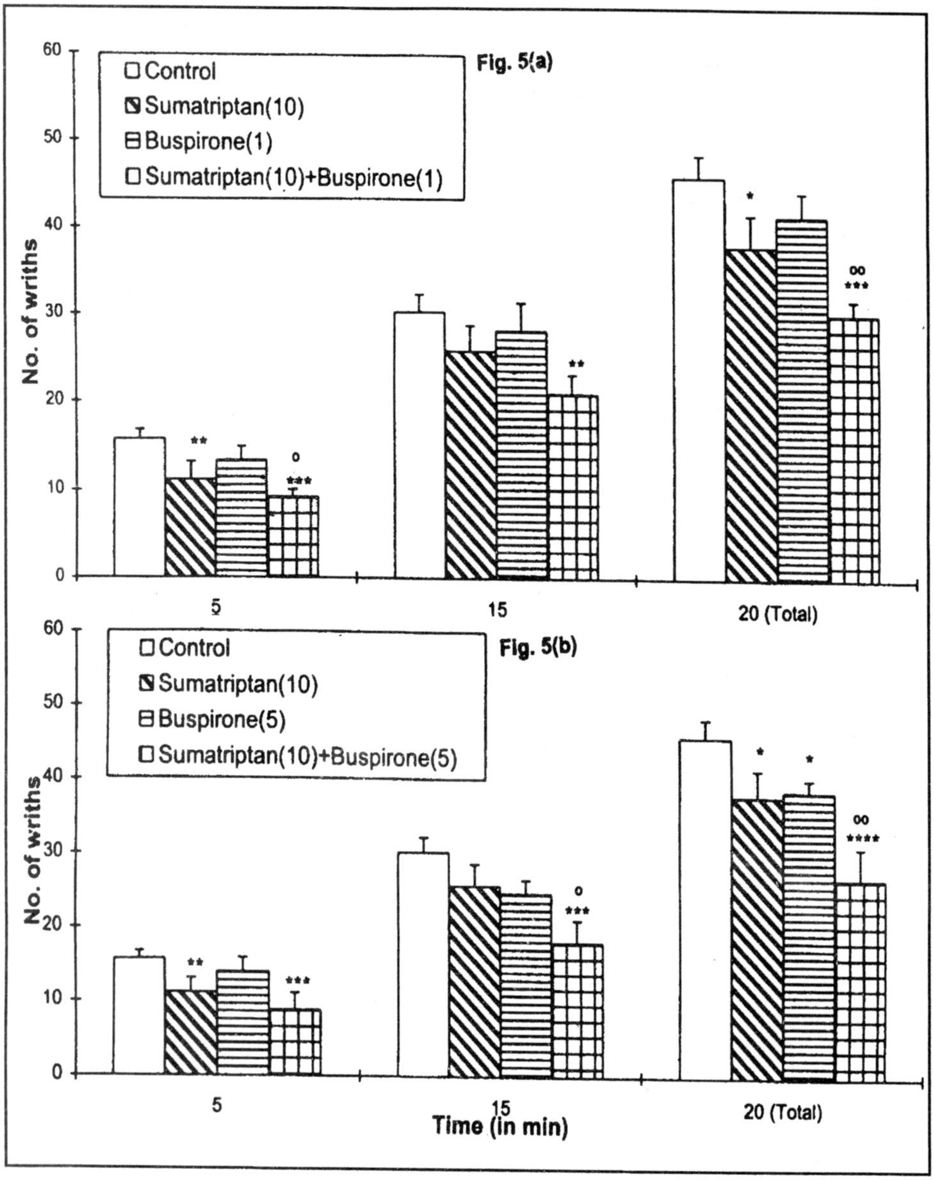

Fig. 5. Potentiation by buspirone of sumatriptan induced antinociception in mouse writhing test (a) buspirone (1 mg/kg) (b) buspirone (5mg/kg). The doses are expressed as mg / kg i.p. or s.c. Vertical lines show mean±S.E. **P* < 0.1 ; ***P* < 0.05 ; ****P* < 0.01 ; compared with controls, °P<0.1; °°P<0.01 compared with buspirone.

REFERENCES

1. Doenicke, A, Brand, J & Perrin, *V L, Lancet*, 1 (1988) 1309.
2. Humphrey, P P A & Feniuk, W, *TIPS*, 12 (1991) 444.
3. Humphrey, P P A & Goadsby, P J, *Cephalagia*, 14 (1991) 444.
4. Dechant, K L & Clissold, S P, *Drugs*, 43-5 (1992) 776.
5. Ghelardini, C, Galeotti, N, Figini, M, Imperato, A, Nicolodi, M, Sicuteri, F, Gessa, G L & Bartolini, A, *J Pharmacol Exp Ther*, 279 (1996) 884.
6. Bianchi, C, Siniscalchi, A & Beani, *L, Br J Pharmacol*, 101 (1990) 448.
7. Hood, D D, Eisenach, J C & Tuttle, *R, Anesthesiology*, 82 (1995) 331.
8. Bartolini, A, Galli, A, Ghelardini, C, Giott, A, Malcangio, M, Aiello, P M & Zucchi, P L, *Br J Pharmacol*, 92 (1987) 711.
9. Bartolini, A, Ghelardini, C, Fantetti, L, Malcangio, M, Malmberg-Aiello, P & Giotti, A, *Br J Pharmacol*, 105 (1992) 105.
10. Koster, R, Anderson, M & De Beer, E J, *Fed Proc*, 18 (1959) 412.
11. Verge, D, Davel, G, Marcinikiewicz, M, Patey, A, El Mestikawy, S, Gozlan, H & Hamon M, *J Neurosci*, 6 (1986) 3474.
12. Desmukh, P P, Yamamura, H I, Woods, L & Nelson, D L, *Brain Res*, 288 (1983) 338.
13. Bianchi, C, Siniscalchi, A & Beani, L, *Br J Pharmacol*, 97 (1989) 213.
14. Siniscalchi, A, Beani, L & Bianchi, C, *Eur J Pharmacol*, 175 (1990) 219.
15. Sharp, T, Bram well, S R & Graham-Smith, D G, *Br J Pharmacol*, 96 (1989a) 283.
16. Sharp, T, Bram well, S R & Graham-Smith, D G, *J Neurochem*, 53 (1989b) 234.
17. Izumi, J, Washizuka, M, Miura, N, Hiraga, Y & Ikeda, Y, *J Neurochem*, 62 (1994) 1804.
18. Mash, D C & Potter, L T, *Neuroscience*, 19 (1986) 551.
19. Pohorecki, R, Head, R & Domino, E F, *J Pharmacol Exp Ther*, 228 (1988) 213.
20. Raiteri, M, Leardi, R & Marchi, M, *J Pharmacol Exp Ther*, 228 (1984) 209.
21. Ghelardini, C, Malmberg-Aiello, P, Giott, A, Malcangio, M & Bartolini, A, *Br J Pharmacol*, 101 (1990) 49.
22. Galeotti, N, Ghelardini, C & Bartolini, *A, Pharmacol Biochem & Behav*, 57 (1997) 835.

Paper Published In:

I.J.E.B. (Vol. 36, October, 1998, pp.973-979)

Index

—•—